Statistical Thinking in Clinical Trials

Recently Published Titles
Cure Models: Methods, Applications, and Implementation
Yingwei Peng, Binbing Yu

Bayesian Analysis of Infectious Diseases: COVID-19 and Beyond
Lyle D. Broemeling

Statistical Meta-Analysis using R and Stata, Second Edition
Ding-Geng (Din) Chen and Karl E. Peace

Advanced Survival Models
Catherine Legrand

Structural Equation Modeling for Health and Medicine
Douglas Gunzler, Adam Perzynski and Adam C. Carle

Signal Detection for Medical Scientists
Likelihood Ratio Test-based Methodology
Ram Tiwari, Jyoti Zalkikar, and Lan Huang

Single-Arm Phase II Survival Trial Design
Jianrong Wu

**Methodologies in Biosimilar Product
Development**
Sang Joon Lee, Shein-Chung Chow (eds.)

Statistical Design and Analysis of Clinical Trials
Principles and Methods, Second Edition
Weichung Joe Shih, Joseph Aisner

Confidence Intervals for Discrete Data in Clinical Research
Vivek Pradhan, Ashis Gangopadhyay, Sandeep Menon, Cynthia Basu, and Tathagata Banerjee

Statistical Thinking in Clinical Trials
Michael A. Proschan

Simultaneous Global New Drug Development
Multi-Regional Clinical Trials after ICH E17
Edited by Gang Li, Bruce Binkowitz, William Wang, Hui Quan, and Josh Chen

Quantitative Methodologies and Process for Safety Monitoring and Ongoing Benefit Risk Evaluation
Edited by William Wang, Melvin Munsaka, James Buchanan and Judy Li

For more information about this series, please visit: https://www.routledge.com/Chapman--Hall-CRC-Biostatistics-Series/book-series/CHBIOSTATIS

Statistical Thinking in Clinical Trials

Michael A. Proschan

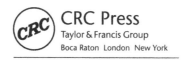

CRC Press
Taylor & Francis Group
Boca Raton London New York

CRC Press is an imprint of the
Taylor & Francis Group, an **informa** business

A CHAPMAN & HALL BOOK

First edition published 2022
by CRC Press
6000 Broken Sound Parkway NW, Suite 300, Boca Raton, FL 33487-2742

and by CRC Press
2 Park Square, Milton Park, Abingdon, Oxon, OX14 4RN

CRC Press is an imprint of Taylor & Francis Group, LLC

Library of Congress Cataloging-in-Publication Data

ISBN: 9781138058590 (hbk)
ISBN: 9781138058569 (pbk)
ISBN: 9781315164090 (ebk)

DOI: 10.1201/9781315164090

Typeset in CMR10 font
by KnowledgeWorks Global Ltd.

Contents

Preface

This book is for biostatisticians intent on learning statistical techniques and intuition for clinical trials. We focus on a relatively small number of statistical principles and many instructive trials such as the Extracorporeal Membrane Oxygenation (ECMO) Trial, the Cardiac Arrhythmia Suppression Trial (CAST), and the Women's Health Initiative. Some principles we present resulted from mistakes made and lessons learned. Other principles allow quick calculation of quantities such as power or sample size with no need for computer programs. For example, the 'EZ' principle shows that there is a single, simple equation that can be used to approximate power, sample size, or detectable effect in many different clinical trial scenarios. All that matters is EZ, the expected value of the z-statistic. Accommodating monitoring is also a snap with the EZ principle.

One difference between our book and other books on statistical aspects of clinical trials is our emphasis on the beauty and simplicity of re-randomization tests. This elegant tool requires almost no assumptions and can be applied in a multitude of settings, including those rare occasions when unexpected events force mid-course changes in design. One such example is the COVID-19 pandemic. Many clinics temporarily closed or curtailed all but essential medical care, resulting in cancellation of routine clinical trial visits. Investigators pondered whether to censor data occurring during periods when patients could not access their scheduled visits, and then restart the clock when the pandemic ended. One trial that originally did not plan to allow early stopping for noninferiority decided to allow it. The most carefully designed trials cannot anticipate emergencies that occur once in a century. Even in non-emergencies, changes might be required because of human error. In one trial, the primary endpoint had to be changed when investigators found that it could not be measured reliably. Is there a valid way to analyze a clinical trial that undergoes unforeseen changes? There is, and re-randomization tests play a pivotal role.

Another feature of the book is extensive coverage of group-sequential monitoring and adaptive methods in clinical trials. There are now amazing tools like the conditional error principle of Müeller and Schäfer (2004), whose applications have only begun to be explored. Adaptive methods have generated considerable controversy. We discuss this controversy and attempt to navigate the reader to 'acceptable' adaptations.

The book is not intended to be a comprehensive reference. Our goal is to engender statistical intuition that can be used in different types of clinical trials. We have included many important references, but omitted others. We assume that the reader is familiar with basic statistical techniques, although Chapter 1 provides a brief review of elementary inference, including Bayesian and frequentist perspectives.

Chapter 1

Evidence and Inference

The reader is expected to be familiar with basic statistical methods involving continuous and binary outcomes, such as t-tests and tests of proportions. Nonetheless, we briefly review classical and Bayesian statistical reasoning.

1.1 Terminology and Paradigm of Inference

Much of elementary statistics involves drawing conclusions about characteristics of populations. For instance, we may be interested in the mean weight μ of all U.S. adults. The outcome Y_i is the weight of person i. The *population* is the set of weights Y_i of all U.S. adults, and the characteristic we are interested in, the mean μ, is the *parameter*. Of course, it would be infeasible to weigh every adult in the U.S., so we use a *sample*, a subset of the population, to help us draw conclusions about the population. The mean $\bar{Y}$ of the sample is an *estimator* of the parameter μ. Weight is an example of a *continuous outcome* because if we could measure it finely enough, weight could take any value in an interval such as $(150, 160)$. Sometimes the outcome of interest is *binary* (also called *dichotomous*). For example, we might be interested in knowing the proportion p of obese individuals among all adults in the U.S. In that case, the outcome Y_i is whether individual i is obese or not, with $Y_i = 0$ or $Y_i = 1$ denoting not obese or obese, respectively. The population is the set of 0s and 1s of all adults in the U.S., and the parameter p is the proportion of 1s in the population. We again take a subset of the population, and estimate p by the proportion $\hat{p}$ of 1s among the subset. The goal is to make inferences about the parameter p from the estimator $\hat{p}$. We are usually interested in comparing two or more populations, in which case the parameter might be the difference in means or proportions between the two populations.

Naturally, the performance of an estimator depends on how the sample was taken. Classical statistical methods assume that samples are *randomly* selected from the population in a way that every possible sample of size n is equally likely. Equivalently, the observations $Y_1, \ldots, Y_n$ in the sample are *independent and identically distributed (iid)* from some probability distribution F, which represents the population. Random sampling from the population allows us to determine how accurately a sample estimator will estimate the parameter. In practice, we never actually take random samples from the population of interest, so the usual basis for inference is shaky. Chapter 6 presents an alternative approach using randomization, rather than random sampling, as the basis for inference.

DOI: 10.1201/9781315164090-1

1.2   Classical Inference

1.2.1   Hypothesis Tests and P-Values

The classical, or *frequentist*, approach to inference uses indirect reasoning. Consider *hypothesis testing*, the testing of statements about parameters. Suppose I claim an ability to correctly guess outcomes of coin flips. Naturally, you are skeptical, and believe that my probability p of a correct guess is 0.5. You conduct an experiment with 500 coin flips. Let Y_i be the indicator that I correctly guess the ith coin flip, $i = 1, \ldots, 500$. That is, $Y_i = 0$ or 1 depending on whether my guess on flip i is incorrect or correct, respectively. The Y_i are 500 independent and identically distributed (iid) *Bernoulli random variables* with probability parameter p. Your position is that my probability of a correct guess is 0.5. This default position, until proven otherwise, is called the *null hypothesis* and denoted by H_0. I want to show the *alternative hypothesis* that my probability of a correct guess exceeds 0.5. Formally, the null and alternative hypotheses are:

$$\begin{aligned} H_0 : p &= 0.5, \\ H_1 : p &> 0.5. \end{aligned} \tag{1.1}$$

I want to reject H_0 in favor of H_1. The number of correct guesses in the sample of 500, $S = \sum_{i=1}^{500} Y_i$, has a *binomial distribution*

$$\text{binom(n, p)} : P(S = s) = \binom{n}{s} p^s (1 - p)^{n-s}, \quad \binom{n}{s} = \frac{n!}{s!(n - s)!},$$

with $n = 500$ trials and probability parameter p. I will reject H_0 and declare a *statistically significant* result, one that defies chance, if my number of correct guesses equals or exceeds a certain *critical value* C. C is selected to make the probability of a *type I error*—rejecting H_0 when it is true—quite small. This probability of a type I error is called the *type I error rate* and denoted by α. Unfortunately, many statisticians confuse type I error with type I error rate; type I error is the error itself and type I error rate is the probability of that error. We often pick $\alpha = 0.05$. To find the critical value C, note that the null probability of 269 or more correct guesses is

$$P(S \geq 269 \,|\, p = 0.5) = \sum_{i=269}^{500} \binom{500}{i} (0.5)^i (1 - 0.5)^{500-i} = 0.049 < 0.05, \tag{1.2}$$

whereas the null probability of 268 or more correct guesses exceeds 0.05. Therefore, $C = 269$. If I correctly guess 269 or more flips, I will reject H_0 and declare that my probability of correctly guessing coin flips exceeds 0.5. The above hypothesis test is known as an *exact test* because the exact distribution of the statistic is used to construct the test.

Remark 1.1. *'Exact test' does not mean that the type I error rate is exactly* 0.05.

We illustrate Remark 1.1 by supposing that the sample size had been $n = 10$ coin flips instead of $n = 500$. Then H_0 is rejected only if $S \geq 9$ because $P(S \geq 9 \,|\, p = 0.5) = 0.011 < 0.05$ but $P(S \geq 8 \,|\, p = 0.5) = 0.055 > 0.05$. The actual type I error rate (called the *size* of the test) is 0.011 instead of 0.05. We could achieve size 0.05, but only by introducing artificial randomness. Specifically, if we reject H_0 for sure if $X \geq 9$, and with probability 0.893 if $X = 8$, the type I error rate is $(0.893)P(X = 8) + P(X \geq 9) = 0.05$. No one would use such a *randomized test*, partly because two different people using the same data could reach different conclusions.

Returning to the 500 coin flips, suppose that I correctly guess 300. To convey that I greatly exceeded the required 269 correct guesses, I argue as follows. If I am really completely guessing (i.e., $p = 0.5$), the probability of 300 correct guesses,

$$P(S = 300 \mid p = 0.5) = \binom{500}{300}(0.5)^{300}(1 - 0.5)^{500-300},$$

is approximately 1.5 in a million. Given that I accomplished what would be nearly impossible if H_0 is true, I conclude that H_0 must be false.

There is a problem with the above reasoning. Under the null hypothesis that $p = 0.5$, even the most likely outcome of 250 correct guesses out of 500 has small probability (0.036) because of the sheer number of possible outcomes. Therefore, I modify my argument as follows. The probability of 300 **or more** correct guesses out of 500 if the null hypothesis is true,

$$P(S \geq 300 \mid p = 0.5) = \sum_{i=300}^{500} \binom{500}{i}(0.5)^{i}(1 - 0.5)^{500-i},$$

is about 4.5 in a million. The *p-value*, the null probability of a result **at least** as extreme (in the direction of the alternative hypothesis) as the observed result, is 4.5 in a million. Either the null hypothesis is false or an incredibly rare event occurred. Note that the p-value circumvents the problem raised above that even the most likely outcome is not very likely; the p-value for the most likely outcome of 250 correct guesses out of 500 is

$$P(S \geq 250 \mid p = 0.5) = \sum_{i=250}^{500} \binom{500}{i}(0.5)^{i}(1 - 0.5)^{500-i} \approx 0.52.$$

P-values indicate whether observed results are consistent with chance.

Remark 1.2. *A tiny p-value does not necessarily imply that the true parameter value is far from the null value. With large sample sizes, we can effectively rule out chance even if the true effect is small.*

For instance, in this coin flipping example, we could have rejected H_0 with an observed proportion of correct guesses as low as $269/500 = 0.54$, which is very close to the null value of 0.50.

Note the indirect reasoning of hypothesis testing: given that results at least as extreme as the observed result would have been very unlikely if H_0 were true, we conclude that H_0 is false.

1.2.2 Confidence Intervals

Having dispelled the notion that $p = 0.5$ in the coin flipping experiment, we might ask what other values of p can be eliminated. For example, is there strong evidence that p exceeds 0.55? We can test a new null hypothesis $H_0 : p = 0.55$ against the alternative hypothesis $H_1 : p > 0.55$ in the same way. The one-tailed p-value for 300 correct guesses out of 500 is now

$$P(S \geq 300 \mid p = 0.55) = \sum_{i=300}^{500} \binom{500}{i}(0.55)^{i}(1 - 0.55)^{500-i} = 0.014.$$

This is still quite unusual, so we are confident that $p > 0.55$. We could use a grid search of values of p_0 until the test of

$$H_0 : p = p_0 \quad \text{versus} \quad H_1 : p > p_0$$

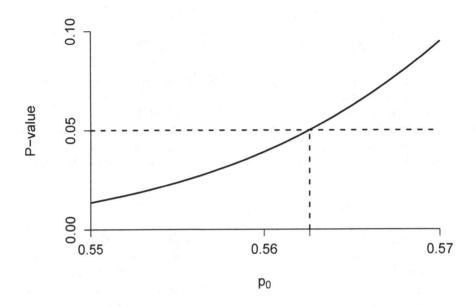

Figure 1.1: Plot of p-values for testing $H_0 : p = p_0$ versus $H_1 : p > p_0$. The p-value is 0.05 when $p_0 = 0.5626$ (dashed vertical line).

produces a p-value at the threshold of what is considered unusual, 0.05.

Figure 1.1 shows that the p-value is 0.05 for the test of $H_0 : p = 0.5626$ versus $H_1 : p > 0.5626$. Therefore, we rule out values of p less than or equal to 0.5626. The one-tailed 95% confidence interval for p is $(0.5626, 1)$. More generally, the $100(1-\alpha)\%$ one-sided confidence interval for p is the set of values p_0 for which the test of $H_0 : p = p_0$ versus $H_1 : p > p_0$ is not statistically significant at level α. This method of constructing a confidence interval is known as *inverting a test* (see section 9.2.1 of Casella and Berger, 2002). We can modify the one-sided interval to get the more common two-sided $100(1-\alpha)\%$ confidence interval for p as follows. Find the lower limit p_L such that the test of $H_0 : p = p_L$ versus $H_1 : p > p_L$ has p-value $\alpha/2$, then find the upper limit p_U such that the test of $H_0 : p = p_U$ versus $p < p_U$ has p-value $\alpha/2$. Then (p_L, p_U) is a $100(1-\alpha)\%$ two-sided confidence interval for p. These exact binomial confidence intervals for p are known as *Clopper-Pearson* exact confidence intervals (see Clopper and Pearson, 1934 or Example 9.2.5 of Casella and Berger, 2002).

Remark 1.3. *Just as 'exact' test does not mean that the type I error rate is exactly α, 'exact confidence interval' does not mean that its coverage probability is exactly $100(1-\alpha)\%$. Instead, the coverage probability is at least $100(1-\alpha)\%$.*

It is important to recognize that, to a classical statistician, the endpoints of the confidence intervals, not the parameter, are random quantities. Imagine repeating the experiment of flipping 500 coins and constructing a 95% confidence interval for p each time. Ninety five percent of such intervals would contain the true, fixed value p. This interpretation in terms of the frequency that confidence intervals cover the parameter accounts for the name *frequentist* statistics.

1.2.3 Criticisms of Classical Methods

The p-value has come under heated attack recently, leading one scientific journal, *Basic and Applied Social Psychology*, to take the drastic, ill-advised measure of banning p-values. One complaint about the p-value is a perceived lack of reproducibility (e.g., Goodman, 1992). Suppose that the test statistic T has continuous distribution function $F(t)$ under H_0 and we reject H_0 for small (resp., large) values of T. Then the p-value $F(T)$ (resp., $1 - F(T)$) has a uniform $(0, 1)$ distribution under H_0. This is easiest to see if F is strictly increasing: with $Y = F(T)$ and $y \in [0, 1]$,

$$P\{Y \leq y\} = P\{F(T) \leq y\} = P\{T \leq F^{-1}(y)\} = F\{F^{-1}(y)\} = y,$$

which is the distribution function of a uniform $(0, 1)$ random variable. Not surprisingly, if H_0 is true, we could easily get a p-value of 0.20 today and 0.80 tomorrow while attempting to replicate the same experiment. That is the nature of the uniform distribution! Therefore, p-values actually behave as they should (Senn, 2001; Senn, 2002; Greenland, 2019). Likewise, under an alternative hypothesis with a small treatment effect, the p-value might be close to uniformly distributed. Again, we should not expect the same value of the p-value from one replication to the next. If we focus instead on whether the p-value meets a typical threshold level like 0.05, there is more consistency. Even then, if the treatment effect is small, we could get a statistically significant effect in one replication, but not the other. However, alternative methods of analyzing the data will be similarly inconsistent under such circumstances.

An understandable criticism of the p-value may be found in the very accessible article by Berger and Berry (1988). They argue that incorporation of probabilities of results more extreme than those observed is strange: why should we consider things that did not happen? Moreover, gauging what is more extreme is not always straightforward. For example, suppose that, in a study that originally planned to examine results only at the end, we stop halfway through because the z-score for treatment benefit is 3.0. What is the p-value? It is not clear what results are more extreme than the observed result. Larger z-scores at the halfway point should certainly be included as more extreme, but we might have also stopped at an even earlier time point if results had been striking enough. For instance, we might have stopped one quarter of the way through the study if the z-score had been 2.8. That might be considered more extreme because it happened at an earlier time point. Retrospectively deciding what is more extreme is problematic. Therefore, computing a p-value or attempting to quantify the type I error rate of an experiment with unplanned changes is simply not possible. Why should we need to worry about what is more extreme than the observed result when we never observe anything more extreme than the observed result?

Another peculiarity of the p-value, noted by Berger and Berry (1988) and discussed extensively by Lindley and Phillips (1976), is that it depends on how data were collected. Consider the following example of what is sometimes called the *binomial negative-binomial paradox*.

Example 1.4. Suppose that the manufacturer of a drug is trying to demonstrate that fewer than 20% of patients experience a certain adverse event (AE). Of 25 people given the drug, exactly 1 experiences the AE. A one-tailed binomial test of $H_0 : p = 0.20$ against the alternative $H_1 : p < 0.20$ is used at $\alpha = 0.025$. The set of results at least as extreme, in the direction of H_1, as the observed result consists of 0 AEs or 1 AE. The p-value is

$$P(\leq 1 \text{ AE} \mid H_0) = \binom{25}{0}(0.20)^0(1 - 0.20)^{25-0}$$
$$+ \binom{25}{1}(0.20)^1(1 - 0.20)^{25-1} = 0.027,$$

which barely misses the pre-specified alpha level of 0.025.

Then the manufacturer points out that the study was actually designed to continue sampling new patients until exactly one experiences the adverse event. That changes everything, argues the manufacturer. The total number of patients with the adverse event is now fixed at 1, and the only randomness lies in the total sample size N. 'At least as extreme' as the observed result now corresponds to N being at least as large as 25. This is equivalent to the first 24 patients not having the AE. Therefore, the actual p-value is

$$P(N \geq 25 \,|\, H_0) = P(\text{none of the first 24 patients experiences the AE} \,|\, H_0)$$
$$= (1 - 0.20)^{24} = 0.005. \tag{1.3}$$

The observed result is now highly statistically significant!

What changed? Regardless of whether the study was designed with a fixed sample size of 25 or a fixed number of patients with the adverse event, 1 patient experienced the AE and 24 did not. Is anything else relevant? What person confronted with this information would even ask how the study was designed? Berger and Berry (1988) facetiously note that if an investigator presented data from a study and died before revealing the design, a classical statistician would have no way to analyze the data!   □

Another complaint against the p-value is that it considers only what happens under the null hypothesis. This issue applies not just to p-values, but to the logic of hypothesis testing more generally, namely that because we observed what would be a rare event if H_0 were true, we conclude that H_0 is false. The observed result might have been unlikely even under the alternative hypothesis, as in the following example illustrating the connection between diagnostic testing and hypothesis testing.

Example 1.5. Consider a diagnostic test for a disease. The test has *specificity* 95%, meaning that if a person does not have the disease, there is a 95% probability that the test will be negative. Think of the diagnostic test as a hypothesis test with null and alternative hypotheses

$$H_0 : \text{The person does not have the disease,}$$
$$H_1 : \text{The person has the disease.} \tag{1.4}$$

We will reject the null hypothesis and declare that the person has the disease if the diagnostic test is positive. The type I error rate of this hypothesis test is

$$P(\text{test is positive} \,|\, \text{does not have disease})$$
$$= 1 - P(\text{test is negative} \,|\, \text{does not have disease})$$
$$= 1 - 0.95 = 0.05. \tag{1.5}$$

Suppose that the diagnostic test is positive. By the reasoning of hypothesis testing, we should be confident that the person has the disease. After all, someone who does not have the disease is unlikely to test positive. But what if the 'diagnostic test' consists of randomly picking a number between 0 and 1 and declaring that the person has the disease if the selected number is in the interval $(0, 0.05)$? The type I error rate of this test is still 0.05 because (1.5) still holds. But the probability of testing positive is only 0.05 whether the person has the disease or not! Therefore, a positive test does not give us **any** information about whether the person has the disease. To be more confident, we must know additional information about the diagnostic or hypothesis test.

We want a diagnostic test to have high probability of testing positive if the person really does have the disease. This probability is called the *sensitivity* of the diagnostic test. If sensitivity is high, say 90%, we should feel more confident about a positive result because a positive result is unlikely if the person does not have the disease and likely if the person does have the disease. Sensitivity in this diagnostic test corresponds to the *power* of the corresponding hypothesis test, namely the probability of rejecting the null hypothesis when it is false. If power is high, then rejecting the null hypothesis is unlikely if H_0 is true and likely if H_0 is false.

Knowing that the diagnostic test has 90% sensitivity and 95% specificity makes us more confident, but other information may be relevant, namely how rare the disease is. Suppose the disease is vanishingly rare, having probability 1 in 1 million. It can be shown that the conditional probability of having the disease given that a person tests positive, called the *positive predictive value* of the diagnostic test, is only 0.00002. This is understandable: even though the error rates of the diagnostic test are relatively low, they pale in comparison to how rare the disease is. Having additional prior information that the disease is extremely rare changes the strength of evidence of the positive diagnostic test. The analog in hypothesis testing of H_0: treatment has no effect versus H_1: treatment has a beneficial effect is having prior information about the treatment effect. We would like to somehow incorporate that information into our conclusion. We would also like to flip the probability calculation like we did with the diagnostic test when we computed positive predictive value instead of sensitivity. The analog in hypothesis testing is computing the probability that the alternative hypothesis is true given that we rejected it, rather than the probability of rejecting the null hypothesis given that the alternative hypothesis is true. We will see that Bayesian methods offer both advantages: they incorporate prior information and they flip the probability calculation. □

1.2.4 Bayesian Approach

A Bayesian views inference differently from a classical statistician. Both view the parameter as a fixed number, but a Bayesian formulates uncertainty about that fixed number using a *prior distribution* for the parameter. After seeing data, the Bayesian updates the prior distribution to a *posterior distribution*, which is the conditional distribution of the parameter given the data. Inference is based on that posterior distribution.

Example 1.6. Return to Example 1.4. To use Bayesian methods, we must specify a prior distribution for p, the probability of experiencing the AE. The beta family of densities, $\pi_{\alpha,\beta}(p) = c(\alpha, \beta)p^{\alpha-1}(1 - p)^{\beta-1}$, where $p \in (0,1)$, $\alpha > 0$, $\beta > 0$, and $c(\alpha, \beta)$ is such that $\int_0^1 \pi_{\alpha,\beta}(p)dp = 1$, is a mathematically convenient and flexible family of prior distributions for a probability parameter. It has a wide variety of different shapes for different values of α and β. The beta distribution is a *conjugate prior distribution* for the binomial, meaning that the posterior distribution of p given the data is also in the beta family.

To see that the beta distribution is a conjugate prior, first imagine that a fixed sample of size n is used rather than sampling to a fixed number of AEs. Let X be the observed number of AEs. The conditional probability mass function of X given p is binomial (n, p). Denote the marginal probability mass function of X by $g(x)$. The posterior density of p given $X = x$ is

$$\pi(p \mid x) = \frac{f(x \mid p)\pi_{\alpha,\beta}(p)}{g(x)} = \frac{\binom{n}{x}p^x(1 - p)^{n-x}c(\alpha, \beta)p^{\alpha-1}(1 - p)^{\beta-1}}{g(x)}$$

$$= k(n, x, \alpha, \beta)p^{x+\alpha-1}(1 - p)^{n-x+\beta-1}, \tag{1.6}$$

where $k(n, x, \alpha, \beta) = c(\alpha, \beta)\binom{n}{x}/g(x)$ does not depend on p. Of course, $k(n, x, \alpha, \beta)$ must be such that $\int_0^1 \pi(p \mid x)dp = 1$. Therefore, the posterior density of p given x is beta with parameters $\alpha + x$ and $\beta + n - x$. The posterior distribution is in the same beta family of distributions, hence the beta distribution is a conjugate prior for the binomial. This relationship between the beta and binomial distribution is called the *beta-binomial distribution*.

We can view the prior information as being comparable to $\alpha + \beta$ Bernoulli observations, α of which are 1 and β of which are 0. The posterior distribution then combines the prior numbers of ones and zeroes with the numbers of ones and zeroes from the data, producing the $\alpha + x$ and $\beta + n - x$ in (1.6).

For example, suppose that the manufacturer considers their prior information to be like 10 prior patients, 1 of whom experiences the AE. That is, the prior is beta ($\alpha = 1$, $\beta = 9$). Recall that in the actual data, $X = 1$ adverse event was observed in $n = 25$ people. The posterior distribution of p given $X = 1$ is beta $(1 + 1, 9 + 25 - 1) = (2, 33)$. We can use this posterior distribution to make inferences about p. For instance, the posterior probability that p is less than 0.20 is

$$\int_0^{0.20} \pi_{2,33}(p)dp = 0.995.$$

The manufacturer can now state, with probability 0.995, that fewer than 20% of patients will experience the AE. $\square$

The manufacturer in Example 1.6 benefits greatly from their prior information, which translates into 10 additional observations. Instead of 25 observations, the manufacturer now has 35. But one way of viewing this Bayesian method is that it makes up data! In a brilliant lecture, Dr. K.K.G. (Gordon) Lan tells the story of two fictitious investigators, one of whom is fired for fabricating data, while the other is lauded for innovative use of a Bayesian method that is mathematically equivalent to the data fabrication of the first investigator!

The above anecdote highlights one danger of Bayesian methods: a prior distribution that assumes a strong treatment benefit requires very little data to confirm the prior opinion. That is why many clinical trialists prefer *skeptical prior* distributions that do not assume that treatment works. To avoid having conclusions depend heavily on the prior distribution, choose small $\alpha + \beta$. That corresponds to a small number of prior observations that are quickly overwhelmed by actual data. One good choice is $\alpha = 1$, $\beta = 1$, the uniform distribution on $(0, 1)$. The prior information in that case is like having only 2 observations, one of which is an AE. Another reasonable choice is *Jeffreys prior*, $\alpha = \beta = 1/2$.

Recall that in Example 1.4, the manufacturer reveals that the actual design was to continue sampling until exactly 1 patient has an AE. For the Bayesian, the same answer results regardless of whether the sample size is fixed or sampling continues to a fixed number of AEs. This is because the conditional distribution of p given x is the same for the two sampling schemes. Note also that only the observed value $x = 1$ was used to calculate the posterior distribution.

Remark 1.7. *With Bayesian methodology, only the observed value of the test statistic matters; there is no computation of probabilities of more extreme results like there is with the p-value.*

1.2.5   Large Sample Inference

When sample sizes are large, inferences become much simpler because many estimators and test statistics are approximately *normally distributed*. Recall that the normal distribution with mean μ and variance σ^2 has density function $f(y; \mu, \sigma^2) = \exp\{-(1/2)(y - $

$\mu)^2/\sigma^2\}/\sqrt{2\pi\sigma^2}$. When $\mu = 0$ and $\sigma^2 = 1$, we say that Y has a *standard normal distribution* and denote its distribution and density functions by $\Phi(y)$ and $\phi(y)$, respectively.

A random variable T_n is said to be *asymptotically normal with mean a_n and variance b_n* if

$$P\left(\frac{T_n - a_n}{\sqrt{b_n}} \leq z\right) \to \Phi(z) \text{ as } n \to \infty$$

for every z. In other words, we can approximate the distribution of T_n with a normal distribution with mean a_n and variance b_n when n is large.

One of the most important theorems in probability, the *central limit theorem*, states that sample means are asymptotically normal under mild conditions:

Theorem 1.8. Central limit theorem (CLT) *Let $Y_1, Y_2, \ldots$ be iid random variables with finite variance σ^2 and let $\bar{Y} = (1/n)\sum_{i=1}^{n} Y_i$. Then $\bar{Y}$ is asymptotically normal with mean μ and variance σ^2/n.*

One of the consequences of the CLT is that $\bar{Y}$ has high probability of being close to μ when n is large because $\bar{Y}$ has mean μ and small variance, σ^2/n.

The central limit theorem applies to the binary outcome setting because a sample proportion $\hat{p}_n$ is just a sample mean of 0s and 1s. The CLT implies that $\hat{p}_n$ is approximately normal with mean p and variance $p(1-p)/n$. Therefore, an approximate test of $H_0 : p = p_0$ treats the z-statistic

$$Z = \frac{\hat{p} - p_0}{\sqrt{p_0(1 - p_0)/n}} \tag{1.7}$$

as standard normal under the null hypothesis. Thus, for a two-tailed test at level α, we would reject H_0 if either $Z < -z_{\alpha/2}$ or $Z > z_{\alpha/2}$, where $z_{\alpha/2}$ is the $(1 - \alpha/2)$th quantile of the standard normal distribution. Note that the denominator of (1.7) is the standard error of $\hat{p}$ under the null hypothesis. Likewise, the CLT implies that a large sample $100(1 - \alpha)\%$ confidence interval for p is

$$\hat{p} \pm z_{\alpha/2}\sqrt{\hat{p}(1 - \hat{p})/n}. \tag{1.8}$$

Note that the standard error in (1.8) uses $\hat{p}$ instead of p_0. Thus, the test statistic and confidence interval use slightly different standard errors.

Similarly, the CLT can be used in the two-sample setting with binary outcomes. The sample proportions $\hat{p}_1$ and $\hat{p}_2$ are independent and each is asymptotically normal by the CLT. Accordingly, the difference $\hat{p}_1 - \hat{p}_2$ is asymptotically normal with mean $p_1 - p_2$ and variance equal to the sum of variances of $\hat{p}_1$ and $\hat{p}_2$. Therefore, a test of $H_0 : p_1 - p_2 = 0$ can be based on the z-statistic

$$Z = \frac{\hat{p}_1 - \hat{p}_2}{\sqrt{\hat{p}(1 - \hat{p})(1/n_1 + 1/n_2)}}, \tag{1.9}$$

where $\hat{p} = (n_1\hat{p}_1 + n_2\hat{p}_2)/(n_1 + n_2)$ is the overall proportion in the two groups combined. This z-statistic is approximately standard normal under the null hypothesis. Likewise, a $100(1 - \alpha)\%$ confidence interval for $p_1 - p_2$ is

$$\hat{p}_1 - \hat{p}_2 \pm z_{\alpha/2}\sqrt{\hat{p}_1(1 - \hat{p}_1)/n_1 + \hat{p}_2(1 - \hat{p}_2)/n_2}. \tag{1.10}$$

Again the test and confidence interval use slightly different standard errors. The test assumes that the null hypothesis is true and uses the best estimate of the common value of p in the two groups, whereas the confidence interval estimates p_1 and p_2 separately.

We sometimes transform an estimator or test statistic to improve the fit of a normal approximation. Consider the setting of a continuous outcome. Although a sample variance

S^2 is asymptotically normal, the distribution of S^2 remains somewhat skewed unless n is extremely large. The distribution of $\ln(S^2)$ is less skewed. Therefore, a better confidence interval for σ^2 is obtained by applying a normal approximation to $\ln(S^2)$, computing a confidence interval (L, U) for $\ln(\sigma^2)$, and then exponentiating the endpoints, $(\exp(L), \exp(U))$.

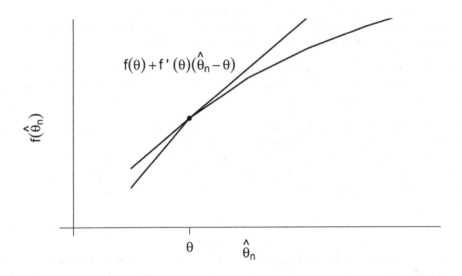

Figure 1.2: The delta method approximates the function $f(\hat{\theta}_n)$ with the tangent line at the true parameter value θ. When n is large, $\hat{\theta}_n$ is close to θ and the linear approximation is accurate.

The key large sample result for dealing with transformations is that if $\hat{\theta}_n$ is asymptotically normal with mean θ and variance tending to 0, then a function $f(\hat{\theta}_n)$ is also asymptotically normal under certain conditions. To see this, note that

$$f(\hat{\theta}_n) \approx f(\theta) + f'(\theta)(\hat{\theta}_n - \theta) \tag{1.11}$$

for large n. This follows from the fact that $\hat{\theta}_n$ will be close to θ because $\hat{\theta}_n$ has mean θ and variance tending to 0. The first-order Taylor series (1.11) will be a good approximation to $f(\hat{\theta}_n)$ for $\hat{\theta}_n$ close to θ (see Figure 1.2). From Equation (1.11), $f(\hat{\theta}_n)$ is approximately a linear function of $\hat{\theta}_n$, and a linear function of a normal random variable is also normal. The precise result is stated in Theorem 1.9, a proof of which can be found on page 118 of Serfling (1980).

Theorem 1.9. Delta method *Let f be a function with nonzero derivative $f'(\theta)$ at the true parameter value θ. Suppose that $\hat{\theta}_n$ is asymptotically normal with mean θ and variance v_n, where $v_n \to 0$ as $n \to \infty$. Then $f(\hat{\theta}_n)$ is asymptotically normal with mean $f(\theta)$ and variance $\{f'(\theta)\}^2 v_n$.*

We illustrate the delta method by computing the asymptotic distribution of $\ln(\hat{p}_n)$, where $\hat{p}_n$ is a sample proportion of n iid Bernoulli observations. Here, $f(\hat{p}_n) = \ln(\hat{p}_n)$, so $f'(p) = 1/p$. Also, $v_n = \text{var}(\hat{p}_n) = p(1-p)/n \to 0$. Therefore, by Theorem 1.9, $\ln(\hat{p}_n)$ is asymptotically normally distributed with mean $\ln(p)$ and variance

$$\{f'(p)\}^2 v_n = (1/p^2)p(1-p)/n = \frac{1-p}{np}.$$

1.3 Robust Methods Are Preferred in Clinical Trials

Statisticians are trained to check assumptions and change the analysis if those assumptions are not met. Clinical trialists, on the other hand, are very leery about changing analyses that were pre-specified in the protocol. A clinical trial is viewed as a definitive experiment. A danger of allowing changes driven by perceived assumption violations is that 'assumption violation' is vaguely defined. A statistician might look at plots of residuals versus predicted values and make a subjective judgment about whether assumptions are satisfied. Furthermore, there are almost always several alternative analysis methods to choose from. If we are allowed to look at observed results, declare in an arbitrary manner that assumptions are violated, and then choose from among several alternative analysis methods, we can get the answer we want rather than the right answer. Clinical trialists prefer *robust methods*, methods that work well even if assumptions are violated. This leads to our first principle.

Principle 1.10. Robustness principle *Robust statistical methods should be used in clinical trials.*

We illustrate robustness in the context of a t-test. The goal of a t-test is to test whether two means, μ_1 and μ_2, are equal. The standard t-statistic is

$$T = \frac{\bar{Y}_1 - \bar{Y}_2}{\sqrt{S_P^2(1/n_1 + 1/n_2)}},$$

where $\bar{Y}_1$ and $\bar{Y}_2$ are sample means of the n_1 and n_2 observations in the two groups, and S_P^2 is the pooled variance estimate. If S_1^2 and S_2^2 are sample variances in the two groups,

$$S_P^2 = \frac{(n_1-1)S_1^2 + (n_2-1)S_2^2}{n_1 + n_2 - 2}$$

is a weighted average of the two sample variances. The assumption is that the population variances σ_1^2 and σ_2^2 in the two groups are equal. But what if they are not? Imagine an extreme situation in which σ_1^2 is much smaller than σ_2^2. If n_1 is larger than n_2, then S_P^2 gives greater weight to the group whose population variance is smaller. This results in a variance estimate that is smaller than it should be. This, in turn, leads to an inflated type I error rate. In other words, the probability of falsely declaring that $\mu_1 \neq \mu_2$ exceeds the desired alpha level when the smaller variance is in the group with the larger sample size.

A simple fix to the above problem uses *Welch's unequal variance t-statistic* (Welch, 1947):

$$T = \frac{\bar{Y}_1 - \bar{Y}_2}{\sqrt{S_1^2/n_1 + S_2^2/n_2}}.$$

Welch's statistic does not have an exact t-distribution under the null hypothesis because $S_1^2/n_1 + S_2^2/n_2$ has only approximately the distribution of a chi-squared random variable divided by its degrees of freedom. To figure out the degrees of freedom ν for this approximation, equate the mean and variance of $S_1^2/n_1 + S_2^2/n_2$ to those of a chi-squared random variable divided by ν and solve for ν. This results in *Satterthwaite's approximation* for the degrees of freedom (Satterthwaite, 1947):

$$\nu = \frac{(S_1^2/n_1 + S_2^2/n_2)^2}{\frac{S_1^4}{n_1^2(n_1-1)} + \frac{S_2^4}{n_2^2(n_2-1)}}.$$

This number is usually not an integer, but that does not matter. There is virtually no down side to Welch's t-test compared to the more common t-test. The two are very similar if $\sigma_1^2 = \sigma_2^2$, but Welch's t-test protects against the possibility that $\sigma_1^2 \neq \sigma_2^2$. By the robustness principle, Welch's t-test is generally preferred to the standard t-test.

Of course, the t-test is based on the assumption that data are normally distributed. If sample sizes are large, the t-test is valid, in the sense of having the right type I error rate, by the central limit theorem. But if the data are quite *skewed* or contain *outliers*, the median may be better than the mean at representing the center. The classic example of out-liers/skewed data is income data. The income of a single individual like Bill Gates can pull the mean dramatically to the right such that a substantial majority of people have incomes below the mean. Additionally, outliers have a profound effect on the standard deviation, which can cause severe loss of power for the t-test. A *nonparametric test*, also called a *rank test*, has much better performance. Nonparametric tests use ranks rather than the original data. For example, the *Wilcoxon rank sum test* combines data from both groups, ranks them, and then determines whether the sum of the ranks in one group is unusually large relative to what would be expected under the null hypothesis of equal distributions in the two groups. Ranks cannot have outliers because they take values $1, 2, \ldots, n$. Consequently, rank tests can be much more powerful than the t-test when data are not normally dis-tributed, and have power close to that of the t-test when data are normally distributed. In other words, nonparametric procedures are robust. Hollander and Wolfe (1973) provide an accessible compendium of nonparametric methods, while Randles and Wolfe (1979) provide a more advanced exposition.

A useful perspective on nonparametric methods is in terms of *monotone transforma-tions* of data, which can be used to reduce skew and permit a t-test to be applied. For example, HIV viral load data, indicating the amount of virus in the plasma, are notori-ously right-skewed because some people can have viral loads in the millions, for example. Base 10 logarithms of viral loads are routinely used to reduce skew. In other settings, we may not know the precise transformation needed, but it is not too much of a stretch to think that there is **some** monotone transformation $f(Y)$ that is normally distributed. The beauty of nonparametric methods is that ranks are unchanged by monotone transforma-tions. Therefore, nonparametric methods can be viewed as not requiring us to know the specific transformation needed to convert the data to normally distributed observations.

One ingenious method called the *van der Waerden normal scores test* (see pages 396-406 of Conover, 1999) explicitly finds the magic transformation of the preceding paragraph. A slightly over-simplified description of the normal scores test is as follows. Combine the data from the two groups, rank them, and replace those ranks with what we would expect if the data followed a standard normal distribution. For example, the smallest and largest ranks are replaced by approximate expected values of smallest and largest order statistics from a standard normal distribution, and so on. Now that we have essentially conjured normally distributed data, we can apply a t-test.

An alternative approach requiring virtually no assumptions is described in Chapter 6.

Exercises

1. Is the p-value the probability that the null hypothesis is true?

2. What does it mean to say that a test is robust? Why is robustness important in clinical trials?

3. Approximate the probability (1.2) using a normal distribution with the same mean and variance as a binomial, namely $\mu = np$ and $\sigma^2 = np(1-p)$. Compare your answer to the exact binomial probability.

4. Show that, in Example 1.4, a Bayesian analysis using a beta prior distribution results in the same answer for the two different sampling schemes. Does the same result hold for any prior distribution?

5. In Example 1.4:

   (a) Do you believe that the level of evidence is the same whether the sample size was fixed at 25 or resulted from continuing until 1 AE occurred? Explain your answer.

   (b) Which of the two p-values (fixed sample or sampling until 1 AE) does the Bayesian analysis tend to support?

6. [1] For iid Bernoulli observations with parameter p, consider the test of $H_0 : p = 1/2$ versus $H_1 : p > 1/2$. Results in two different datasets are: (1) 20 successes out of 20 and (2) 576 successes out of 1,000.

   (a) Show that the p-value is approximately the same for each dataset.

   (b) Compute the 95% upper confidence limit for p for each dataset.

   (c) Which dataset do you think shows stronger evidence against H_0?

7. **The $3/n$ rule** Suppose that among n people given a drug, none has a serious adverse event. Calculate the one-tailed Clopper-Pearson 95% upper confidence limit for p, the probability of experiencing an AE, if:

   (a) $n = 50$.

   (b) $n = 500$

   Compare your upper confidence limit to $3/n$.

8. Do you think the frequentist and Bayesian analyses of binary data (using the beta prior) should be quite similar if the sample size is large and $\alpha = \beta = 1$? Explain your reasoning.

1.4 Summary

1. Hypothesis tests and confidence intervals are useful and complementary tools.

   (a) Hypothesis tests reflect the strength of evidence for one hypothesis versus another. They can answer the question of whether a treatment has any benefit.

   (b) Confidence intervals provide a plausible range of values for the parameter being estimated. They can quantify the size of the treatment effect.

---

[1] This example is motivated by an example in Potter (2020), a fascinating article arguing against the use of the fragility index in clinical trials.

2. The p-value is the null probability of results at least as extreme as the observed result. It is useful for determining whether observed data are inconsistent with chance, but a p-value has limitations:

    (a) It is computed only under the null hypothesis; the observed result could be unusual even under the alternative hypothesis.

    (b) A small p-value need not mean a large effect. If the sample size is large enough, even a small effect will be statistically significant.

3. The contrasts between frequentist and Bayesian methods are as follows:

    (a) Bayesians specify a prior distribution reflecting uncertainty about the parameter, which allows computation of posterior probabilities about the parameter.

    (b) Frequentists use indirect reasoning that does not require quantifying initial uncertainty about the parameter.

    (c) Frequentists compute the probability of results **at least as extreme** as the observed result, whereas Bayesians use only the observed result in calculations; they do not have to think about what constitutes more extreme results.

4. The central limit theorem and delta method are essential tools for large sample inference.

5. Robustness is important in clinical trials; post-hoc changes because of assumption violations are frowned upon.

Chapter 2

2 × 2 Tables

2.1 Measures of Treatment Effect

Table 2.1: 28-day mortality in the Partnership for Research on Ebola Virus in Liberia II (PREVAIL II) trial in Ebola virus disease in Western Africa.

	Dead	Alive	
SC+ZMapp	8	28	36
SC	13	22	35
	21		71

Binary data from two groups are often summarized using a 2 × 2 table. For example, Table 2.1 presents 28-day mortality from the Partnership for Research on Ebola Virus in Liberia II (PREVAIL II) trial randomizing patients with Ebola virus disease in Liberia, Sierra Leone, and Guinea in Western Africa to either standard care (SC) or standard care plus the triple monoclonal antibody product ZMapp (SC+ZMapp). Standard care includes fluid replacement, treatment of fever and other symptoms, and so on. The trial was designed to have 100 patients in each group, but was terminated early because the Ebola epidemic in Western Africa ended. Denote SC + ZMapp as group 1 and SC alone as group 2. Let $\hat{p}_i = X_i/n_i$, $i = 1, 2$ be the sample proportions of people in the two groups who die by day 28. The two groups can be compared in at least three different ways:

$$\hat{p}_1 - \hat{p}_2, \tag{2.1}$$

$$\hat{p}_1/\hat{p}_2, \text{ or} \tag{2.2}$$

$$\frac{\hat{p}_1/(1 - \hat{p}_1)}{\hat{p}_2/(1 - \hat{p}_2)}. \tag{2.3}$$

Equations (2.1), (2.2), and (2.3) are known as the sample *risk difference, relative risk,* and *odds ratio*, respectively, of treatment 1 relative to treatment 2. In this Ebola example, (2.1), (2.2), and (2.3) are $8/36 - 13/35 = -0.149$, $(8/36)/(13/35) = 0.598$, and $\{(8/36)/(1-8/36)\}/\{(13/35)/(1-13/35)\} = 0.484$, respectively. These quantities estimate their population counterparts obtained by replacing sample proportions by population proportions (probabilities) in (2.1), (2.2), and (2.3). Treatment 1 is preferred to treatment 2 if the risk difference is negative, which is equivalent to the relative risk being less than 1, which in turn is equivalent to the odds ratio being less than 1.

DOI: 10.1201/9781315164090-2   15

Remark 2.1. *Although our discussion of the three measures focuses on death as the outcome of interest, any binary outcome can be used.*

Many people prefer the risk difference as a measure of treatment effect because of its interpretation: if N people get treatment 1 and N get treatment 2, the expected numbers of deaths in the two groups are Np_1 and Np_2. Accordingly, $Np_1 - Np_2 = N(p_1 - p_2)$ is the difference in expected numbers of deaths in the two groups. For example, if 100 people are given treatment 1 and 100 are given treatment 2 and $p_1 = 0.02$ and $p_2 = 0.05$, we expect $100(0.02) = 2$ and $100(0.05) = 5$ deaths in groups 1 and 2. Then $100(p_1 - p_2) = -3$, indicating that 3 fewer people will die with treatment 1 than with treatment 2 if 100 people are given each treatment.

A measure closely related to the risk difference is the *number needed to treat*. Assume that group 1 is receiving an active treatment and group 2 is not, so we hope that $p_1 < p_2$. The *number needed to treat (NNT)* is

$$N = \frac{1}{p_2 - p_1}. \tag{2.4}$$

Formula (2.4) is obtained by equating the number saved by treatment relative to no treatment, $N(p_2 - p_1)$, to 1 and solving for N. That is, the NNT is the number of people needing to receive the treatment to save one of them (relative to receiving no treatment). If the NNT is a small number like 5, treatment will have a big impact because only 5 people need to be treated before one life is saved. On the other hand, if the NNT is 500, then 500 people must be treated before one life is saved. The NNT reflects both the effectiveness of the treatment and the deadliness of disease. If p_1 and p_2 are both tiny, then the NNT will be small even if the **relative** benefit of treatment is large.

The relative risk, RR, also has an attractive interpretation because $100(1 - RR)$ is the percentage reduction in mortality for treatment 1 relative to treatment 2. For example, a relative risk of 0.75 is a relative reduction of $100(1 - 0.75) = 25\%$. If the same number of people are given treatment 1 and treatment 2, then the number of deaths on treatment 1 will be 25% smaller than on treatment 2. When interest centers on combining results from different trials of the same interventions (called *meta-analysis*), the relative risk may be preferred to the risk difference because it is more likely to be constant across trials. For example, suppose that the control event rate is 0.10 in one trial and 0.50 in another. If the risk difference of treatment to control is -0.20 in the second trial, then it necessarily differs from the risk difference in the first trial, which can be no smaller than $0 - 0.10 = -0.10$. A disadvantage of the relative risk is that it can be large even in situations in which the treatment will benefit almost no one. For example, consider an incredibly rare disease affecting only 10 people in the world. Even if a new treatment is 100% effective (that is, the relative risk is 0), only 10 people in the entire world will be saved!

The odds ratio is also a relative measure of treatment effect. Gamblers are familiar with odds because of their interpretation in terms of payoffs of bets: someone placing a $1 bet on a horse with 50 : 1 odds receives $50 if the horse wins. In biostatistics, odds and odds ratios seem more difficult to interpret than probabilities and relative risks. However, there are several reasons for thinking in terms of odds and odds ratios. The first is that the odds ratio is a reasonable measure regardless of whether the study samples a fixed number of people with and without a risk factor and compares the proportions with a given disease (*cohort study*), or samples a given number of people with and without a disease and compares the proportions with a given risk factor (*case control study*). The odds ratio for a given 2 × 2 table does not depend on the type of study, and remains unchanged if rows and columns are switched. This is not true for the other two measures.

Another reason for using the odds ratio is that it facilitates extension of regression techniques to binary data. If the outcome variable Y takes value 0 or 1, then fitting a linear

model of the form

$$Y = \beta_0 + \beta_1 x_1 + \ldots + \beta_k x_k \qquad (2.5)$$

to covariates $x_1, \ldots, x_k$ makes no sense because the left side of (2.5) is binary, but the right side is not. We could make the left side continuous by replacing Y by $P(Y = 1)$, but then the left side is restricted to be in the interval $[0, 1]$, but the right side is not. We could take another step in the right direction by replacing the left side of (2.5) by the odds, $P(Y = 1)/\{1 - P(Y = 1)\}$. The advantage is that the odds can take any nonnegative value. Still, the right side of (2.5) can be negative. The final step, called *logistic regression*, replaces the left side of (2.5) by the natural logarithm of the odds. Taking logs serves two purposes: (1) the log odds can take any negative or positive value, and (2) the log odds is invariant to whether we model the probability of an event E or its complement. To understand the second point, suppose that the event is death. The odds of death being $1/2$ is the same as the odds of survival being $2/1$, and yet $1/2$ and $2/1$ are not equidistant from the 'as likely as not' odds value of 1.

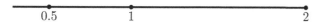

$$
\begin{array}{ccc}
\bullet & \bullet & \bullet \\
0.5 & 1 & 2
\end{array}
$$

Therefore, if we model the odds of death, we could get a different answer than if we model the odds of survival. However, the logs of $1/2$ and $2/1$ are equal distances in opposite directions from the 'as likely as not' log odds value of 0.

$$
\begin{array}{ccc}
\bullet & \bullet & \bullet \\
\ln(0.5) & 0 & \ln(2)
\end{array}
$$

Therefore, the answer will be the same whether the log odds of death or survival is used. With logistic regression, if x is the indicator of treatment 1, then the coefficient β corresponding to x is the log odds ratio of treatment 1 relative to treatment 2.

Equation (1.10) shows how to obtain a large sample confidence interval for the risk difference. We can obtain large sample confidence intervals for the relative risk or odds ratio using the delta method applied to the logarithmic function. For instance, we showed after Theorem 1.9 that $\ln(\hat{p})$ is asymptotically normal with mean $\ln(p)$ and variance estimated by $(1 - \hat{p})/(n\hat{p})$. Therefore, $\ln(\hat{p}_1/\hat{p}_2) = \ln(\hat{p}_1) - \ln(\hat{p}_2)$ is asymptotically normal with mean $\ln(p_1/p_2)$ and variance estimated by

$$v_{RR} = \frac{1 - \hat{p}_1}{n_1 \hat{p}_1} + \frac{1 - \hat{p}_2}{n_2 \hat{p}_2}. \qquad (2.6)$$

We construct a $100(1 - \alpha)\%$ large sample confidence interval for $\ln(\hat{p}_1/p_2)$ and then exponentiate the endpoints to obtain the following large sample confidence interval for the relative risk, $RR = p_1/p_2$:

$$100(1 - \alpha)\% \text{ CI for } RR := \left(\exp\left\{ \ln(\widehat{RR}) - z_{\alpha/2}\sqrt{v_{RR}} \right\}, \right.$$

$$\left. \times \exp\left\{ \ln(\widehat{RR}) + z_{\alpha/2}\sqrt{v_{RR}} \right\} \right)$$

$$= \left(\widehat{RR}e^{-z_{\alpha/2}\sqrt{v_{RR}}}, \widehat{RR}e^{z_{\alpha/2}\sqrt{v_{RR}}} \right). \qquad (2.7)$$

The same approach shows that the log odds ratio has variance estimated by

$$v_{OR} = \frac{1}{n_1 \hat{p}_1 (1 - \hat{p}_1)} + \frac{1}{n_2 \hat{p}_2 (1 - \hat{p}_2)}, \qquad (2.8)$$

so the large sample confidence interval for the odds ratio, $OR = \{p_1/(1-p_1)\}/\{p_2/(1-p_2)\}$, is

$$100(1 - \alpha)\% \text{ CI for } OR := \left(\exp\left\{ \ln(\widehat{OR}) - z_{\alpha/2}\sqrt{v_{OR}} \right\}, \right.$$
$$\times \exp\left\{ \ln(\widehat{OR}) + z_{\alpha/2}\sqrt{v_{OR}} \right\} \Big)$$
$$= \left(\widehat{OR}e^{-z_{\alpha/2}\sqrt{v_{OR}}}, \widehat{OR}e^{z_{\alpha/2}\sqrt{v_{OR}}} \right). \tag{2.9}$$

We close this subsection with another estimator of the log odds ratio. Table 2.2 shows a generic 2 × 2 table. Treat

Table 2.2: Typical 2 × 2 table.

	Event	No event	
Group 1	X_1		n_1
Group 2	X_2		n_2
	s_1	s_2	n

Treat the row and column totals n_1, n_2, s_1, and s_2 as fixed constants. Under the null hypothesis that treatment does not change the probability of an event, the proportion of people with events in the treatment arm should be roughly the overall proportion of people with events, s_1/n. Therefore, the null expected number of treatment patients with events is

$$E = n_1(s_1/n) = \frac{n_1 s_1}{n}.$$

Likewise, the expected number in row i and column j of the table is the product of the ith row and jth column totals divided by the overall total. There is no loss in focusing only the upper left cell because the other cells are determined by the constraint of fixed row and column totals. Let O be the observed number of people in the upper left cell. We have seen that its conditional mean is $E(O) = n_1 s_1/n$. Its conditional variance is

$$V = \frac{n_1 n_2 s_1 s_2}{n^2(n-1)}.$$

It is by no means obvious, but

$$\frac{O - E}{V}$$

is actually a good estimator of the log odds ratio when sample sizes are fairly large. For example, consider the data of Table 2.1. The conditional mean and variance of the upper left cell are $E = (36)(21)/71 = 10.648$ and $V = (36)(35)(21)(50)/\{(71)^2(70)\} = 3.749$. Therefore,

$$\frac{O - E}{V} = \frac{8 - 10.648}{3.749} = -0.706.$$

Now exponentiate to estimate the odds ratio: $\exp(-0.706) = 0.494$. Earlier, we directly calculated the odds ratio as 0.484. The advantage of the $(O - E)/V$ method is that its variance can be computed easily. Again we fix row and column totals, which fixes E and V. Then

$$\text{var}\left(\frac{O - E}{V} \right) = (1/V^2)\text{var}(O - E) = (1/V^2)\text{var}(O) = V/V^2 = 1/V. \tag{2.10}$$

We use the mnemonic device *O minus E except after V* to summarize:

Principle 2.2. O minus E except after V *In a 2×2 table, $(O - E)/V$ estimates the log odds ratio with (conditional) variance $1/V$.*

We will extend the O minus E except after V principle to survival analysis in Chapter 7.

2.2 Exact Tests and Confidence Intervals

2.2.1 Fisher's Exact Test

Comparing two groups is more complicated than dealing with a single group. With a single group, there is only one parameter, whereas with two groups, there are two. When sample sizes in the two groups are large, we can rely on the asymptotic test (1.9) and confidence interval (1.10). We could also use the *contingency table method* based on the chi-squared statistic $\chi^2 = \sum(\text{Observed}_{ij} - \text{Expected}_{ij})^2/\text{Expected}_{ij}$, where the sum is over the four cells in the 2×2 table. Here, the 'Expected' cell count in cell ij is obtained by multiplying the row i and column j totals and dividing by the overall total. The chi-squared test generalizes to arbitrary $R \times C$ contingency tables, where the chi-squared statistic is referred to a chi-squared distribution with $(R - 1) \times (C - 1)$ degrees of freedom to test whether there is an association between the row factor and column factor. In the 2×2 setting, the z and chi-squared tests are mathematically equivalent because the chi-squared statistic is the square of the z-statistic. But the z/chi-squared test is valid only with large sample sizes. A common rule of thumb is not to trust the method unless all expected cell counts are at least 5. We prefer to use an exact test.

Table 2.3: Typical 2×2 table.

	Event	No event	
Group 1	X_1		n_1
Group 2	X_2		n_2
	S		

One way to simplify matters in the two-sample case is to eliminate one parameter by conditioning on the total number of deaths, $S = X_1 + X_2$ (see Table 2.3). This method, called *Fisher's exact test*, is valid regardless of sample sizes. Once S is fixed, knowledge of one cell reveals all four cells. For example, consider the PREVAIL II Ebola trial in Table 2.1. Knowing that the sample sizes are 36 and 35, the total number of deaths is 21, and the upper left cell is 8 tells us that the upper right cell is $36 - 8 = 28$, the lower left cell is $21 - 8 = 13$, and the lower right cell is $35 - 13 = 22$. We say that there is only 1 *degree of freedom* in the table. Any cell can be treated as the random variable, but it is customary to use the upper left cell, X_1. The Appendix at the end of this chapter shows that

$$P(X_1 = x_1 \mid S = s) = \frac{\binom{n_1}{x_1}\binom{n_2}{s-x_1}\theta^{x_1}}{\sum_j \binom{n_1}{j}\binom{n_2}{s-j}\theta^j}, \tag{2.11}$$

where $\theta = \{p_1/(1 - p_1)\}/\{p_2/(1 - p_2)\}$ is the odds ratio of treatment 1 to treatment 2. Formula (2.11) is the *noncentral hypergeometric* probability mass function. Note that the conditional distribution of the test statistic depends on p_1 and p_2 only through the odds ratio θ. The fact that the odds ratio arises naturally from the mathematics is another reason for its popularity.

Under the null hypothesis $H_0 : p_1 = p_2$, the odds ratio θ is 1 and (2.11) reduces to the *central hypergeometric* probability mass function

$$P_{\theta=1}(X_1 = x_1 \mid S = s) = \frac{\binom{n_1}{x_1}\binom{n_2}{s-x_1}}{\binom{n_1+n_2}{s}}. \qquad (2.12)$$

To see this, note first that the numerators of (2.11) and (2.12) are clearly equivalent when $\theta = 1$. Also, when $\theta = 1$, the denominator of (2.11) becomes $\sum_j \binom{n_1}{j}\binom{n_2}{s-j}$. Think of the total number of ways of forming a committee of size s from n_1 men and n_2 women. On the one hand, this number is simply $\binom{n_1+n_2}{s}$. On the other hand, there are $\binom{n_1}{x_1}\binom{n_2}{s-x_1}$ ways to pick x_1 men from the n_1 men and $x_2 = s - x_1$ women from the n_2 women. Summing over all possible x_1 gives us the total number of ways to pick s people from the $n_1 + n_2$ people. Equating expressions from the two different ways of viewing the combinatorics equation, we see that the denominators of (2.11) and (2.12) are equivalent when $\theta = 1$. This completes the argument that (2.11) and (2.12) are equivalent when $\theta = 1$.

To obtain a p-value, sum relevant hypergeometric probabilities. For example, to test $H_0 : p_1 = p_2$ against $H_1 : p_1 < p_2$ or $H_1 : p_1 > p_2$, compute

$$\text{p} - \text{value} = \sum_{i \le x_1} \frac{\binom{n_1}{i}\binom{n_2}{s-i}}{\binom{n_1+n_2}{s}} \quad \text{or} \quad \text{p-value} = \sum_{i \ge x_1} \frac{\binom{n_1}{x_1}\binom{n_2}{s-x_1}}{\binom{n_1+n_2}{s}},$$

respectively. For instance, the two one-tailed p-values for the PREVAIL II data in Table 2.1 are

$$\text{p} - \text{value} = \sum_{i \le 8} \frac{\binom{36}{i}\binom{35}{21-i}}{\binom{71}{21}} = 0.132 \quad \text{and} \quad \text{p-value} = \sum_{i \ge 8} \frac{\binom{36}{i}\binom{35}{21-i}}{\binom{71}{21}} = 0.950,$$

respectively. The standard method of computing a two-tailed p-value is to sum the probabilities of values of X_1 whose probabilities are less than or equal to the probability of the observed value of X_1, 8. That yields a two-tailed p-value of 0.200 in this example. We will see in Section 2.2.3 that this method of computing a two-tailed p-value can lead to irregularities.

2.2.2   Exact Confidence Interval for Odds Ratio

The $100(1 - \alpha)\%$ confidence interval for the odds ratio is obtained by inverting two one-tailed tests, as we did in Section 1.2.2 for the Clopper-Pearson confidence interval for a single proportion. For the lower limit, we consider one-tailed tests of

$$H_0 : \theta = \theta_0 \text{ versus} \qquad (2.13)$$
$$H_1 : \theta > \theta_0. \qquad (2.14)$$

For instance, suppose we want to test whether 0.10 is a reasonable value of θ. Using (2.11), find the one-tailed p-value

$$\sum_{x_1=8}^{21} \frac{\binom{36}{x_1}\binom{35}{21-x_1}\theta_0^{x_1}}{\sum_{j=0}^{21}\binom{36}{j}\binom{35}{21-j}\theta_0^{j}}, \qquad (2.15)$$

where $\theta_0 = 0.10$. The resulting p-value of 0.004 is far less than the conventional one-tailed level of 0.025, showing that 8 or more deaths in the SC+ZMapp arm would be very unusual if the true odds ratio were as low as 0.10. We can rule out θ_0 values less than 0.10. To see what other values θ_0 can be ruled out, equate the p-value (2.15) for the one-tailed test of

(2.13) against (2.14) to 0.025 and solve for θ_0. This yields $\theta_0 = 0.147$. We can confidently conclude that θ exceeds 0.147.

Likewise, the upper limit is obtained by equating the one-tailed p-value for testing

$$H_0 : \theta = \theta_0 \text{ versus} \tag{2.16}$$

$$H_1 : \theta < \theta_0 \tag{2.17}$$

to 0.025 and solving for θ_0. Solving

$$\sum_{x_1=0}^{8} \frac{\binom{36}{x_1}\binom{n_2}{21-x_1}\theta_0^{x_1}}{\sum_{j=0}^{21}\binom{36}{j}\binom{35}{21-j}\theta_0^{j}} = 0.025$$

for θ_0 yields 1.538. Therefore, the 95% confidence interval from inverting two Fisher exact tests is $(0.147, 1.538)$.

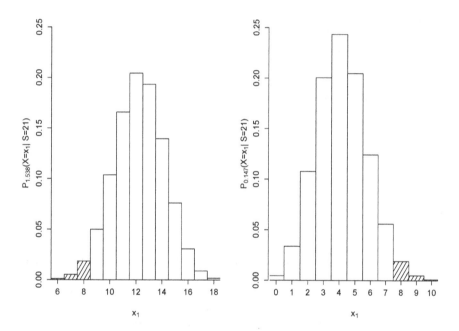

Figure 2.1: When $\theta = \theta_U = 1.538$, the one-tailed p-value $P_{\theta_U}(X_1 \leq 8 \mid S = 21)$ (area of shaded bars in left plot) for testing $H_0 : \theta = \theta_0$ versus $H_1 : \theta < \theta_0$ is 0.025. When $\theta = \theta_L = 0.147$, the opposite one-tailed p-value $P_{\theta_L}(X_1 \geq 8 \mid S = 21)$ (area of shaded bars in right plot) for testing $H_0 : \theta = \theta_0$ versus $H_1 : \theta > \theta_0$ is 0.025. The 95% confidence interval for θ is $(0.147, 1.538)$.

2.2.3 Oddities of Fisher's Exact Test and Confidence Interval

We mentioned exact tests and confidence intervals in connection with a single sample of Bernoulli observations in Sections 1.2.1 and 1.2.2, and in connection with two samples of Bernoulli observations in Sections 2.2.1 and 2.2.2. The advantage of exact tests is clear: they are valid whether sample sizes are large or small. Nonetheless, the reader should be aware that exact tests can sometimes exhibit unexpected behavior. An excellent reference for the oddities arising from Fisher's exact test is Fay and Hunsberger, 2021.

We noted in Section 1.2.1 that the actual type I error rate of an exact test can be far from the target, and this can lead to other oddities such as power decreasing when sample size is increased. To see this, return to the coin-flipping example in Section 1.2.1, but change two things. First, use alpha level 0.001 instead of 0.05. Second, flip the coin only 10 times. The null hypothesis can be rejected only if all 10 flips are correctly guessed because $P(S \geq 10 \,|\, p = 0.5) = (0.5)^{10} < 0.001$, but $P(S \geq 9) = 0.011 > 0.001$. Suppose we increase the sample size by flipping the coin 11 times. Now all 11 coin flips must be correctly guessed to reject the null hypothesis that $p = 0.5$ because $P(S \geq 11 \,|\, p = 0.5) = (0.5)^{11} = 0.0005 < 0.001$ but $P(S \geq 10 \,|\, p = 0.5) = 0.006 > 0.001$. If the actual probability of a correct guess is $p > 0.5$, power is p^{10} with 10 coin flips and p^{11} with 11 coin flips. Because $p^{11} < p^{10}$, power actually **decreases** when the sample size increases from 10 to 11. The same thing happens when testing $H_0 : p = p_0$ versus $H_1 : p > p_0$ for any p_0. Note that this problem occurs because of the discreteness of the distribution of the number of correct guesses, which prevents us from achieving the targeted alpha level without using a randomized test.

A similar phenomenon can occur with Fisher's exact test. For example, consider a tiny study, study 1, with only 3 people per group (avoid such studies!) and a one-tailed alpha of 0.05. Fisher's exact test is statistically significant only if all 3 treatment patients survive and all 3 controls die. In that case, the p-value is exactly 0.05. Now consider study 2 with 4 treatment patients and 3 controls. Fisher's exact test in study 2 is statistically significant only if all 4 treatment patients survive and all 3 controls die. Let pow_1 and pow_2 denote power in studies 1 and 2. Then

$$\mathrm{pow}_1 = P(\text{all 3 treatment patients survive and all 3 controls die}) = (1 - p_T)^3 p_C^3$$

and

$$\mathrm{pow}_2 = P(\text{all 4 treatment patients survive and all 3 controls die}) = (1 - p_T)^4 p_C^3.$$

As $\mathrm{pow}_2/\mathrm{pow}_1 = 1 - p_T < 1$ for all $p_T \neq 1$ and all $p_C \neq 0$, power in study 2 is smaller even though the sample size in study 2 is larger! Again, the culprit is the inability to achieve the correct alpha level because of discreteness with exact tests.

Fisher's exact test has a quirk related to the computation of a two-tailed p-value. The standard method of computing a two-tailed p-value sums probabilities of X_1 values whose probabilities are less than or equal to that of the observed value. A disadvantage of this method is that the test does not necessarily match the confidence interval, which is computed by inverting two one-tailed tests. Many two-tailed tests have the property that they are significant at level α precisely when the corresponding $100(1 - \alpha)\%$ confidence interval for the parameter excludes the null value. This is not true for Fisher's exact test with the standard method of computing a two-tailed p-value. Table 2.4 yields a two-tailed p-value of $0.044 < 0.05$, yet the 95% confidence interval for the odds ratio is $(0.039, 1.056)$, which includes the null value of 1.

Table 2.4: A 2 × 2 table with a two-tailed p-value of $0.044 < 0.05$, yet the 95% confidence interval $(0.039, 1.056)$ for the odds ratio contains the null value of 1.

	Event	No event	
Treatment	6	12	18
Control	12	5	17
	18		

A statistical colleague once encountered another quirk of the standard method of computing a two-tailed p-value for Fisher's exact test. He was presented with results of a small experiment comparing a treatment to a control (Table 2.5). The two-tailed p-value of 0.054 narrowly missed the level of 0.05 required to declare statistical significance. The clinical colleague conducting the experiment wondered whether results would reach statistical significance if an additional control patient were added and had an event. Ignore the impropriety of modifying the design of a trial after observing results. If we simply add another patient to the control arm, and that patient has an event, the two-tailed p-value slightly **increases** to 0.055!

Table 2.5: A 2 × 2 table whose two-tailed p-value of 0.054 narrowly misses statistical significance, yet if another control patient is added and has an event, the p-value **increases** to 0.055.

	Event	No event	
Treatment	1	18	19
Control	7	16	23
	8		

The problems in the preceding two paragraphs are eliminated if we use an alternate method of computing a two-tailed p-value. Double the smaller of the two one-tailed p-values. If this exceeds 1, replace it by 1. This alternative method ensures that results of a two-tailed level α test match the corresponding $100(1 - \alpha)\%$ confidence interval. We recommend use of this alternative two-tailed p-value with Fisher's exact test.

2.2.4   Unconditional Tests As Alternatives to Fisher's Exact Test

Some statisticians oppose conditioning on the total number of people with events, like Fisher's exact test does, on the grounds that it severely limits the number of possible tables. This is what causes Fisher's exact test to be overly conservative, leading to the problems of Section 2.2.3. Alternative *unconditional tests* such as *Barnard's test* (Barnard, 1945) and *Boschloo's test* (Boschloo, 1970) determine whether the observed data are consistent with **any** common value of p in the two groups. These tests do not restrict the set of tables to those producing the same marginal totals as the observed table. Consequently, their distribution is less coarse. On the other hand, because they consider all possible values of the common mortality probability in the two groups and essentially compute the maximum p-value, one might surmise that unconditional tests are more conservative than Fisher's exact test. However, the advantage of a less coarse distribution for the test statistic more than compensates for the disadvantage of having to maximize over all possible values of p, and unconditional tests generally have superior power to Fisher's exact test. An advantage of Fisher's exact test is that the parameter is the odds ratio, which facilitates supplemental analyses that adjust for covariate differences between groups using logistic regression. Unconditional tests are not commonly used in clinical trials, but provide an attractive alternative to Fisher's exact test when sample sizes are small.

To understand the difference between an unconditional and conditional test, consider a small study with 1 out of 4 people dying in group 1 and 3 out of 3 people dying in group 2. Consider a one-tailed test to try to show that the probability of death is lower in group 1. Boschloo's test starts by computing the one-tailed p-value from Fisher's exact test, which is 0.1143. If we were using Fisher's exact test, this would be the end, but this is only the beginning for Boshloo's test. We now consider every table t with 4 people in group 1 and 3 in group 2, without fixing the total number of deaths at 4 like we would for Fisher's exact

Table 2.6: Mortality data from a small study.

	Dead	Alive	
Group 1	1	3	4
Group 2	3	0	3
	4		7

test. There are now more tables to consider. For example, one table has 0 deaths in each group, while another has 4 deaths in group 1 and 2 deaths in group 2. For each table t, compute Fisher's one-tailed p-value. A table t is considered at least as extreme as Table 2.6, if its Fisher's exact p-value is less than or equal to the Fisher exact p-value for Table 2.6, namely 0.1143. The two tables at least as extreme as Table 2.6 are Table 2.6 itself and Table 2.7. Let E denote this set of at least as extreme tables. Because we are no longer

Table 2.7: More extreme result than in Table 2.6.

	Dead	Alive	
Group 1	0	4	4
Group 2	3	0	3
	3		7

conditioning on the total number of deaths, the null probability of a table t is

$$\binom{4}{x_{1t}}\binom{3}{x_{2t}}p^{x_{1t}+x_{2t}}(1-p)^{7-x_{1t}-x_{2t}},$$

where p is the true, common probability of death in the two groups and x_{it} is the number of deaths in group i for table t. Sum the probabilities of tables in E:

$$\sum_{t\in E}\binom{4}{x_{1t}}\binom{3}{x_{2t}}p^{x_{1t}+x_{2t}}(1-p)^{7-x_{1t}-x_{2t}}.$$

Substituting the numbers in Tables 2.6 and 2.7 gives a sum of

$$\binom{4}{1}\binom{3}{3}p^4(1-p)^3+\binom{4}{0}\binom{3}{3}p^3(1-p)^4=p^3(1-p)^3(3p+1).$$

The only problem is that we do not know p. To be conservative, we compute the maximum over all $p\in[0,1]$:

$$\begin{aligned}
\text{Boschloo's p} - \text{value} &= \sup_{p\in[0,1]}\sum_{t\in E}\binom{4}{x_{1t}}\binom{3}{x_{2t}}p^{x_{1t}+x_{2t}}(1-p)^{7-x_{1t}-x_{2t}}\\
&= \sup_{p\in[0,1]}\{p^3(1-p)^3(3p+1)\}\\
&= 0.0402.
\end{aligned} \tag{2.18}$$

Note that Boschloo's p-value of 0.0402 is smaller than the Fisher exact p-value of 0.1143. This is no accident. It is not difficult to show that Boschloo's one-tailed p-value is **always** less than or equal to that of Fisher's exact test, so Boschloo's test is *always* more powerful than Fisher's exact test (Boschloo, 1970). This is very important, especially in small studies.

Boschloo's test can also be used to test a nonzero null hypothesis $H_0 : p_1 - p_2 = \delta$ against $H_1 : p_1 - p_2 < \delta$ using a similar approach. When we invert Boschloo's test, we get a confidence interval for $p_1 - p_2$. Thus, inverting Fisher's exact test and Boschloo's test produces confidence intervals for the odds ratio and risk difference, respectively.

Exercises

1. Give an example where the risk difference is more appropriate than the relative risk, and another example in which the relative risk is more appropriate than the risk difference.

2. Why are unconditional tests like Boschloo's test more attractive than Fisher's exact test when sample sizes are very small?

3. For the data of Table 2.4:

   (a) Compute the risk difference, relative risk, and odds ratio.

   (b) Estimate the odds ratio using the 'O minus E except after V' method and compare your answer to the odds ratio in part (a).

4. Suppose that 40 out of 500 patients in the control arm and 58 out of 506 patients in the treatment arm die within 1 year. Compute a 95% large sample confidence interval for the treatment-to-control odds ratio. Compare your interval to the exact confidence interval from Fisher's exact test, which is $(0.080, 0.428)$.

5. In a trial in which none of the 10 treated patients die and all of the 8 control patients die, what is the one-tailed p-value to show that treatment is superior using Fisher's exact test?

6. In a trial with n people per arm, what is the most extreme one-tailed p-value possible using Fisher's exact test?

7. Show that the following are equivalent: (1) risk difference is negative, (2) relative risk is less than 1, (3) odds ratio is less than 1.

8. Use the delta method to verify that the asymptotic variance of the log odds ratio, $\ln[\{\hat{p}_1/(1 - \hat{p}_1)\}/\{\hat{p}_2/(1 - \hat{p}_2)\}]$, is $1/\{n_1 p_1(1 - p_1)\} + 1/\{n_2 p_2(1 - p_2)\}$. Note that $\ln\{\hat{p}_1/(1-\hat{p}_1)\}$ and $\ln\{\hat{p}_2/(1-\hat{p}_2)\}$ are independent, so it suffices to sum the variances of log odds within each arm.

2.3   Appendix: $P(X_1 = x_1 \mid S = s)$ in Table 2.3

Before conditioning on $S = X_1 + X_2$, the X_i are independent and have binomial distributions with probability mass functions

$$P(X_i = x_i) = \binom{n_i}{x_i} p_i^{x_i}(1 - p_i)^{n_i - x_i} = \binom{n_i}{x_i}(1 - p_i)^{n_i}\{p_i/(1 - p_i)\}^{x_i}, \quad i = 1, 2. \quad (2.19)$$

Bayes formula shows that the conditional probability mass function of X_1 given $S = s$ is

$$P(X_1 = x_1 \mid S = s) = \frac{P(X_1 = x_1 \cap S = s)}{P(S = s)} = \frac{P(X_1 = x_1 \cap X_2 = s - x_1)}{P(S = s)}. \quad (2.20)$$

By (2.19) and independence of X_1 and X_2, the numerator of (2.20) is

$$\binom{n_1}{x_1}(1-p_1)^{n_1}\{p_1/(1-p_1)\}^{x_1}\binom{n_2}{s-x_1}(1-p_2)^{n_2}\{p_2/(1-p_2)\}^{s-x_1}$$

$$=\binom{n_1}{x_1}\binom{n_2}{s-x_1}(1-p_1)^{n_1}(1-p_2)^{n_2}\{p_2/(1-p_2)\}^s\theta^{x_1}, \tag{2.21}$$

where $\theta=\{p_1/(1-p_1)\}/\{p_2/(1-p_2)\}$ is the odds ratio of treatment 1 to treatment 2.
The denominator of (2.20) is

$$\sum_j P(X_1=j,X_2=s-j)=\sum_j\binom{n_1}{j}\binom{n_2}{s-j}(1-p_1)^{n_1}(1-p_2)^{n_2}\{p_2/(1-p_2)\}^s\theta^j.$$

Therefore, (2.20) becomes

$$P(X_1=x_1\,|\,S=s)=\frac{\binom{n_1}{x_1}\binom{n_2}{s-x_1}(1-p_1)^{n_1}(1-p_2)^{n_2}\{p_2/(1-p_2)\}^s\theta^{x_1}}{\sum_j\binom{n_1}{j}\binom{n_2}{s-j}(1-p_1)^{n_1}(1-p_2)^{n_2}\{p_2/(1-p_2)\}^s\theta^j}$$

$$=\frac{\binom{n_1}{x_1}\binom{n_2}{s-x_1}\theta^{x_1}}{\sum_j\binom{n_1}{j}\binom{n_2}{s-j}\theta^j}. \tag{2.22}$$

2.4   Summary

1. Three useful treatment effect estimators are the risk difference, relative risk, and odds ratio.

   (a) The risk difference is easy to interpret: multiply it by n to get the number saved if n people are treated.

   (b) The relative risk is more likely to be constant across trials with different baseline risk.

   (c) The odds ratio arises naturally from the mathematics of 2 × 2 tables (see appendix), is appropriate for either a case-control or cohort study, and arises in logistic regression: $\ln(\text{odds})=\beta_0+\beta_1 x_1+\ldots+\beta_k x_k$.

2. A useful estimator of the log odds ratio can be obtained from the 'O minus E except after V' principle: $(O-E)/V\approx\ln(OR)$.

3. Large sample confidence intervals for the 3 treatment effect estimators are derived using the delta method.

4. Fisher's exact test:

   (a) conditions on the row and column totals of the 2 × 2 table,

   (b) gives a valid p-value regardless of sample sizes,

   (c) can be quite conservative when sample sizes are small,

   (d) can be inverted to produce an exact confidence interval for the odds ratio.

5. Exact unconditional methods like Barnard's and Boschloo's tests tend to be more powerful than Fisher's exact test.

Chapter 3

Introduction to Clinical Trials

Progress in medicine follows the paradigm of the scientific method: observations lead to hypotheses that are tested with carefully designed experiments. Early-stage experiments occur in a highly controlled environment, e.g., preclinical testing of compounds in a laboratory. For example, an experiment may demonstrate that an antibiotic kills bacteria in vitro. Next, experimentation in more complicated settings is essential. For example, the compound might be tested in animals. Attempts are made to ensure comparability of the animals given the compound and control animals. Nonetheless, it is not possible to control or even know which characteristics predict treatment benefit. Final testing occurs in humans, in a *controlled clinical trial*. Studies in humans represent an exceedingly complex setting, with limited ability to enforce the kinds of scientific controls available in a laboratory setting. The inability to control all influencing factors fundamentally alters the evidentiary requirements for hypothesis testing. Whereas a laboratory experiment with duplication of results under identical conditions leads to conclusive evidence, clinical trials require an experimental design that attempts to balance uncontrollable but potentially influential factors. In a clinical trial, this is addressed by including a *control group*, a group of people who do not receive an experimental treatment. Precise balancing of all possible influencing factors between the control and experimental group would "wash out" these effects and isolate the effect of treatment. However, this is practically impossible in clinical research. Instead, randomization attempts to equalize the groups. A *randomized controlled trial (RCT)* assigns people to different groups, called *arms*, at random. The control arm may receive an inert substance called a *placebo* that is expected to have no therapeutic effect. Alternatively, the control arm may receive an established treatment against which we compare one or more experimental treatments. Random assignment is what separates randomized controlled trials from all other studies, rendering RCTs the gold standard of medical evidence. This book is devoted to the study of methodology used in clinical trials.

Example 3.1. Hormone Replacement Therapy To understand why clinical trials are needed, consider the case of hormone replacement therapy (HRT) in post-menopausal women. Women have a much lower rate of heart disease than men until they reach menopause. After that, their risk increases dramatically, and becomes comparable to that of men. Researchers hypothesized that hormones might protect against heart disease. Observational evidence on the association of HRT with heart disease was available because the FDA approved hormones in the 1940s to treat menopause symptoms. Hormones were also used to increase bone density and protect against fractures, leading to an upsurge of HRT in the 1960s. The conjecture that HRT protects against heart disease was buoyed by at least 30 observational studies, including the 1985 Nurse's Health Study (Stampfer et al., 1985) of more than 100,000 women with nearly 93 percent follow-up. In that study, women

DOI: 10.1201/9781315164090-3

taking estrogen had 67 percent fewer heart attacks. Based on this evidence, many concluded that replacing women's hormones following menopause protects against heart disease. Then came placebo-controlled clinical trials of HRT.

The first placebo-controlled trial casting doubts about the cardiac benefit of HRT was the Heart and Estrogen/Progestin Replacement Study (HERS) in 2,763 women (Hulley et al., 1998). Not only was no benefit observed, but there was a suggestion of increased risk of heart attack soon after HRT. The Women's Health Initiative followed, and randomized approximately 16,000 women to HRT or placebo (Writing Group for the Women's Health Initiative Investigators, 2002). In this trial, the hazard ratio for coronary heart disease was 1.29, 95% confidence interval (1.02, 1.63). In other words, not only were large or even small benefits ruled out, but there was a statistically significant increase in coronary heart disease events.   □

How could this happen? The observational evidence appeared to be strong, and the logic seemed solid:

1. Observational evidence suggests that the loss of hormones may increase the risk of heart disease in women.

2. Observational evidence indicates that post-menopausal women undergoing HRT have less heart disease than post-menopausal women not undergoing HRT.

3. Conclusion: HRT following menopause protects against heart disease.

Closer examination suggests that the cause and effect relationship implied by points 1-3 may be wrong. For point 1, the fact that women's heart disease risk increases after menopause does not mean that it is the loss of hormones that increases the risk. One obvious confounder is age; post-menopausal women are older than pre-menopausal women, and older age increases the risk of heart disease. Another explanation is that menopause causes changes other than hormonal that affect heart disease risk. In other words, an association between loss of hormones and increased risk of heart disease does not necessarily imply causation.

What about the Nurse's Health Study and other studies showing that post-menopausal women undergoing HRT have a lower heart disease risk? In these studies, we cannot be confident that women who choose HRT therapy are comparable to those who do not. The HRT women may be more health-conscious in general, exercising more, eating a better diet, being more diligent about health care visits, etc. These factors may be causing the difference in heart disease between those who choose and do not choose HRT. If we knew all of the variables that might differ between the two groups, we could attempt to adjust for them in a statistical model. But we will not be able to identify all of the factors differentiating the groups. For example, what if the people choosing HRT are more likely to have some unknown gene or combination of genes that cause them to have lower heart disease rates?

Contrast observational studies like the Nurse's Health Study with a randomized controlled trial like the Women's Health Initiative. Because the decision to undergo HRT is made essentially by the flip of a coin, the two groups tend to be comparable on factors that might influence heart disease. This is true of known factors like diet and exercise, but also unknown factors such as genetic factors. Therefore, any differences in heart disease are not likely to be explained by anything other than HRT.

Even if we concede a cause and effect relationship between loss of hormones and cardiac events, that does not necessarily imply that HRT will reduce this risk in post-menopausal women. Suppose, hypothetically, that loss of these hormones quickly causes irreparable damage to the heart. In that case, replacing hormones may have no benefit. Furthermore, any agent may have negative effects in addition to any positive effects. For instance, some antiarrhythmic drugs also have pro-arrhythmic effects, and the arrhythmias they cause may be more dangerous than those they prevent. Thus, even if loss of hormones causes the increased heart risk in post-menopausal women, that does not imply that taking pills to replace hormones will lower that risk. In fact, one of the explanations offered for the discouraging results of the Women's Health Initiative is that the HRT occurred too long after menopause. Proponents of this theory argue that had the HRT been given soon after menopause, results would have been different. Implicit is the assumption that prolonged loss of hormones leads to harm that cannot be reversed by HRT. Regardless of whether one believes different explanations for results of the Women's Health Initiative (WHI), one thing is clear: the conclusion that HRT decreases heart disease risk following menopause is not supported by the strongest form of medical evidence–a randomized controlled trial.

In addition to potential lack of comparability between groups, biases can plague observational studies. For example, events may be discovered more frequently in one group because of more frequent or detailed scrutiny. This is called *ascertainment bias*, and can result from the perception that one group is at higher risk. For instance, suppose that doctors become convinced from a study like the Nurse's Health Study that HRT protects against heart disease. They may monitor women on HRT less frequently out of the belief that they are protected. Also, if they see two women with the same symptoms, only one of whom is on HRT, they may be more likely to interpret symptoms as being a heart attack in the woman not using HRT. One consequence of perceived differences in risk between groups is that doctors may give them different treatments. For example, they may be more likely to give cholesterol-lowering medications to women who are not on HRT. This is called *background treatment bias*. Other biases of observational studies can be more subtle, as in the following example.

Example 3.2. When to Start ART Antiretroviral therapy (ART) allows patients with HIV, the virus that causes AIDS, a lifespan comparable to that of people without HIV. HIV attacks CD4 'helper' T-cells, so CD4 count is a measure of how advanced HIV is. Many doctors initially believed that deferring antiretroviral treatment until a patient's CD4 count drops to 200 would improve outcomes. However, a body of observational data suggested early treatment would be better. Conclusions based on observational studies about when to start ART are particularly problematic because many people starting ART early do so in response to other clinical manifestations, such as a serious infection. Therefore, early starters of ART may be doing so because of an emergency, so they may be more likely to have a poor outcome.

Another type of bias in observational studies of when to start ART is more subtle. Suppose we are trying to determine whether it is better to start ART when the CD4 count drops to 500 versus 350. We would study a group starting at 500 and another group starting at 350 and record the time to death or an AIDS-defining event. But when does the clock start, when patients reach 500 or when they reach their separate start times, 500 and 350? It seems fairest to start at 500 for everyone. After all, even if starting ART early had no effect on delaying the time to death/AIDS, the time from reaching 350 to AIDS/death would still tend to be shorter than the time from reaching 500 to AIDS/death (because one must necessarily reach 500 before reaching 350). However, if we start the clock when everyone reaches 500, we have a problem: everyone in the 350 group must necessarily have survived from 500 to 350, whereas some people in the 500 group may die before reaching 350. This dilemma is known as *lead-time bias*.

The when to start question was resolved definitively by the Strategic Timing of Anti-Retroviral Treatment (START) clinical trial randomizing patients with HIV and CD4 counts above 500 to either starting ART immediately or deferring until CD4$\leq$ 350 (INSIGHT START Study Group, 2015). All events following randomization were included, so there was no lead-time bias. START showed that immediate commencement of antiretroviral therapy reduced the combination of serious AIDS and serious non-AIDs events.   □

The WHI and START are at two ends of the spectrum; the WHI contradicted observational studies, while START corroborated them. The WHI scenario is relatively uncommon. More commonly, results of observational studies and clinical trials are roughly consistent, though the size of the clinical benefit tends to be smaller in clinical trials. For this reason, many researchers tend to believe only relatively large effects seen in observational studies. A risk reduction of 30 percent or less in observational studies is easily attributable to biases.

Exercises

1. The 1976 vaccination against H1N1 (swine flu) was linked to Guillain-Barré syndrome, a very rare neurodegenerative disorder. Explain which of the following observational studies seems better to study whether the relationship is real? (1) Compare recipients of the H1N1 vaccine to unvaccinated people in the same year, or (2) compare recipients of the H1N1 vaccine to recipients of the ordinary flu vaccine in the same year.

2. In an observational study in patients with Ebola virus disease, one might expect that patients with longer times from diagnosis to enrollment should have higher mortality because the disease has had more time to inflict damage.

    (a) Give one explanation for why the opposite trend might occur, i.e., longer times from diagnosis might actually predict better survival.

    (b) It would be unethical to conduct a clinical trial randomizing patients with Ebola virus disease to either start treatment immediately or delay treatment by 3 days, but if we could conduct such a trial, would you expect to see better mortality in the delay group?

3. In HIV vaccine studies, there can be a *disinhibition effect* whereby patients who know they are receiving a vaccine may engage in riskier behaviors because they believe they will be protected.

    (a) Explain how, in an observational study, this could wrongly lead to the conclusion that the vaccine is ineffective.

    (b) Explain why this is not as problematic in a blinded clinical trial.

4. One of many conditions from which patients can spontaneously recover is sudden idiopathic sensorineural hearing loss. Some doctors have concluded that if the condition is caught early enough, it can be successfully treated with steroids.

    (a) Explain why it is problematic to conclude that early treatment cured the patient.

    (b) Explain how a randomized clinical trial could end the controversy.

3.1   Summary

1. Observational studies can provide supportive evidence of the effectiveness of interventions, but they are prone to bias, especially selection bias.

2. Several features of a clinical trial tend to minimize bias:

    (a) Randomization eliminates bias resulting from preferentially offering treatment to the sickest or least sick patients, a phenomenon known as *selection bias*.

(b) Keeping patients blinded to treatment assignment tends to equalize the power of positive thinking (the so-called *placebo effect*) on patient outcomes across arms. It also minimizes a form of *background treatment bias* whereby patients assigned to placebo compensate by instituting other treatments or behaviors.

(c) Keeping the staff who interact with patients blinded minimizes *background treatment bias.*

(d) Keeping staff who adjudicate events blinded minimizes *adjudication bias,* namely a greater tendency to judge a given set of evidence as an event in one arm than another.

3. Randomized controlled trials are considered the gold standard of medical evidence.

Chapter 4

Design of Clinical Trials

4.1 Different Phases of Trials

Trials are categorized by phases. In a *Phase I* trial, the safety of one or more doses of a drug is evaluated. There may or may not be a placebo arm. In cancer, one assumes that higher doses will be more effective, but also more toxic. Therefore, phase I cancer trials are in cancer patients, and the goal is often to find the highest dose that is associated with no more than a given level of toxicity, say 30%. In other diseases, phase I trials are often conducted in healthy volunteers rather than patients when the perceived risk is low.

The best dose or doses from a phase I trial may then be used in a *phase II* trial. These are often randomized trials with a control arm. The goal of a phase II trial is to show that a treatment has activity under ideal conditions. Investigators may restrict the population to those who will receive the maximum benefit. For example, they may weed out people who are unlikely to adhere to treatment. This might be accomplished by using a *run-in* prior to randomization in which patients undergo conditions similar to what will follow during the subsequent randomized trial. Only patients who adhere during the run-in period are randomized. Similarly, investigators may further restrict the population to those whose disease is thought to be most susceptible to treatment. Moreover, the primary outcome for a phase II trial might be an intermediate outcome. For instance, even though the ultimate goal may be to show benefit on serious events like heart attacks, the first step may be to show that the treatment reduces cholesterol. Therefore, the outcome for a phase II trial might be change in cholesterol from beginning to end of the study. Trials such as these aimed at finding treatment benefit on an outcome thought to be necessary for longterm benefit are called *efficacy trials.* If benefit cannot be shown under such ideal conditions, the treatment may be abandoned; there is no reason for a much larger and more expensive definitive trial.

If phase I and II trials demonstrate that a treatment is safe and works under ideal conditions, it is time for *phase III*, namely a large definitive trial with a clinical endpoint to show benefit under real world conditions. Phase III trials often include a broader population than do phase II trials. The primary outcome of a phase III trial involves serious outcomes like heart attacks or deaths. Trials aimed at showing benefit under real-world conditions are called *effectiveness trials* as opposed to *efficacy trials.*

Certain design aspects are beneficial in all clinical trials regardless of phase. These include blinding, baseline assessment, controls, choice of primary endpoint, and reduction of variability. We cover each of these topics.

DOI: 10.1201/9781315164090-4

4.2   Blinding

One key aspect of clinical trials is blinding of treatment assignments to patients and staff. As pointed out in Chapter 3, blinding equalizes the power of positive thinking and prevents differential background treatment in different arms. Trials can be either *single blind* or *double blind*. Single blind means that patients, but not staff, are blinded to treatment assignments. Double blind means that both patients and staff are blinded to treatment assignments. Blinding in a medicine trial is accomplished by making a placebo that appears identical to treatment. Double blinding in a medicine trial is achieved as follows. Each medication bottle is given a unique number. A secret list matching bottle numbers to their contents (active drug versus placebo) is locked away. When a patient arrives and is determined eligible to be randomized, that patient is assigned a unique identification (ID) number. A computer program randomly assigns patients to bottle numbers. Personnel dispensing, and patients receiving, medication know the bottle number, but not its contents. Consequently, they are blinded to treatment assignment. When it is time to analyze data from the trial, the secret list is consulted to match bottle numbers to treatment assignments.

How far should one go to maintain blinding? If treatment is an injection, one could easily prepare a placebo injection as well, but what if the treatment is surgery? Should sham surgery be used as a placebo? Sham brain surgery was used in trials of Parkinson's disease (Freeman et al., 1999), sham arthroscopic knee surgery was used in a trial of osteoarthritis of the knee (Moseley, et al., 2002), and sham back surgery was used in a trial of osteoporotic spinal fractures (Kallmes, Comstock, and Heagerty, 2009). Investigators in these trials clearly felt that maintaining blinding was paramount. The trials demonstrate that blinding can be achieved even in difficult settings. The Partnership for Research on Ebola Virus in Liberia II (PREVAIL II) trial in Ebola virus disease (The Prevail II Writing Group, 2016) was *open-label* (unblinded) partly because of a perceived lack of acceptability of blinding among afflicted communities in Western Africa. Some investigators later lamented that blinding would have helped medical personnel maintain impartiality and reduce guilt and stress caused by knowing which patients received the experimental treatment ZMapp. Even in trials in which side effects may unblind some patients, it is better to have partial blinding than no blinding. There should be a very strong justification for using an unblinded trial; convenience is **not** a strong justification.

Regardless of whether a trial is unblinded, single blinded, or double blinded, personnel who determine whether a patient has had a given outcome must be blinded. Bias could easily be introduced if they know the treatment assignment of the patient.

4.3   Baseline Variables

One very important component of clinical trials is measurement of key baseline variables. *Baseline variables*, also called *baseline characteristics,* are variables measured prior to randomization to reflect the patient's demographic characteristics (e.g., age, gender, race) and health (e.g., size of tumors, blood pressure, amount of virus in plasma) at the beginning of the trial. There are several reasons for measuring baseline characteristics: (1) to document that patients have the disease under study and to characterize how sick they are, (2) to observe the natural progression of the disease over time in the placebo arm, (3) to document that randomization balanced baseline characteristics across arms, so any between-arm differences in outcome can be attributed to treatment rather than to baseline differences, and (4) to allow calculation of change from baseline to end of study as an outcome variable. For instance, a trial of hepatitis C or other viral diseases might use as outcome the change in log viral load, the base 10 logarithm of the amount of virus in plasma. Therefore, there are many good reasons for collecting baseline variables in a clinical trial.

It is crucial to distinguish baseline from post-randomization covariates. We often adjust the treatment effect for differences in **baseline** covariates, but we do not adjust for **post-randomization** covariates in the primary analysis of a clinical trial. Such variables might be influenced by treatment, making interpretation very difficult. A classic example is analyzing results of a clinical trial by level of compliance to treatment. This is very natural. After all, how can a patient derive benefit if he/she does not receive the treatment? Nonetheless, compliance is measured after randomization, and is therefore not a baseline variable. The following example illustrates the problems this can cause.

Example 4.1. The Coronary Drug Project (CDP) investigated mortality rates for five different lipid lowering drugs in men aged 30-64 with a prior myocardial infarction. One of the arms was clofibrate, a member of the fibrate class. Investigators examined 5-year mortality rates of patients in the clofibrate arm broken down by whether patients exhibited less than, versus greater than or equal to, 80% pill compliance (The Coronary Drug Project Research Group, 1980).

Table 4.1: Five-year mortality rate in the clofibrate arm of the Coronary Drug Project broken down by compliance.

Compliance< 80%	Compliance≥ 80%
24.6 ± 2.3	15.0 ± 1.3

Table 4.1 shows that the 5-year mortality rate of patients who were at least 80% compliant was substantially lower (15%) than that of patients who were less than 80% compliant (24.6%). One would naturally assume that the treatment works; people who take it derive benefit. But Table 4.2 augments Table 4.1 with data in the placebo arm broken down by compliance. Amazingly, a very similar pattern was seen in placebo patients; those who took at least 80% of placebo pills had substantially lower mortality than those who took fewer than 80% of placebo pills. How can this be? The placebo should have no effect on mortality. The lesson here is that people who are compliant are very different from those who are not. They may engage in other health conscious behaviors such as consuming a better diet, exercising more, being more diligent about medical checkups, etc. Investigators attempted to adjust the above analysis for 40 baseline variables, but mortality differences between compliers and noncompliers remained. Some of these differences may be intangible. For example, those who comply may be the ones who are convinced that they are receiving active treatment. The power of positive thinking may lead to improved survival. Psychological characteristics differentiating those with and without the power of positive thinking are not likely to be recorded in a clinical trial. Also, some noncompliers may not be able to tolerate the drug, and may therefore differ from those who can tolerate it in ways that may be difficult to measure.

Table 4.2: Five-year mortality rate in the placebo arm of the Coronary Drug Project broken down by compliance.

Compliance< 80%	Compliance≥ 80%
28.2 ± 1.5	15.1 ± 0.8

One might argue that we should compare compliers on clofibrate with compliers on placebo, but what assurances do we have that these two groups are comparable? Clofibrate might produce side effects that make compliance difficult. If so, then patients complying with clofibrate might differ from those complying with placebo. If we had infinite knowledge at the start of a trial, we could partition patients into those likely to comply with: (A) placebo or clofibrate, (B) placebo, but not clofibrate, (C) clofibrate, but not placebo, or (D) neither placebo nor clofibrate. For each category, we could ensure equal numbers of people in the two arms. That is what randomization tends to do. Consequently, the randomized arms **are** likely to be comparable.   □

The CDP and other examples have led to one of the most influential principles of clinical trials, the *intention-to-treat principle.*

Principle 4.2. Intention-to-treat (ITT) *The primary comparison in a clinical trial should be of treatments to which patients were randomized, not of treatments actually received.*

Another way to phrase the ITT principle is that one should analyze according to how one intended to treat the patients regardless of whether they received treatment, hence the name, intention-to-treat.

Remark 4.3. *Two important consequences of the ITT principle are:*

1. *One should never stop following patients who do not comply with their randomized treatment.*

2. *Missing data threaten the integrity of a clinical trial by making it difficult to compare the original randomized groups.*

The ITT principle is a tough pill to swallow, so to speak. For instance, the ITT principle implies that in a surgery trial, patients who refuse surgery should nonetheless be counted in the surgery arm. This seems completely counter-intuitive to people not familiar with clinical trials. Arguments in favor of the ITT principle include (1) the randomized arms tend to be balanced with respect to important covariates, but the same cannot be said of groups determined by compliance or other post-randomization covariates, (2) analysis by randomized groups irrespective of compliance tells what will happen in the real world if we attempt to treat patients, and (3) knowledge that trials will be analyzed in accordance with the intention-to-treat principle will encourage trial staff to obtain follow-up data on all patients randomized, not just those who comply with treatment. Opponents of the ITT principle counter the second point above with the argument that compliance during the trial and outside the trial are two different things. If the trial shows that the intervention works, that will likely lead to better compliance in the real world. It has also been argued that a more modern re-analysis of the CDP trial yields a different conclusion. The CDP analyses, although state-of-the-art at the time, are primitive compared to newer techniques like inverse probability weighting. Much of the difference between compliers and noncompliers in the CDP trial is explained if one uses more sophisticated analysis techniques (Murray and Hernán, 2016). Nonetheless, many clinical trialists do not like to rely on complicated, model-dependent techniques to demonstrate treatment benefit. Often, the data required to validate model assumptions is lacking, raising concerns if conclusions depend on those assumptions. Any benefit should be made manifest through simple methods whose validity depends on randomization alone. Accordingly, we emphasize throughout the book that anything interfering with the ability to compare randomized groups must be avoided whenever possible.

There have been major breaches of the ITT principle. The following is an example.

Example 4.4. The Danish Breast Cancer Cooperative Group (DBCG) trial (Blichert-Toft et al., 1992) randomized women with invasive breast cancer to either mastectomy (removal of the breast, the standard treatment at the time) or breast conservation therapy (removal of only part of the breast). The final manuscript reported, "From January 1983 to March 1989, the trial accrued a total of 1153 women... 905 patients (79%) were randomly assigned to one of the two treatment options, whereas 248 patients (21%) did not accept randomization...This latter nonrandomized group are not reported in this presentation." It is ironic that they refer to the group who refused to follow the randomized assignment as the nonrandomized group. In truth, the randomized group included 1153 women, 905 who accepted randomization and $1153 - 905 = 248$ who did not. Reporting on only the 905 compliers is a violation of the ITT principle. Even though results of the DBCG trial were consistent with those of other trials showing no survival benefit of mastectomy compared to breast conservation therapy, failure to follow the ITT principle led to controversy (see the penultimate paragraph of the discussion section of Jatoi and Proschan, 2005). □

The fact that the ITT principle is widely followed has implications on other design aspects of a trial. The following is a good example.

Example 4.5. The Asymptomatic Cardiac Ischemia Pilot (ACIP) study randomized patients with cardiac ischemia (not enough blood getting to parts of the heart) to one of three arms: (1) an angina-guided arm in which medication was given when the patient had heart pain, (2) an angina/ischemia-guided arm in which medication was given when the patient had either heart pain or evidence of ischemia on a heart monitor, or (3) a revascularization arm in which the patient got either bypass surgery or balloon angioplasty (at the interventionist's discretion). In the third arm, patients had to first undergo an invasive procedure called an angiogram to make sure they were eligible for revascularization. Two options were debated for ACIP. Option 1 randomizes first, and performs angiograms on only those randomized to revascularization. Option 2 performs angiograms on everyone before randomization, and randomizes only patients who would be eligible to be revascularized. Proponents of option 1 argued that recruitment would be better if patients did not have to commit to an angiogram upfront. But if a patient would not be willing to enter the trial under option 2, then imagine that patient under option 1 if randomized to revascularization. Under option 1, when the patient is randomized to revascularization and refuses to have the required angiogram, the patient will not be revascularized but must nonetheless be counted in the revascularization arm by the ITT principle. This will introduce bias that could have been eliminated if option 2 had been used. Therefore, option 2 is preferred. □

We are not saying that post-randomization covariates should never be analyzed. Indeed, some trials supplement the primary ITT analysis with a lower tier analysis by level of compliance. Also, the nature of some questions arising in clinical trials requires the use of post-randomization covariates to answer, as the following example illustrates.

Example 4.6. The Antihypertensive and Lipid-Lowering treatment to prevent Heart Attack Trial (ALLHAT) compared three different newer blood pressure lowering classes of medicines to an older class with respect to cardiovascular events like heart attack and stroke (The ALLHAT Officers and Coordinators for the ALLHAT Collaborative Research Group, 2002). The idea was to try to lower blood pressure by the same amount in different arms to see if it mattered how one lowered blood pressure. However, some agents lowered blood pressure more effectively than others. Despite the fact that the protocol called for increasing the dose if needed, the achieved blood pressure differed by arm. The primary analysis in ALLHAT used ITT. However, an exploratory analysis adjusted for achieved blood pressure using a Cox model with blood pressure as a time-varying covariate (Proschan et al., 2013).

The blood pressure actually achieved is, of course, a post-baseline covariate, but a necessary one to answer the question.   □

It is sometimes possible to cleverly use baseline variables to predict later response and thereby avoid the dangers of adjusting for post-randomization covariates. We offer an example.

Example 4.7. In some trials, investigators have eliminated early deaths on the grounds that these patients were simply too ill to derive benefit from a given intervention. Clearly, elimination of early deaths is a breach of the ITT principle because survivors in one arm may not be comparable to survivors in another arm. If treatment causes early deaths, eliminating them is a form of scientific obstruction of justice. An alternative method preserving the randomized groups is *principal stratification*. The idea is attributed to Frangakis and Rubin (2002), although Hallstrom et al. (2001) used the same idea a year earlier in the context of a clinical trial. One uses baseline characteristics to develop an equation for the probability of early death. One can then examine the effect of treatment within the subgroup of patients who are at low risk of early death. This approach was used in the PREVAIL II trial in Ebola virus disease (The Prevail II Writing Group, 2016). Logistic regression was used to relate baseline variables to early death. The treatment effect was examined separately in those at low and high risk of early death.   □

One must sometimes think carefully about what is and is not a baseline variable, as the next example demonstrates.

Example 4.8. Legitimate and illegitimate baseline variables In Example 3.2, we discussed the START trial involving the CD4 count at which a patient with HIV should begin antiretroviral therapy. Recall that HIV patients with CD4 counts above 500 were randomized to start immediately or defer until the CD4 count dropped to 350 or below. One interesting alternative design would involve asking the treating physician to specify a CD4 trigger value X_i at which he/she intended to begin CD4 therapy for patient i. Enroll patients with $X_i > 500$, and randomize them to start therapy either at CD4 count X_i or 350. Then use X_i as a continuous, rather than binary covariate. Suppose that this design had been selected. Even though the doctor may have specified an intended CD4 trigger level X_i, the CD4 count X_i' at which patient i actually started therapy might differ from X_i. It seems preferable to use X_i' in the analysis, but that is not a legitimate baseline variable. X_i is a legitimate baseline variable because it is specified by the treating physician **before** randomization. On the other hand, X_i' would undoubtedly be influenced by the health of the patient **after** randomization. For instance, a serious infection would likely result in starting ART earlier than intended. This would make interpretation of results very difficult.   □

4.4   Controls

Is a control arm really needed? Why not simply treat sick patients and measure the change from before to after treatment? One problem is that people may have been recruited when their disease was at its worst, in which case they may have been on the verge of recovery even without any treatment. Without a control group, we might wrongly ascribe benefit to treatment. In contrast, in a randomized trial, the distribution of illness progression will be similar across arms. If we see no difference between arms, we will correctly conclude that treatment is not beneficial.

4.4.1 Regression to the Mean

There is another factor interfering with our ability to attribute to treatment a beneficial change from beginning to end of study. We often study people with high or low values of a marker of health: people with high cholesterol or blood pressure, or low values of estimated glomerular filtration rate (eGFR), a measure of kidney function. When we require extreme values to qualify for a study, the next value will tend to be less extreme. This phenomenon is known as *regression to the mean*.

One of several ways to view regression to the mean is as follows. For simplicity, assume that the measured systolic blood pressures Y_i of patients in some population are normally distributed with mean 130. To qualify for the study, a patient must have $Y_i > 140$. If the same patient is measured again after no intervention, the second measurement Y_i' need not exceed 140. By this simple fact, the mean of the second measurement tends to be smaller than the mean of the first (Figure 4.1).

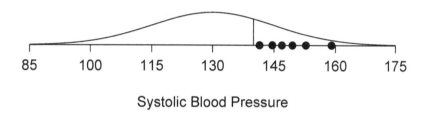

Systolic Blood Pressure

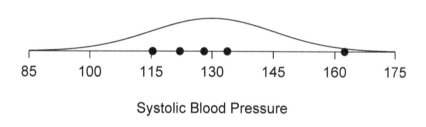

Systolic Blood Pressure

Figure 4.1: Regression to the mean when the baseline systolic blood pressure measurements (dots in top plot) are constrained to exceed 140 (vertical line). The follow-up measurements (dots in bottom plot), which are not constrained to exceed 140, tend to be lower, on average.

We can further dissect the above example as follows. Patient i's measurement Y_i decomposes into $T_i + \epsilon_i$, where T_i is the patient's true value if we could measure without error, and ϵ_i is a mean 0 measurement error independent of T_i. Study entry requires $T_i + \epsilon_i > 140$. Even though ϵ_i has mean 0 across all participants screened for the trial, the ϵ_i of patients who actually qualify is strictly positive (Figure 4.2).

Although regression to the mean is often explained using the bivariate normal distribution, it is far more general. Whenever entry criteria require the baseline measurement to exceed a given cutpoint, the follow-up measurement tends to be smaller. Likewise, whenever entry criteria require the baseline measurement to be smaller than a given cutpoint, the follow-up measurement tends to be larger.

The following is a fascinating example of regression to the mean.

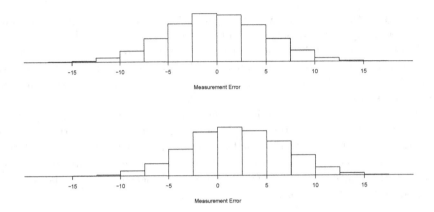

Figure 4.2: Histograms of error distributions for all patients screened (top panel) and all patients meeting entry criteria of systolic blood pressure > 140 (bottom panel). The latter error distribution has positive mean.

Example 4.9. In a trial of approximately 1700 patients, there was a kidney substudy of patients whose baseline eGFR was less than 60. Figure 4.3 shows the eGFR by time from randomization, along with 95% confidence intervals. Note that baseline values had to be less than 60, whereas there was no such restriction at later time points. There is a substantial increase in eGFR of follow-up compared to baseline measurements. Investigators theorized that patients may have been dehydrated at baseline, resulting in the relatively lower eGFR measurements.

To prove that much of the difference between baseline and follow-up measurements is attributable to regression to the mean, we tried an experiment. We pretended that substudy eligibility was determined by **1-month**, rather than baseline, values. From all patients in the main study, we selected the subset whose 1-month eGFR was less than 60. We computed mean values for these selected patients at other time points (Figure 4.4). Notice that there is a big jump in eGFR even when we go backwards in time from 1 month to baseline. Under the hypothesis that patients were dehydrated before starting the trial, baseline eGFR should be lower, not higher, than 1-month eGFR. The correct explanation for Figure 4.4 is regression to the mean.   □

In a randomized controlled trial, regression to the mean will be present in both arms. If treatment has no effect, the regression to the mean effects in the two arms will cancel out.

4.4.2   Appropriate Control

Many different controls are possible in a clinical trial. Often, the control arm receives a placebo that matches the treatment in appearance. For instance, in a trial evaluating the effect of fish oil on cardiac arrhythmias, olive oil was used as a placebo. In trials with non-pharmacologic interventions, determination of an appropriate control can be challenging. For example, if the intervention is cognitive behavioral therapy, part of the effect of treatment may simply be added attention. To see whether cognitive behavioral therapy has benefit beyond simply attention, we need to ensure that the control arm also has an attention component. Likewise, in a trial evaluating temperature biofeedback for treatment of Raynaud's disease, a different form of biofeedback (electromyograph biofeedback) was used as a control (Raynaud Treatment Study Investigators, 2000).

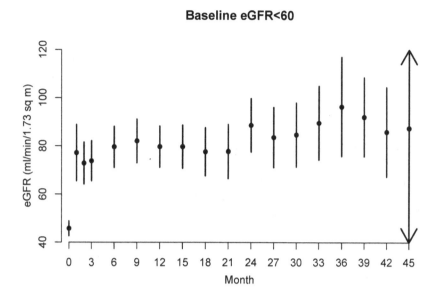

Figure 4.3: eGFR over time in a kidney substudy of a trial. Patients were required to have eGFR< 60 at baseline. eGFR increased substantially in subsequent months.

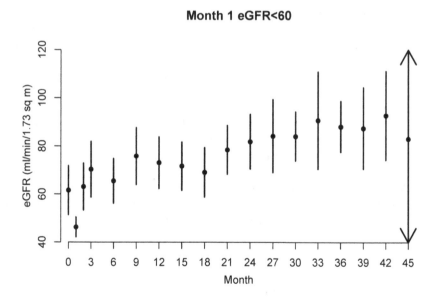

Figure 4.4: EGFR over time if entry criteria had been based on eGFR< 60 at **month 1**. Note that eGFR increases as we go **backwards** in time from month 1 to baseline.

Giving only a placebo is unethical in a serious disease when there is a known effective treatment or treatment mechanism. For instance, in the ALLHAT trial of Example 4.6, it was already known that lowering blood pressure among hypertensive patients reduces the risk of stroke and other cardiovascular events. It would have been unethical to give only a placebo to patients at elevated cardiovascular risk. Instead, ALLHAT used a diuretic (Chlorthalidone) as an *active control*. Other times, the control arm is standard of care, the standard treatment given for a disease. In the PREVAIL II Ebola trial of Example 4.7, the control group was standard care.

4.5   Choice of Primary Endpoint

In a clinical trial, we want to answer many questions, but we often choose one *primary endpoint* (also called *primary outcome*), the outcome upon which the benefit of treatment will be judged. The reason for choosing only one primary endpoint is the scourge of multiplicity (see Chapter 7). The *familywise error rate (FWE)*, namely the probability of at least one false positive conclusion among multiple comparisons, can be quite high if the type I error rate for each comparison is 0.05. To control the familywise error rate, we must use a more stringent criterion for each comparison. Instead, clinical trialists often pick one primary endpoint and several *secondary endpoints*.

Remark 4.10. *Multiplicity concerns do not arise in phase I safety trials whose main goal is to have some confidence that one can safely proceed to the next phase to try to demonstrate efficacy. In such trials, we want to avoid missing a true safety signal. Consequently, null hypotheses of no between-arm difference in the probability of each of many adverse events (e.g., liver or kidney toxicity, etc.) are assessed with no adjustment for multiple comparisons.*

In a phase II trial, the primary endpoint may be an intermediate outcome that the treatment is thought to work through. For example, the ultimate goal of a cholesterol lowering drug is to reduce cardiovascular events like heart attacks and strokes, but the mechanism of action is through cholesterol lowering. The first step is to demonstrate that the drug has an effect on the change in cholesterol from baseline to end of study. This is called a *surrogate endpoint*, an endpoint other than the one of ultimate interest, but thought to be the main mechanism of action through which the treatment confers benefit on the ultimate endpoint. Other surrogate endpoints include blood pressure when the ultimate goal is to reduce strokes, change in HIV viral load or CD4 T-cell count when the ultimate goal is to reduce serious AIDS infections and death, and culture conversion (based on a sputum test) when the ultimate goal is to cure tuberculosis. Although drugs are sometimes approved on the basis of a surrogate endpoint (such as hemoglobin A1c in diabetes trials), there are also examples in which treatment produced a benefit on the surrogate endpoint and no benefit on the ultimate endpoint. For instance, culture conversion is now considered necessary, but not sufficient, to cure tuberculosis. The following is a classic example showing that there may even be benefit on a surrogate endpoint and harm on the serious clinical endpoint.

Example 4.11. The Cardiac Arrhythmia Suppression Trial (CAST)   Contractions in the normal heart occur with a specific timing, beginning with the top and proceeding systematically down the heart to produce efficient pumping of blood to the rest of the body. Cardiac arrhythmias are disruptions of that normal timing. Patients who have had a heart attack and experience cardiac arrhythmias are at increased risk of cardiac arrest and sudden death. As a result, doctors routinely prescribed antiarrhythmic medication for such patients. CAST tested the hypothesis that suppression of cardiac arrhythmias in patients with a heart attack and arrhythmias would reduce cardiac arrests and sudden arrhythmic deaths (see CAST Investigators, 1989 or Moore, 1995). Patients with at least 80% suppression of their arrhythmias through some drug were randomized to receive either that drug or a matching placebo. It was a classic case of trying to show that improvement in a surrogate endpoint, cardiac arrhythmias, would translate to improvement in a serious clinical endpoint, sudden arrhythmic death and cardiac arrest. Unfortunately, the opposite occurred. The trial stopped early because, although the drugs decreased the number of arrhythmias, they increased the rate of sudden death and cardiac arrest. The fact that there can be improvement on a surrogate endpoint and harm on a serious clinical endpoint is one of many lessons from CAST that we will study throughout the book. □

As a result of CAST and other trials, surrogate endpoints must satisfy rigorous criteria to be considered validated for phase III trials. It is not sufficient for the surrogate endpoint S to be correlated with the 'true' endpoint T within each arm. Baker and Kramer (2003) show for continuous endpoints that S and T can have correlation 1 within each arm, but the slope relating S and T may differ by arm in a way that makes S higher and T lower in the treatment arm compared to control. In other words, a surrogate can perfectly predict the true outcome within each arm, but the between-arm difference in the surrogate may not predict the between-arm difference in the true endpoint in the manner expected.

Prentice (1989) offered criteria intended to show that the effect of the intervention on the binary true endpoint is entirely through its effect on the binary surrogate. The idea is that the true outcome T and treatment assignment Z should be independent precisely when the surrogate endpoint S and Z are independent. One shows that (1) treatment affects S, (2) treatment affects T, (3) the conditional distribution of T given S depends on S, and (4) the conditional distribution of T given S and Z depends only on S. Condition (4) says that the effect of treatment on the true outcome is entirely through its effect on the surrogate.

Many regard the Prentice criteria as too stringent (Fleming et al, 1994). After all, if we could really establish condition (2) in a trial using a surrogate endpoint, there would be no need to use the surrogate! Also, most surrogate endpoints explain some, but not all, of the effect of treatment. Freedman et al (1992) expanded on the Prentice approach by computing the proportion of effect on the clinical endpoint explained by the surrogate.

Perhaps the best way to validate a surrogate is with data from a *meta-analysis*, a formal synthesis of results of different clinical trials. In that case, one can see if the effect of treatment on the surrogate endpoints predicts the effect on the true endpoint. Meta-analyses have made a strong case for using progression-free survival as a surrogate for overall survival in certain cancers. Buyse et al (2000) review methods of validating a surrogate and extend them to the setting of a meta-analysis.

In a phase III trial, the primary endpoint is a very serious event. For instance, the primary endpoint in the CAST trial of Example 4.11 was sudden arrhythmic death or cardiac arrest. This combination of different events is called a *composite endpoint*. A common composite endpoint in cancer is progression of disease or death. In HIV trials, the primary outcome is often a composite of any serious opportunistic infection. The standard approach with composite endpoints is to analyze time to the first event in the composite. Thus, if a CAST patient had a cardiac arrest at 1 year and died suddenly 6 months later, the time to event would be 1 year. One reason for using a composite endpoint is that treatment is expected to affect different related outcomes to a similar degree, so including multiple outcomes increases the number of events and power. For example, treatments that reduce cholesterol are expected to reduce the number of heart attacks and cardiovascular deaths. HIV drugs should reduce the incidence of serious AIDS-related infections. Note that the components of a composite endpoint should all be serious. For example, it would be a mistake in an HIV trial to include **all** infections, serious or not; minor infections would inappropriately dominate the composite.

One very important principle when deciding the primary endpoint of a clinical trial is the following.

Principle 4.12. Measurement Principle   *The process of measurement of the primary endpoint should not be influenced by treatment.*

Of course the **value** of the measurement will be influenced by an effective treatment, but **how it is measured** should not be. One obvious violation of the measurement principle occurs when an event can only occur in one arm. For instance, in a trial in which patients in only one arm receive an organ transplant, it would not make sense for the primary endpoint to include rejection of the organ. These events can occur only in the transplant arm. The null hypothesis of no difference between arms is patently false. Another violation of the measurement principle occurs if the amount of monitoring for events differs by arm. Other violations of the measurement principle are more subtle, as the following two examples show.

Example 4.13. A vaccine can have two possible benefits: (1) to prevent a disease or (2) to lessen the severity of a disease. Therefore, one could compare the proportions of people getting the disease in the two arms, or the disease severity (e.g., the amount of virus) among people who get the disease. The latter analysis is problematic because the people in whom it is measured differ in the two arms. For example, if the vaccine protects some people from getting the disease, whereas the placebo does not, then only the most susceptible people may get the disease in the vaccine arm. In other words, the process of measurement of the endpoint can be influenced by the treatment, violating the measurement principle. This can lead to misleading conclusions. For instance, suppose that the vaccine actually **causes** a mild form of the disease. Then the average viral load among people getting the disease may be lower in the vaccine arm than in the control arm, but that is a moot point if the vaccine actually causes the disease! The comparison of proportions with the disease does not have this problem. For each person randomized, we will have a 1 or 0 denoting disease or no disease. We are comparing the entire randomized arms. Therefore, the primary endpoint in a vaccine trial is usually occurrence of disease.   □

Example 4.14. In heart disease trials, angiograms are used to measure the blockage of coronary arteries. Arteries are divided into sections, and the minimum diameter in each section is compared between baseline and end of study. A smaller minimum diameter at the end of the study would signify disease progression. A problem is that many segments may have no blockage, so we will be averaging many 0s, which may 'water down' any effect. Many feel that the average change should therefore be computed only across segments that were blocked at baseline. But what if there are segments that were not blocked at baseline but became blocked at the end of the study? Shouldn't they be counted? After all, one of the benefits of treatment may be to prevent these new lesions. Therefore, it seems advantageous to average changes over segments that were blocked either at baseline or the end of the study. Michael Proschan argued in favor of including segments blocked at either baseline or the end of the study in the Women's Angiographic Vitamin and Estrogen (WAVE) trial. He now believes that this was a mistake because it violates the measurement principle; the set of lesions over which the average is calculated can depend on the effect of treatment. For a given patient, a section that would not have been included if the patient had been assigned to placebo would be included if the patient had been assigned to treatment. This has the potential to produce misleading results akin to those of Example 4.13 (see Exercise 12).

□

4.6 Reducing Variability

Another very important aspect of clinical trials is minimizing variability. Statistical tests comparing means of a continuous outcome in different arms are often based on a properly standardized ratio of between-arm to within-arm variability. A large value of this ratio results in a statistically significant result.

Principle 4.15. Variability ratio principle *Reducing within-arm variability increases the ratio of between- to within-arm variability and increases power.*

4.6.1 Replication and Averaging

One way to deal with variability is through averaging. For example, blood pressure may vary from day to day because of stressful events on some days, among other reasons. Which days are stressful varies from one patient to the next. To account for day-to-day variability, we average, for each patient, blood pressure taken over several days. This average blood pressure has smaller variance than a single measurement, leading to a smaller variance of the treatment effect estimate. If the treatment effect estimate $\hat{\delta}$ is the difference between treatment and control sample means with n observations per arm, then $\text{var}(\hat{\delta}) = 2\sigma^2/n$, where σ^2 is the common within-arm variance. But σ^2 depends on the number of days over which we average for each patient. Averaging over an unlimited number of days essentially eliminates the day-to-day variability component of σ^2. This illustrates that we diminish random variability by replication and averaging. The larger the variability, the greater the replication and averaging needed. Patients are often the largest source of variability in a clinical trial, so to reduce the variance of the treatment effect estimate, we need to average over many patients. There is much less variability of blood pressure measurements taken minutes apart than taken days apart. Consequently, averaging two blood pressure measurements taken a few minutes apart reduces variability much less than averaging blood pressure measurements on two consecutive days.

We can express the above facts using the following mixed model for the blood pressure Y_{ijk} for patient i on day j on replication k (Figure 4.5):

$$Y_{ijk} = \mu + P_i + D_{ij} + \epsilon_{ijk}. \tag{4.1}$$

Here, μ is a fixed effect representing the mean blood pressure in the population, and P_i, D_{ij}, and ϵ_{ijk} are statistically independent, mean 0 random effects representing deviations due to patient, day, and other error, respectively. The "other error" component includes measurement error, short-term fluctuations, and anything else not accounted for by patient-to-patient and day-to-day components. If we randomly select a patient, day, and replication, the variance of Y_{ijk} will be

$$\text{var}(Y_{ijk}) = \sigma_P^2 + \sigma_D^2 + \sigma_\epsilon^2, \tag{4.2}$$

where σ_P^2, σ_D^2, and σ_ϵ^2 are variances of the respective random effects. For instance, if the patient-to-patient, day-to-day, and within-day variances are $15^2 = 225$, $5^2 = 25$, and $2^2 = 4$, respectively, the variance of a single measurement on a single day from a single patient is $225 + 25 + 4 = 254$.

Now suppose that we average blood pressure over I people, J days, and K measurements per day. We denote this average using 'dot' notation, where the dots denote the indices over

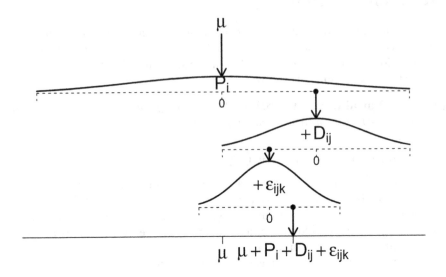

Figure 4.5: Patient-to patient, day-to-day and within-day variability of blood pressure. A given measurement is an overall mean μ plus the sum of these 0 random fluctuations.

which we average:

$$
\begin{aligned}
\bar{Y}_{...} &= \frac{\sum_{i=1}^{I}\sum_{j=1}^{J}\sum_{k=1}^{K} Y_{ijk}}{IJK} = \frac{\sum_{i=1}^{I}\sum_{j=1}^{J}\sum_{k=1}^{K}(\mu + P_i + D_{ij} + \epsilon_{ijk})}{IJK} \\
&= \frac{(IJK)\mu + JK\sum_{i=1}^{I} P_i + K\sum_{i=1}^{I}\sum_{j=1}^{J} D_{ij} + \sum_{i=1}^{I}\sum_{j=1}^{J}\sum_{k=1}^{K}\epsilon_{ijk}}{IJK} \\
&= \mu + \frac{1}{I}\sum_{i=1}^{I} P_i + \frac{1}{IJ}\sum_{i=1}^{I}\sum_{j=1}^{J} D_{ij} + \frac{1}{IJK}\sum_{i=1}^{I}\sum_{j=1}^{J}\sum_{k=1}^{K}\epsilon_{ijk} \\
&= \mu + \bar{P}. + \bar{D}.. + \bar{\epsilon}....
\end{aligned}
\tag{4.3}
$$

Accordingly,

$$
\text{var}(\bar{Y}_{...}) = \sigma_P^2/I + \sigma_D^2/(IJ) + \sigma_\epsilon^2/(IJK).
\tag{4.4}
$$

Note that each variance component is divided by the number of observations for that component. For example, the total number of days is the product of the number of patients and the number of days per patient, so the variance component σ_D^2 is divided by IJ. In the above example in which $\sigma_P^2 = 225$, $\sigma_D^2 = 25$, and $\sigma_\epsilon^2 = 4$, the variance of a single patient's average over 5 days, 2 measurements per day, is $225/1 + 25/5 + 4/10 = 230.4$.

The smallest source of variability in the above example is within-day variability. Therefore, increasing the number of measurement per day has a minimal effect on reducing variability. Even letting $K \to \infty$ eliminates only the within-day variability term in (4.4). Therefore, we reduce the variance by only 4. Averaging blood pressure over multiple days has a larger effect for two reasons. First, day-to-day variability is larger than within-day variability. Second, letting $J \to \infty$ eliminates both the day-to-day and within-day variance terms in (4.4). Averaging over many patients reduces variance the most. Letting $I \to \infty$ eliminates all three variance terms in (4.4).

In summary:

Principle 4.16. Replication principle *Sources with the largest random variability require the most replication.*

4.6.2 Differencing

The end of the preceding section discussed blood pressure, a variable whose patient-to-patient variability usually dwarfs other sources of variability. One way of dealing with this large variability is to average over many patients, but another strategy is to eliminate patient-to-patient variability altogether by computing a within-patient difference from baseline to end of study. Essentially, each patient is acting as his/her own control. To illustrate, we simplify Model (4.1) slightly by subsuming day-to-day and within-day variability into a single category, within-patient variability. Let Y_{ij} be the measurement for patient i at time j in a given arm, with $j = 0$ and $j = 1$ denoting baseline and end of study, respectively. A reasonable model is

$$Y_{ij} = \mu_0 + P_i + j\Delta + \epsilon_{ij}, \tag{4.5}$$

where μ_0 and Δ are fixed effects representing the mean baseline blood pressure and mean blood pressure change from baseline to end of study, respectively. The terms P_i and ϵ_{ij} are mean 0 random effects; P_i is the difference between patient i's true baseline value (if we could measure it without error) and the mean baseline value μ_0 over all patients, and the ϵ_{ij} are within-patient deviations. Suppose we use, as outcome for patient i, the blood pressure at the end of the study. Then

$$\mathrm{var}(Y_{ij}) = \sigma_P^2 + \sigma_\epsilon^2, \tag{4.6}$$

where σ_P^2 and σ_ϵ^2 are between-patient and within-patient variances, respectively. We can eliminate between-patient variance by using as outcome for patient i the difference

$$Y_{i1} - Y_{i0} = \mu_0 + P_i + \Delta + \epsilon_{i1} - (\mu_0 + P_i + \epsilon_{i0}) = \Delta + \epsilon_{i1} - \epsilon_{i0}.$$

Then

$$\mathrm{var}(Y_{i1} - Y_{i0}) = \mathrm{var}(\Delta + \epsilon_{1j} - \epsilon_{0j}) = 2\sigma_\epsilon^2. \tag{4.7}$$

Notice going from (4.6) to (4.7) eliminates the patient-to-patient variability σ_P^2 but adds another σ_ϵ^2. In other words, we traded a σ_ϵ^2 for a σ_P^2. This is a good trade if $\sigma_P^2 > \sigma_\epsilon^2$. Between-patient variance usually exceeds within-patient variance, so Expression (4.7) is smaller than Expression (4.6). That is, change from baseline is more efficient than end of study measurement if $\sigma_P^2 > \sigma_\epsilon^2$.

We can express the efficiency of differencing in an equivalent way in terms of the correlation between the two measurements comprising the difference. If Y_0 and Y_1 are two measurements with the same variance σ^2, then

$$\begin{aligned}
\mathrm{var}(Y_1 - Y_0) &= \mathrm{cov}(Y_1 - Y_0, Y_1 - Y_0) \\
&= \mathrm{cov}(Y_1, Y_1) - \mathrm{cov}(Y_1, Y_0) - \mathrm{cov}(Y_0, Y_1) + \mathrm{cov}(Y_0, Y_0) \\
&= \sigma^2 - 2\,\mathrm{cov}(Y_0, Y_1) + \sigma^2 = 2\sigma^2 \left\{ 1 - \frac{\mathrm{cov}(Y_0, Y_1)}{\sigma^2} \right\} \\
&= 2\sigma^2(1 - \rho), \tag{4.8}
\end{aligned}$$

where $\rho = \mathrm{cor}(Y_0, Y_1)$ is the correlation between the two measurements. Therefore, the difference has smaller variance than the single measurement Y_1 precisely when $2(1 - \rho) < 1$ (equivalently, $\rho > 1/2$). We have derived the following result that will be used in several different clinical trial contexts.

Proposition 4.17. Efficiency of differencing *If Y_0 and Y_1 have the same variance, the difference $Y_1 - Y_0$ has smaller variance than the single measurement Y_1 precisely when the correlation between Y_0 and Y_1 exceeds $1/2$.*

In relatively short duration trials with a continuous outcome, the correlation between baseline and end of study measurements can be quite high, say 90%. This correlation tends to increase as trial duration decreases. For example, one's cholesterol level today should be extremely highly correlated with one's cholesterol level tomorrow. When the correlation is very high, the gain in efficiency from using a change from baseline instead of an end of study measurement is enormous.

Another scenario in which differencing can be very efficient is when there is a strong effect of the interventionist. For example, the effectiveness of counseling surely depends on the counselor. Suppose we are comparing psychotherapy to cognitive behavioral therapy. Having the same counselor provide both types of therapy allows a within-counselor comparison, thereby eliminating the counselor effect. That begs the question, why not use just one counselor in the entire trial? Likewise, because the effect of surgery depends on the surgeon, why not eliminate the surgeon effect by having a single surgeon perform all surgeries? That is exactly what happened in the following example.

Example 4.18. Moseley et al. (2002) evaluated the effect of arthroscopic surgery for osteoarthritis of the knee. They used sham surgery as a placebo, and concluded that real arthroscopic surgery was no more effective than sham surgery. The same surgeon performed all actual and sham surgeries. Our understanding is that this surgeon had an impeccable reputation, and procedures were standardized to try to ensure high quality. Nonetheless, having only one surgeon for the entire trial is extremely problematic because it is not possible to know for sure whether (1) arthroscopic surgery does not work or (2) arthoscopic surgery **performed by this surgeon** does not work. By contrast, a trial of vertebroplasty for osteoporotic spinal fractures, which also incorporated a simulated surgery as a control, used multiple surgeons (Kallmes, Comstock, and Heagerty, 2009). Having multiple surgeons performing sham and actual surgeries allows determination of whether the effect of surgery differs appreciably from one surgeon to the next.   □

The lesson from the Moseley et al. study can be summarized in the following principle.

Principle 4.19. Generalizability Principle *When the effect of treatment may depend on a random factor such as counselor, surgeon, etc. (i.e., there is an interaction between treatment and the random factor), replication of the random factor is essential for assessing generalizability of effect across the random factor.*

4.6.3   Stratification

Another way of dealing with variability is to stratify the analysis by the given factor. We compute the treatment effect separately in each subgroup and then combine those treatment effects in an optimal way.

Before getting into the details, we illustrate graphically why stratification can be so helpful, namely by reducing the variance of the treatment effect estimator. Suppose that we are comparing an intervention to placebo with respect to end of study weight. Note that, without using stratification, weight change rather than end of study weight is more prudent, but this example is solely to illustrate the effect of stratification. Men and women have very different baseline weights, as depicted in the first two boxplots of Figure 4.6. Within each stratum, variability is not large, but if we lump the two gender strata, variability is much larger (rightmost boxplot of Figure 4.6). The same is very likely to hold for end of study

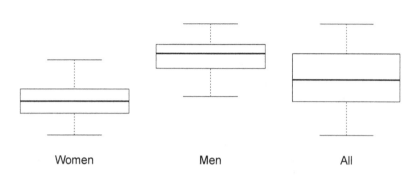

Figure 4.6: Illustration of the advantage of stratification. Men and women with very different baseline values of a variable like weight. If we lump men and women, the variability is much larger (rightmost boxplot).

weight. Therefore, end of study weight lumped across genders will be highly variable, as will the treatment effect estimate. Instead of lumping the two genders, we should compute treatment effect estimates $\hat{\delta}_M$ and $\hat{\delta}_W$ separately in men and women, and then combine them. This treatment effect estimator will be less variable than the one computed in the entire group. For example, suppose the sample sizes within each of the four gender by treatment groups is the same, but the variance within men and within women is half of the overall variance. Then the variance of the stratified treatment effect estimator will be half the variance of the unstratified treatment effect estimator.

What is the optimal way to combine the two independent treatment effect estimates? We can gain insight by splitting a random sample $Y_1, \ldots, Y_n$ of independent and identically distributed (iid) random variables into two strata of sizes n_1 and n_2. Let $\bar{Y}_1$ and $\bar{Y}_2$ be the separate sample means. The variance of $\bar{Y}_i$ is $v_i = \sigma^2/n_i$, $i = 1, 2$. Consider a weighted combination $w_1\bar{Y}_1 + w_2\bar{Y}_2$, $w_1 + w_2 = 1$. It is clear that when all observations are iid, we cannot do better than the sample mean of all n observations, which results by taking weight $w_i = n_i/(n_1 + n_2)$, $i = 1, 2$. These weights can be written as $w_i = (1/v_i)/(1/v_1 + 1/v_2)$, $i = 1, 2$. This gives us the clue that for general independent estimators $\hat{\delta}_1$ and $\hat{\delta}_2$ with finite variances v_1 and v_2, the weighted combination $\hat{\delta} = w_1\hat{\delta}_1 + w_2\hat{\delta}_2$ minimizing variance is $w_i = (1/v_i)/(1/v_1 + 1/v_2)$, $i = 1, 2$. The variance of this optimal weighted combination is

$$
\begin{aligned}
\operatorname{var}(w_1\hat{\delta}_1 + w_2\hat{\delta}_2) &= w_1^2 v_1 + w_2^2 v_2 \\
&= \frac{(1/v_1)^2 v_1 + (1/v_2)^2 v_2}{(1/v_1 + 1/v_2)^2} = \frac{1/v_1 + 1/v_2}{(1/v_1 + 1/v_2)^2} \\
&= \frac{1}{1/v_1 + 1/v_2}.
\end{aligned}
\tag{4.9}
$$

This generalizes to more than two strata, as we now see.

Theorem 4.20. *(Gauss-Markov) Let $\hat{\delta}_1, \ldots \hat{\delta}_k$ be statistically independent, unbiased estimators of a parameter δ with respective finite variances $v_1, \ldots, v_k$. The weighted linear* combination $\hat{\delta} = \sum w_i \hat{\delta}_i$, $\sum_{i=1}^{n} \hat{w}_i = 1$, *with smallest variance uses inverse variance weights:*

$$w_i = \frac{1/v_i}{\sum_{j=1}^{k} 1/v_j}, \quad i = 1, \ldots, k.$$

The variance of this optimally weighted linear combination $\hat{\delta}_{\text{opt}}$ is $1/\sum_{i=1}^{k}(1/v_i)$.

The same idea of running separate analyses within subgroups and then combining treatment effect estimates across subgroups can be employed with binary or time to event analyses as well. The motivation for doing so is not quite the same as with continuous outcomes because an outcome variable that takes values 1 or 0 with probabilities p and $1 - p$ has variance $p(1-p)$. Stratifying generally does not markedly affect variance in this setting. But the other major advantage of stratification in either a binary or continuous outcome setting is that it can fix accidental imbalances in baseline variables. Suppose that the treatment arm contains a higher proportion of men than the control arm. Because men are generally heavier than women, the treatment minus control difference in weight will likely be positive even if treatment has no effect on weight. Stratifying eliminates the effect of this accidental imbalance because the difference between treatment and control is computed within weight strata.

One stratified analysis with a binary outcome uses the O minus E except after V principle (Principle 2.2 in Section 2.1). Suppose there are k subgroups. Within subgroup i, we estimate the log odds ratio λ_i by $\hat{\lambda}_i = (O - E)/V$. The variance of $\hat{\lambda}_i$ (conditioned on the row and column totals of the 2×2 table) is $1/V$. Therefore, if we use inverse variance weights w_i, then $w_i = 1/(1/V_i) = V_i$. The stratified estimator of the log odds ratio is

$$\hat{\theta} = \frac{\sum_{i=1}^{k} w_i(O_i - E_i)/V_i}{\sum_{i=1}^{k} w_i} = \frac{\sum_{i=1}^{k} V_i\{(O_i - E_i)/V_i\}}{\sum_{i=1}^{k} V_i} = \frac{\sum_{i=1}^{k}(O_i - E_i)}{\sum_{i=1}^{k} V_i}. \tag{4.10}$$

The estimated variance of the stratified estimator of the log odds ratio is, from the Gauss-Markov theorem (Theorem 4.20),

$$\text{var}(\hat{\theta}) = \frac{1}{\sum_{i=1}^{k} w_i} = \frac{1}{\sum_{i=1}^{k} V_i}.$$

The z-score for testing whether the common log odds ratio is 0 is obtained by dividing $\hat{\theta}$ by its estimated standard error:

$$Z = \frac{\sum_{i=1}^{k}(O_i - E_i)/\sum_{i=1}^{k} V_i}{1/\sqrt{\sum_{i=1}^{k} V_i}} = \frac{\sum_{i=1}^{k}(O_i - E_i)}{\sqrt{\sum_{i=1}^{k} V_i}}. \tag{4.11}$$

We refer z to a standard normal distribution if the sample sizes in the different trials are large. This test is not as the *Mantel-Haenszel test*. Likewise, a $100(1 - \alpha)\%$ confidence interval for the log odds ratio λ is

$$\frac{\sum_{i=1}^{k}(O_i - E_i)}{\sum_{i=1}^{k} V_i} \pm \frac{z_{\alpha/2}}{\sqrt{\sum_{i=1}^{k} V_i}}.$$

We then exponentiate the lower and upper limits of this confidence interval to get the confidence interval for the odds ratio θ:

$$95\% \text{ CI for odds ratio } \theta: \quad \exp\left[\frac{\sum_{i=1}^{k}(O_i - E_i)}{\sum_{i=1}^{k} V_i} \pm \frac{z_{\alpha/2}}{\sqrt{\sum_{i=1}^{k} V_i}}\right]. \tag{4.12}$$

Incidentally, given that the z-score (4.11) is called the Mantel-Haenszel statistic, you might assume that the estimator (4.10) is called the Mantel-Haenszel estimator, but the Mantel-Haenszel estimator is different. In the generic 2×2 table, ad should approximately equal θbc, where θ is the population odds ratio. With multiple tables, let the four cells of table i be $a_i, b_i, c_i,$ and d_i. Because different tables may have drastically different sample sizes, we would like to use a weighted combination of results from the different tables. Using the same reasoning, the weighted combination $w_i a_i d_i$ should be approximately $\theta w_i b_i c_i$. Accordingly,

$$\sum_{i=1}^{k} w_i a_i d_i \approx \theta \sum_{i=1}^{k} w_i b_i c_i; \quad \theta \approx \frac{\sum_{i=1}^{k} w_i a_i d_i}{\sum_{i=1}^{k} w_i b_i c_i}.$$

Example 4.21. The Pamoja Tulinde Maishe (PALM) trial in the Democratic Republic of the Congo randomized patients with Ebola virus disease to one of four interventions. The primary outcome was 28-day mortality. Randomization was stratified by whether patients had high or low viral load (defined as a cycle threshold of ≤ 22 or > 22, respectively). At the end of the trial, the numbers of deaths in the REGN-EB3 and ZMapp arms in the two subgroups were as shown in Table 4.3.

Table 4.3: Deaths by 28 days in the REGN-EB3 and ZMapp arms of the PALM trial, stratified by low viral load (left) and high viral load (right).

Low VL

	Dead	Alive	Total
REGN EB3	10	79	89
ZMapp	24	74	98
Total	34	153	187

High VL

	Dead	Alive	Total
REGN EB3	42	24	66
ZMapp	60	11	71
Total	102	35	137

O, E and V values for the two viral load strata are shown in Table 4.4. For example, in the low viral load stratum, $O_i = 10$, $E_1 = (89)(34)/187 = 16.1818$, and $V_1 = (89)(98)(34)(153)/\{(187^2)(186)\} = 6.9757$.

The $(O - E)/V$ estimator and confidence interval for the log odds ratio are

$$(52 - 65.3205)/(13.5295) = -0.9846; \quad 95\% \text{ CI: } -0.9846 \pm \frac{1.96}{\sqrt{13.5295}}$$

$$= (-1.5175, -0.4517).$$

Table 4.4: O_i, E_i, and V_i in the two viral load strata and overall in the PALM trial.

	O_i	E_i	V_i	$(O_i - E_i)/V_i$
Low VL	10	16.1818	6.9757	-0.8862
High VL	42	49.1387	6.5538	-1.0892
Total	52	65.3205	13.5295	-0.9846

The corresponding estimator and confidence interval for the odds ratio are

$$\hat{\theta} = \exp(-0.9846) = 1.37; \quad 95\% \text{ CI: } (\exp(-1.5175), \exp(-0.4517)) = (0.22, 0.64).$$

The Mantel-Haenszel estimate of the odds ratio is very similar: 0.35.

4.6.4   Regression

Another way to deal with variability is through a regression model. Let D_i, z_i, and s_i be change in blood pressure from baseline to end of study, treatment assignment ($z_i = 0$ for control, $z_i = 1$ for treatment), and stratum indicator ($s_i = 0$ for normal baseline blood pressure, $s_i = 1$ for baseline hypertension) for participant i. Consider the model

$$D_i = \mu_0 + \delta z_i + \tau s_i + \epsilon_i, \tag{4.13}$$

where ϵ_i are iid random errors with mean 0 and variance σ_ϵ^2. It is always helpful when modeling to construct a table with different cells and the expected value of the outcome within each cell. Table 4.5 shows the 4 treatment by baseline blood pressure cells and the expected value of Y_i within each cell. For example, in the treatment group of the baseline normotensive stratum, we substitute $z_i = 1$ and $s_i = 0$ into (4.13) and eliminate the ϵ_i, yielding $\mu_0 + \delta$. Notice that the difference in means between treatment and control is $\mu_0 + \delta - \mu_0 = \delta$

Table 4.5: Within-cell means under Model (4.13).

	Control ($z = 0$)	Treatment ($z = 1$)
Baseline normotensive ($s = 0$)	μ_0	$\mu_0 + \delta$
Baseline hypertensive ($s = 1$)	$\mu_0 + \tau$	$\mu_0 + \delta + \tau$

for baseline normotensives and $\mu_0 + \delta + \tau - (\mu_0 + \tau) = \delta$ for baseline hypertensives. That is, Model (4.13) assumes that the treatment effect is the same number δ within baseline blood pressure strata. The model also implies that the variances of observations in the four blood pressure by treatment groups are the same, namely σ_ϵ^2. The treatment effect estimators in the two strata will have different variances only because of different sample sizes. Therefore, it seems that Model (4.13) should yield results similar to a stratified analysis. In fact, if in our stratified analysis, we also assume equal variances within each treatment by baseline blood pressure stratum, then the treatment effect estimator is the same using model (4.13) or using a stratified analysis. The regression program estimates the treatment effect δ using the same stratified analysis described in Section 4.6.3.

We may not want to assume that the variances are the same in the two baseline blood pressure by treatment groups. In fact, variances of changes from baseline could easily be larger for those with higher baseline blood pressure. This phenomenon was observed in the Dietary Approaches to Stop Hypertension (DASH) trial (Appel et al., 1997) comparing blood pressure changes from baseline among three different dietary patterns. To accommodate the possibility of unequal variances, we could run the models $D_i = \mu_0 + \delta_N z_i + \epsilon_i$ and $D_i' = \mu_0' + \delta_H z_i + \epsilon_i'$ separately within normotensive and hypertensive strata. The treatment effects among normotensives and hypertensives are δ_N and δ_H, respectively, estimated by $\hat{\delta}_N$ and $\hat{\delta}_H$. Because we are running separate models in different subgroups, the variances within each subgroup are not constrained to be equal. Let $\hat{v}_N$ and $\hat{v}_H$ be the estimated variances of $\hat{\delta}_N$ and $\hat{\delta}_H$. We use our familiar stratified estimator $\hat{\delta}$ for the overall treatment effect and its estimated variance $\hat{v}$:

$$\hat{\delta} = \frac{(1/\hat{v}_N)\hat{\delta}_N + (1/\hat{v}_H)\hat{\delta}_H}{1/\hat{v}_N + 1/\hat{v}_H} \quad \text{and} \quad \hat{v} = \frac{1}{1/\hat{v}_N + 1/\hat{v}_H}.$$

We can use this to construct approximate tests and confidence intervals if the sample size is large. For example, for testing $H_0 : \delta = 0$, refer $\hat{\delta}/\sqrt{\hat{v}}$ to a standard normal distribution. This stratified approach would give a different answer than Model (4.13) because Model (4.13) assumes equal variances and the stratified approach does not. An advantage of Model (4.13) is that if the variances really are equal, Model (4.13) estimates that common variance more efficiently by using all of the data. However, if the variances are different in the separate treatment by stratum groups, Model (4.13) could be misleading and lead to an inflated type I error rate. In that sense, the stratified approach is more robust than the simple model (4.13). The robustness principle (Principle 1.10) suggests that a stratified analysis is preferred unless there is very good a priori reason to believe equal variances in treatment by stratum groups.

Of course, Model (4.13) is very basic, and we might want to include other covariates. One specific regression model is called *analysis of covariance (ANCOVA)*. ANCOVA is simply a regression model that includes the baseline value of the outcome variable. In its simplest case with no other covariates, the model is expressed as

$$Y_i = \beta_0 + \beta_1 x_i + \beta_2 z_i + \epsilon_i, \tag{4.14}$$

where x_i and Y_i are baseline and end of study outcome values, respectively, for patient i, and the ϵ_i are iid errors with mean 0 and variance σ_ϵ^2. Note that σ_ϵ^2 is the conditional variance of Y_i given the baseline value $X_i = x_i$. Model (4.14) implies that the relationship between baseline and end of study values is linear with the same slope in both arms. The model also assumes that the variability of outcomes about the regression line is the same in the two arms. The treatment effect estimate is

$$\hat{\beta}_2 = \bar{Y}_T - \bar{Y}_C - \hat{\beta}_1(\bar{x}_T - \bar{x}_C). \tag{4.15}$$

The estimate $\hat{\beta}_1$ of the common slope relating Y to x is obtained by first computing within-arm slope estimates and then combining them using inverse variance weights. Note that inverse variance weights keep arising! If we had not included the baseline value x_i in Model (4.14), the treatment effect estimator would have equaled the unadjusted treatment effect estimator $\bar{Y}_T - \bar{Y}_C$. ANCOVA corrects the unadjusted estimate for any between-arm differences in x. For example, suppose that the unadjusted treatment effect $\bar{Y}_T - \bar{Y}_C$ is -5, but the mean baseline blood pressure is 2 units lower in the treatment arm than in the control arm. Suppose that the common slope relating baseline and end of study blood pressure is 0.9. Then the adjusted treatment effect (4.15) will be a $-5 - 0.9(-2) = -3.2$. That is, the adjusted treatment effect is attenuated compared to the unadjusted treatment effect.

It is helpful to view ANCOVA in the following way. Assume that we knew the true slope β_1. Imagine using $Y' = Y - \beta_1 x$ instead of Y as the primary outcome of the trial. This makes sense; Y' is the part of the end of study value that is not already explained by the baseline value. If we did a simple t-test comparing arms on the new outcome $Y' = Y - \beta_1 x$, the treatment effect estimate would be

$$\overline{(Y - \beta_1 x)_T} - \overline{(Y - \beta_1 x)_C} = \bar{Y}_T - \bar{Y}_C - \beta_1(\bar{x}_T - \bar{x}_C).$$

This is the same as Formula (4.15) except it has β_1 instead of $\hat{\beta}_1$. Of course, we do not really know β_1, so we are forced to estimate it. If the sample size is large, $\hat{\beta}_1$ will be very close to β_1. Furthermore, the estimate of σ_ϵ^2 using Model (4.14) will be very close to the pooled variance estimate for a t-test comparing arms on outcome $Y' = Y - \beta_1 x$.

Remark 4.22. *When the sample size is large, the t-statistic for the treatment effect using ANCOVA is nearly identical to the two-sample t-statistic comparing the two arms on the modified outcome $Y' = Y - \hat{\beta}_1 x$. This holds whether or not Model (4.13) is correct.*

Up to now we have taken the usual regression approach of conditioning on $X = x$. When we do that, the mean of the ANOVA treatment effect estimate is

$$E\{(\bar{Y}_T - \bar{Y}_C) - \hat{\beta}_1(\bar{x}_T - \bar{x}_C)\} = E(\bar{Y}_T - \bar{Y}_C) - \beta_1(\bar{x}_T - \bar{x}_C). \tag{4.16}$$

This adjusted treatment effect estimate differs from the unadjusted treatment effect $E(\bar{Y}_T - \bar{Y}_C)$. But we can also take an unconditional viewpoint by treating the baseline value X as a random variable. When we do that, the expected value of the ANCOVA treatment effect estimate is obtained by replacing $\bar{x}_T$ and $\bar{x}_C$ in Expression (4.16) by the random variables $\bar{X}_T$ and $\bar{X}_C$ and taking the expectation over the distribution of $\bar{X}_T - \bar{X}_C$. Because X is a baseline covariate, the expectation of $\bar{X}_T - \bar{X}_C$ is 0. The resulting unconditional mean of treatment effect estimator (4.15) is

$$E\{(\bar{Y}_T - \bar{Y}_C) - \beta_1(\bar{X}_T - \bar{X}_C)\} = E(\bar{Y}_T - \bar{Y}_C) - \beta_1 \cdot 0 = E(\bar{Y}_T - \bar{Y}_C).$$

We have shown the following.

Remark 4.23. *From an unconditional viewpoint, $\bar{Y}_T - \bar{Y}_C$ and the ANCOVA adjusted estimator (4.15) estimate the same thing,* **whether the model is correct or not,** *because* $E(\bar{X}_T - \bar{X}_C) = 0$.

We now visualize the efficiency gain of ANCOVA over a t-test on the end of study value Y. With a t-test, the within-arm variance is the variance of end of study values about a horizontal line, the sample mean in that arm. With ANCOVA, the within-arm variance is the variance of end of study values about the best fitting lines (Figure 4.7). If Model (4.14) holds, these variances are $\beta_1^2\sigma_X^2 + \sigma_\epsilon^2$ and σ_ϵ^2, respectively. The difference between the two variances, namely $\beta_1^2\sigma_X^2$, becomes larger as $|\beta_1|$ increases. This example of the variability ratio principle (Principle 4.15) shows that ANCOVA can be considerably more efficient than a t-test on end of study values. We can apply similar reasoning to see the efficiency gain of ANCOVA to a t-test on change from baseline. Simply let Y be the change from baseline instead of end of study value.

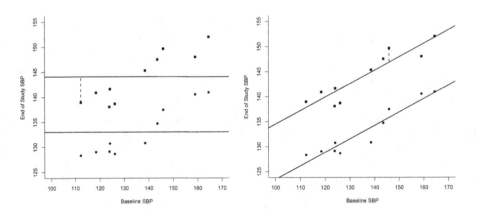

Figure 4.7: Within-arm variability is about horizontal (left) versus best fitting lines (right) for the t-test versus ANCOVA.

Even though ANCOVA is fairly robust to assumption violations, there are even more robust methods. For example, the semiparametric approach of Tsiatis et al. (2008) allows separate regression models to be used in different arms, obviating the need for conventional assumptions such as equal variances. Flexible modeling has also been proposed by Vermuelen, Thas, and Vansteelandt (2015) in the context of an extension of a Mann-Whitney U-test. More recently, Benkeser et al. (2020) showed how flexible modeling is more efficient than unadjusted analysis methods for binary, ordinal, and survival endpoints.

4.7 Different Types of Trials

4.7.1 Superiority Versus Noninferiority

Most trials are intended to show that one treatment is superior to placebo or to another treatment. These are called *superiority trials*. Occasionally, the goal instead is to show that a new treatment is almost as good as a standard treatment. These are called *noninferiority trials*. For example, the standard treatment for a disease may be very invasive or onerous. A new treatment may be much easier to take. Even if it is almost, but not quite as good as the standard, it may be considered a superior option. One example is in the setting of tuberculosis, where patients must undergo treatment for a long duration. If we can shorten the duration without materially compromising effectiveness, we would like to do so. Another reason for using a noninferiority trial is to show that a new treatment is superior to placebo in a circumstance where it is unethical to include a placebo. For example, if there is a known effective treatment for a serious disease, it would not be ethical to randomize a patient to receive a new treatment or placebo. We could give everyone the known effective treatment, and then randomly add either a placebo or the new drug. Such an *add-on trial* would answer the question of whether the new drug provides additional benefit over the known effective drug. But there are many circumstances in which an add-on trial is not appropriate. For example, consider the setting of antibiotics. We do not necessarily expect that an experimental antibiotic provides additional benefit under background treatment with the standard antibiotic. Still, if the experimental antibiotic provides benefit compared to a placebo, the experimental antibiotic may be an attractive option for people with infections that are resistant to the standard antibiotic.

A noninferiority trial leverages information from previous trials about how much better the standard treatment S is compared to placebo P, together with results of the noninferiority trial of the new treatment N versus S, to show that N would have beaten P. For example, suppose that from an earlier trial, the mortality rate on S is 0.10 lower than on P. If we demonstrate that the mortality rate on N is not more than 0.05 higher than on S, we have de facto shown that the mortality rate on N is at least 0.05 lower than P. More generally, we specify a *noninferiority margin M* (0.05 in this example), and declare the new treatment noninferior to the standard if the upper limit of a confidence interval for the difference in mortality probabilities, $p_N - p_S$ is less than or equal to M. The choice of noninferiority margin can be difficult and controversial.

4.7.2 Parallel Arm Trials

The most common trial design is a *parallel arm trial* in which each patient is randomized to only one treatment. This is a clean design with independent data for different arms. Any observed difference between arms could be explained either by a true treatment effect or because of patient-to-patient variability within arms. This variability could cause a chance imbalance whereby patients assigned to the treatment arm are healthier than those assigned to the control. To rule this out, we need a large number of patients, in accordance with the replication principle (Principle 4.16). Most of this book considers parallel arm trials.

4.7.3 Crossover Trials

Crossover trials assign each patient to all treatments in a randomly selected order. For simplicity, we focus on two treatments, called T and C. Each patient is assigned to either C followed by T or T followed by C, so we are able to compute a treatment difference within each patient. Note that the term 'crossover' is sometimes used to describe a participant who 'crosses over' from control to treatment or vice versa, but not by design. This section does not consider such unplanned crossovers. Crossover trials are typically used in relatively short duration trials with a continuous outcome. They were thought not to be appropriate in trials with serious outcomes like death because a patient who dies in period 1 is not available in period 2. However, Nason and Follmann (2010) have challenged this view. Crossover trials gain efficiency for two reasons. First, each patient is like two patients in a parallel arm trial. Second, by computing a treatment difference in each patient, we eliminate the patient-to-patient component of variance, which is often large. In accordance with the variability ratio principle (Principle 4.15), the variance of the treatment effect estimate is reduced. Consequently, the sample size for a crossover trial is substantially smaller than for a parallel arm trial.

One disadvantage of a crossover design is that there may be a *carryover effect*, meaning that the effect of a treatment continues to be felt even after it is discontinued. This leads to a biased treatment effect estimator. For instance, suppose that placebo has no effect on blood pressure, whereas treatment T lowers systolic blood pressure by 6 mmHG. Suppose, however, that its effect continues even after it is discontinued. The expected treatment minus placebo change in blood pressure in a crossover trial is −6 for patients assigned to placebo followed by treatment, and 0 for patients assigned to treatment followed by placebo (because the effect of treatment carries over into the placebo period). When we average over the two possible orders, we get −3, half of the actual treatment effect. Carryover effects can sometimes be mitigated by incorporating a *washout period* of no treatment between successive intervention periods. This gives the effect of the previous intervention time to wear off before the next intervention has its effect. Nonetheless, some effects of interventions may be long-lasting. For this reason, crossover trials should not be used if carryover effects are expected.

A crossover trial can also have *period effects*, which are different from carryover effects. A period effect occurs when there is a systematic difference between observations in different time periods. This can occur, for example, if patients are more used to being measured in the second period compared to the first, causing their blood pressure to be lower in the second period. Period effects do not cause a problem in crossover trials (see Exercise 17).

4.7.4   Cluster-Randomized Trials

Sometimes treatment is applied not to individuals, but to clusters such as communities. For example, the Rapid Early Action for Coronary Treatment (REACT) trial (Luepker et al., 2000) addressed whether a public education campaign would decrease the delay time from onset of symptoms of a heart attack to arrival at the emergency department. The intervention consisted of televised public service announcements and pamphlets telling people to call 911 if they experience chest pain consistent with a heart attack. The intervention was applied to entire communities. Communities, not individuals, were randomized to the education campaign or no intervention. A summary measure was computed in each community, namely the slope of the line relating delay times to calendar time.

Because entire communities are randomized, there is an analogy between communities in a community-randomized trial and patients in a patient-randomized trial. Power in a community-randomized trial is dictated more by the number of communities than by the number of people in a community. For instance, a study randomizing only two communities cannot possibly be convincing, even if there are hundreds of millions of people in each. For example, suppose that a community-randomized trial includes only two communities, Russia and the United States. Russia is assigned to treatment and the United States is assigned to control. Any observed difference could just as easily be explained by differences in the two countries rather than by treatment. A much more convincing trial would randomize many communities within Russia and within the United States to treatment and control.

A very important principle with implications for cluster-randomized trials is the following.

Principle 4.24. Balanced block principle *Suppose that data from a trial of n/arm consists of independent blocks of size k, and within any block, each pair of observations has correlation $\rho > 0$. The variance $\text{var}(\bar{Y}_T - \bar{Y}_C)$ of a difference in sample means is smallest when exactly half of each block is assigned to treatment, and largest when all members of the block are assigned to the same treatment.*

Remark 4.25. *The balanced block principle says in no uncertain terms that cluster randomized trials are inefficient. Randomizing clusters means that everyone in a cluster receives the same treatment. Principle 4.24 says that it is more efficient to randomize individuals within clusters such that half of the cluster receives treatment and half control. Therefore, cluster-randomized trials should be avoided unless the intervention is necessarily applied to entire clusters rather than individuals.*

4.7.5 Multi-Arm Trials

Evaluating multiple new treatments in a single trial gains efficiency and shortens the time to approval of products. Many people argue for adjustment for multiple comparisons to protect the integrity of all declarations made in a trial. Such adjustments are discussed in Chapter 10, but we now briefly touch on this topic in connection with two different types of multi-arm trials. Rothman (1990) argues that no one would adjust for multiple comparisons if they were made in separate trials, so why should there be any such adjustment if comparisons are made in the same trial? By this reasoning, if a trial consists of statistically independent comparisons, as would be the case in separate trials, a multiplicity adjustment may not be necessary. A *factorial trial* can be viewed as combining two or more trials in a way that is analogous to separate trials. Factorial trials are employed in two different settings: (1) when no treatment interaction is expected (i.e., the treatment effects are *additive*) and (2) when the goal is specifically to test whether treatment effects are additive. We consider the first scenario.

The simplest case is a 2×2 factorial of treatments A and B. Patients are randomized to one of four conditions: placebo A and placebo B, placebo A but active B, active A but placebo B, or active A and active B. An example is the Women's Angiographic Vitamin and Estrogen (WAVE) trial in which postmenopausal women with heart disease were randomized to active or placebo antioxidants and active or placebo hormone replacement therapy (HRT) (Waters et al., 2002). The primary outcome was a measure of the change in the degree of blockage of coronary arteries from baseline to end of study, as measured by coronary angiograms. The two interventions were originally planned to be studied in separate trials, and they were combined into one for logistic/efficiency reasons. Moreover, the t-statistics for the effects of antioxidants and HRT are nearly statistically independent. If we knew the population variances and substituted them for their estimates in the denominators of the t-statistics, the test statistics would be completely independent. The analogy with separate clinical trials is strong. Consequently, no multiple comparison adjustment was made for the two comparisons.

Factorial trials can have more than two levels of each factor or more than two factors. For example, if the WAVE trial had included 3 levels of antioxidants (placebo, dose 1, and dose 2) and two levels of HRT, it would have been a 3×2 factorial. If it had instead combined a trial of another factor such as diet A versus diet B, it would have been a $2 \times 2 \times 2$ factorial trial.

Table 4.6: The Women's Angiographic Vitamin and Estrogen (WAVE) trial was a 2×2 factorial trial of antioxidants and hormone replacement therapy (HRT) in postmenopausal women with heart disease. Women were randomized in equal proportions to the four cells.

	Placebo HRT	Active HRT
Placebo antioxidant		
Active antioxidant		

A different multi-arm design compares k treatments to the same control arm. An example is the Antihypertensive and Lipid-Lowering treatment to reduce Heart Attack (ALLHAT) trial described in Example 4.6. Three newer classes of antihypertensive drugs were compared to a diuretic with a longer track record. Here, the $k = 3$ comparisons with the diuretic are not statistically independent because the same control arm is used for all comparisons. A randomly 'bad' control arm might increase the probability of a false positive for each comparison. For this reason, clinical trialists have traditionally made a multiple comparison adjustment in this type of trial, as opposed to in a factorial trial. That thinking began to change in the era of emerging infectious diseases like Ebola virus disease and COVID-19. One reason is that in a deadly pandemic, there is an urgent need to find something that works. Adhering to an arguably unnecessary, austere level of rigor is counterproductive. Moreover, pharmaceutical companies would have no incentive to join a multi-armed trial that adjusts for multiple comparisons when they can perform their own trial with no multiplicity adjustment. Still, if more than one dose of the same drug is compared to a control, a multiple comparison adjustment is in order if a claim of efficacy could be made based on at least one dose being beneficial. The simplest and most conservative multiple comparison adjustment is the *Bonferroni method* with significance level α/k for each of the k comparisons. This is based on the *Bonferroni inequality* $P\{\cup_i A_i\} \leq \sum_i P(A_i)$ for any events $A_1, A_2, \ldots$ Chapter 10 contains more powerful alternative methods.

Another thing to bear in mind for comparisons with the same control arm is that the sample size in the control arm is often made larger than the sample size in each other arm. A heuristic explanation is as follows. If a patient is assigned to one of the other arms, power for the comparison of that arm with control is increased, but if the patient is assigned to the control arm, power for each comparison with control is increased. Of course, there is a limit to how large the control arm should be; if all patients are assigned to control, there are no comparisons! Likewise, if almost all patients are assigned to control, power is poor.

We can determine the allocation ratio that maximizes power for each comparison with control as follows. Suppose that N patients are randomized to k comparator arms plus a control (a total of $k+1$ arms) in a trial comparing means. Let n_0 and n denote the sample sizes in the control and each of the other arms, respectively. The constraint is that

$$n_0 + kn = N. \tag{4.17}$$

Assume a common known variance σ^2 in the different arms. Power for the comparison of arm i to control (arm 0) is a decreasing function of $\text{var}(\bar{Y}_i - \bar{Y}_0) = \sigma^2(1/n + 1/n_0)$. We would like to choose the control sample size minimizing $1/n + 1/n_0$. From Equation (4.17), $n = (N - n_0)/k$. Therefore, we want to choose n_0 to minimize $k/(N - n_0) + 1/n_0$. Even though n_0 must be an integer, replace it with a variable x that can take any value, and minimize

$$\frac{k}{N - x} + \frac{1}{x} \tag{4.18}$$

with respect to x. Differentiating with respect to x and equating to 0 gives $(N-x)/x = k^{1/2}$ which, after substituting n_0 for x and using the constraint (4.17), leads to

$$n_0 = \sqrt{k}\,n. \tag{4.19}$$

That is, $\text{var}(\bar{Y}_T - \bar{Y}_C)$ is minimized (and power is maximized) when the sample size is larger in the control arm than in each other arm by a factor of the square root of the number of non-control arms. In practice, there may be interest in comparisons between active arms as well. For fixed total sample size, enlarging the control sample size compromises power for comparisons of active arms. Therefore, some trials make n_0/n larger than 1, but not as large as $k^{1/2}$, to increase power for control comparisons while maintaining reasonable power for comparisons of active arms.

It may seem paradoxical, but increasing the control sample size n_0 actually decreases the correlation between the test statistics comparing different arms to control (again assuming known common variance). The only reason these test statistics are correlated is because they share the control arm, so increasing n_0 seems like it would increase the correlation. Think instead about the fact that a larger n_0 makes $\bar{Y}_0$ closer to a constant, namely its expectation μ_0. If $\bar{Y}_0$ were exactly μ_0, the test statistics would be completely independent.

Other multi-arm designs are more popular for phase II trials to determine which interventions have the most promise for a more definitive phase III trial. Multi-arm multi-stage (MAMS) designs begin with several arms, but drop arms that do not meet a certain minimum level of benefit compared to the control (see, for example, Royston, Parmar, and Qian, 2003; Barthel, Parmar, and Royston, 2009; Magirr et al. 2012; Wason and Jaki, 2012). A simple example would be to drop any arm whose standardized z-score for comparison with control is less than 0. It might seem that dropping bad arms should require comparable multiple comparison adjustment to selecting the best treatments. However, this is not the case. The amount of statistical adjustment required to control the familywise error rate is much less when dropping arms not meeting a minimal level of efficacy.

Bayesian multi-arm designs are often used in *platform trials*, extensive duration trials comparing multiple arms to a control. Bayesian trials use a different criterion for dropping arms, often the posterior probability that an arm is best, or among the best, given data observed thus far. See Section 9.7 for a brief discussion of Bayesian monitoring of clinical trials. Bayesian platform trials are often accompanied by *response-adaptive randomization (RAR)*. See Section 5.7 for more details of RAR.

Exercises

1. A trial was conducted in heart patients with implantable cardiac defibrillators (ICDs), devices implanted in the heart that record and correct life-threatening arrhythmias. Patients were randomized to fish oil versus olive oil, and the mean number of arrhythmias per patient were obtained from the ICDs and compared across arms. The principal investigator decided not to follow patients who discontinued treatment. What is the problem with this?

2. Which of the following is true in a truly blinded, two-armed trial?

   (a) There will be no power of positive thinking in either arm.

   (b) There will be no placebo effect in the placebo arm.

   (c) The power of positive thinking could invalidate the result.

   (d) The power of positive thinking should be the same in the two arms.

3. Some trials use what is called *modified intention-to-treat (MITT)* in which some randomized patients are not included. Which of the following MITT strategies is more acceptable? Explain.

    (a) You eliminate patients who never start treatment because, after finding out what they would receive, they refused to take it.

    (b) A laboratory test required to determine eligibility for the trial takes a week for results to be available, so you randomize patients immediately, and later eliminate those who are not eligible.

4. Consider an HIV trial of patients with baseline CD4 T-cell count > 500 randomized to one of two arms. One arm starts antiretroviral treatment immediately, while the other defers treatment until the CD4 count drops below 350. Which of the following would be a legitimate baseline variable?

    (a) The CD4 count just prior to randomization.

    (b) The CD4 count just prior to starting antiretroviral therapy.

    (c) The CD4 count just prior to a serious AIDS-related event.

    (d) The change in CD4 count from randomization to start of antiretroviral therapy.

5. Determine whether using an end of study value or change from baseline to end of study is more efficient with a continuous outcome measure in each of the following settings.

    (a) The correlation between baseline and end of study measurements is 0.72.

    (b) The correlation between baseline and end of study measurements is 0.30.

6. Suppose that in a blood pressure trial, the patient-to-patient, day-to-day, and measurement variances in a population are 400, 25, and 5, respectively.

    (a) Randomly pick a patient and day and measure blood pressure. What is its variance?

    (b) Randomly pick a patient and average that patient's blood pressure over 5 days. What is the variance of that average?

    (c) If we average over a huge number of days for a given patient, approximately how low will the variance of that average be?

    (d) If we average over 100 people, taking one measurement per patient, what will the variance of that average be?

7. Laboratory values can vary substantially depending on the technician. Consider a clinical trial using change from baseline as outcome. For a given patient, would you use the same technician or different technicians for the baseline and follow-up measurements? Explain. Would you expect to see a technician-by-treatment interaction the way there might be a surgeon-by-treatment interaction in Example 4.18?

8. Consider the Asymptomatic Cardiac Ischemia Pilot Study (ACIP) of Example 4.5.

    (a) If ACIP had randomized first and performed an angiogram only on those randomized to revascularization (option 1), should they exclude from the analysis those patients who refused revascularization? Explain.

(b) Patients had to have at least two episodes of ischemia at baseline to qualify for ACIP. At the end of the trial, some people concluded that all 3 arms were effective at reducing ischemia because the number of ischemic episodes decreased from baseline to the end of the study in all 3 arms. Explain what is wrong with this conclusion.

9. Suppose that in a clinical trial, the primary outcome is the difference between the baseline value and the average value of all post-randomization measurements. Tell whether this makes sense under each of the following circumstances.

   (a) The post-randomization measurements are at pre-specified time points that are the same in both arms.

   (b) Extreme results trigger repeat measurements to confirm the extreme values, and repeat measurements are included in the post-randomization average.

10. Suppose that a new treatment emerges that could potentially alter the effectiveness of the intervention you are testing. Which of the following two strategies is better and why?

    (a) Stratify the analysis by whether patients received the new medication or not at any time during follow-up.

    (b) Stratify the analysis by whether patients were recruited before or after the new intervention became available.

11. Suppose that an HIV trial compares a strategy of continuous antiretroviral (ART) treatment versus intermittent ART. Would it make sense to include, in a composite primary outcome, "treatment failure," defined as an elevated level of HIV while on treatment? Explain.

12. In the WAVE trial of Example 4.14, explain how a misleading answer can result if treatment causes very small new lesions (see Example 4.13).

13. Suppose the primary endpoint for a clinical trial is death within 28 days of randomization. At an interim analysis, some patients have not yet reached 28 days of follow-up, but have died. An argument is made that these patients will remain dead when they reach 28 days of follow-up, so they should be included in the interim analysis as dead by 28 days. Suppose these deaths are included in the numerator and denominator of the proportion dead by 28 days, but people who have not reached 28 days of follow-up and are alive are not included in either the numerator or denominator. Will the 28-day mortality probability be underestimated, overestimated, or accurately estimated?

14. Verify Figure 4.2 with the following simulation experiment. Simulate true systolic blood pressure values T_i as 1000 independent and identically distributed normals with mean 130 and standard deviation 15. Now generate measurement errors as 1000 independent normals with mean 0 and standard deviation 5. The observed blood pressures of people screened for the trial are $T_i + \epsilon_i$, $i = 1, \ldots, 1000$. The entry criterion is $T_i + \epsilon_i > 140$.

    (a) Make a histogram of the ϵ_i of all patients screened.

    (b) Make a histogram of the ϵ_i of patients meeting the entry criterion. What is the mean of the error distribution for patients meeting the entry criterion?

    (c) Now repeat the experiment, but use error standard deviation 10 instead of 5. What happens to the mean of the error distribution for patients meeting the entry criterion?

15. Consider a randomized trial in which patients in one arm receive a specific antiarrhythmic drug. If that drug fails, another specific drug is tried. If that drug also fails, a defibrillator is implanted in the heart. The other arm receives no intervention. Halfway through the trial, there is an innovation in the technique for implanting defibrillators. The protocol is changed such that patients get a defibrillator implanted even if just 1 drug fails. As a result, many more patients have a defibrillator implanted after the innovation. Which of the following is the best way to show that implanting a defibrillator is what made the intervention effective? Explain.

    (a) Compare randomized arms before and after the innovation occurred.

    (b) Compare patients who had a defibrillator implanted to all placebo patients.

    (c) Compare patients who had a defibrillator implanted to those who received only drugs.

16. Consider the analysis of covariance model $Y = \beta_0 + \beta_1 x + \beta_2 z + \epsilon$, where x is the baseline value and z is the treatment indicator. The slope estimates in the control and treatment arm are

$$\hat{\beta}_{1C} = \frac{\sum_{i \in C}(x_i - \bar{x}_C)Y_i}{\sum_{i \in C}(x_i - \bar{x}_C)^2} \quad \text{and} \quad \hat{\beta}_{1T} = \frac{\sum_{i \in T}(x_i - \bar{x}_T)Y_i}{\sum_{i \in T}(x_i - \bar{x}_T)^2},$$

    with variances (conditional on the x values) estimated by

$$v_C = \frac{\hat{\sigma}_\epsilon^2}{\sum_{i \in C}(x_i - \bar{x}_C)^2} \quad \text{and} \quad v_T = \frac{\hat{\sigma}_\epsilon^2}{\sum_{i \in T}(x_i - \bar{x}_T)^2},$$

    where $\hat{\sigma}_\epsilon^2$ is an estimate of the residual variance (treat $\hat{\sigma}_\epsilon^2$ as a constant). What is the stratified estimator $\hat{\beta}_1$ of the common slope β_1 that best combines $\hat{\beta}_{1C}$ and $\hat{\beta}_{1T}$?

17. Consider a crossover trial with no carryover effect. Perform the following steps to show that a period effect does not bias the treatment effect estimator. Consider a patient whose normal blood pressure is 130, but readings in period 1 tend to be 3 points higher than in period 2. Assume that the true treatment effect is -4 (i.e., treatment reduces blood pressure by 4).

    (a) What is the expected treatment minus control difference if the patient is assigned to C followed by T? What if the patient is assigned to T followed by C?

    (b) What is the expected treatment minus control difference averaged over the two possible treatment assignment orders?

18. You have a new HIV vaccine that you want to test in Africa. Your idea is that if enough people in a given community get the vaccine, there will not be many people who can transmit the disease, and that will help protect even people who do not get the vaccine. This is called an *indirect effect* of vaccination. Which of the following designs makes the most sense to evaluate the total effect (direct plus indirect) of vaccine? Explain your answer.

    (a) Pick a community and randomize HIV uninfected individuals within that community to vaccine or placebo. Compare the percentages with HIV by the end of the trial in the two randomized arms.

    (b) Pick many communities with similar HIV rates and randomize half of them to an intervention that offers and encourages everyone to receive a free HIV vaccine, and the other half to no intervention. At the end of the trial, compare the mean percentage with HIV among intervention communities to the mean percentage with HIV among non-intervention communities.

19. Consider a multi-armed trial comparing k arms to a placebo (arm 0) with fixed total sample size N. Let $\hat{\delta}_1 = \bar{Y}_1 - \bar{Y}_0$ and $\hat{\delta}_2 = \bar{Y}_2 - \bar{Y}_0$. Show that $\hat{\delta}_1$ and $\hat{\delta}_2$ become less correlated as the control sample size increases.

20. If treatment B is superior to treatment A, and treatment C is superior to treatment B, is treatment C superior to treatment A? If treatment B is noninferior to treatment A, and treatment C is noninferior to treatment B, both using noninferiority the same margin M, is treatment C noninferior to treatment A using margin M? Explain.

4.8 Appendix: The Geometry of Stratification

Finding the weighed combination of stratum-specific treatment effect estimates that minimizes the variance can be viewed geometrically as follows. The variance of the linear combination $\sum_{i=1}^{k} w_i \hat{\delta}_i$ of independent, unbiased estimators $\hat{\delta}_i$, $i = 1, \ldots, k$, is $\sum w_i^2 v_i$. The goal is to minimize $\sum w_i^2 v_i$ subject to $\sum w_i = 1$. Equivalently, maximize

$$\frac{1}{\sqrt{\sum_{i=1}^{k} w_i^2 v_i}} = \frac{\sum_{i=1}^{k} w_i}{\sqrt{\sum w_i^2 v_i}} \quad \left(\text{because } \sum_{i=1}^{k} w_i = 1 \right)$$

$$= \frac{\sum_{i=1}^{k} \lambda_i (1/\sqrt{v_i})}{\sqrt{\sum_{i=1}^{k} \lambda_i^2}}, \quad \text{where } \lambda_i = w_i \sqrt{v_i}$$

$$= \frac{(1\sqrt{v_1}, \ldots, 1/\sqrt{v_k}) \cdot \boldsymbol{\lambda}}{||\boldsymbol{\lambda}||}, \tag{4.20}$$

where $\cdot$ denotes dot product and $||\boldsymbol{\lambda}||$ denotes length of the vector λ. Geometrically, (4.20) is the length of the projection of the vector $(1/\sqrt{v_1}, \ldots, 1/\sqrt{v_k})$ onto the vector $\boldsymbol{\lambda}$ (Figure 4.8). The longest length is $(1/\sqrt{v_1}, \ldots, 1/\sqrt{v_k})$, which occurs when $\boldsymbol{\lambda}$ is in the same direction as $(1/\sqrt{v_1}, \ldots, 1/\sqrt{v_k})$. Because $\lambda_i = w_i \sqrt{v_i}$, this means that w_i is proportional to $1/v_i$. $\quad \square$

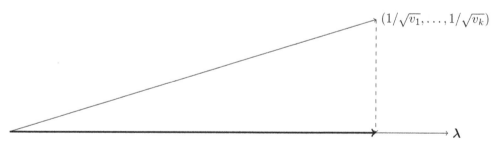

Figure 4.8: (4.20) is the length of the darkened vector, the projection of $(1/\sqrt{v_1}, \ldots, 1/\sqrt{v_k})$ onto the vector $\boldsymbol{\lambda}$. The longest length+ is $(1/\sqrt{v_1}, \ldots, 1/\sqrt{v_k})$, occurring when $\boldsymbol{\lambda}$ is in the same direction as $(1/\sqrt{v_1}, \ldots, 1/\sqrt{v_k})$.

4.9 Summary

1. There are several phases of clinical trials:

   (a) Phase I: safety and dose-finding.

   (b) Phase II: efficacy—ideal conditions, intermediate outcome.

(c) Phase III: effectiveness—real world conditions, major clinical outcomes.

2. As much blinding as possible should be used: double blinding (patients and staff) and blinding of event adjudication staff.

3. Baseline assessment is important to (1) verify that patients met eligibility criteria, (2) evaluate the natural history in the control arm, (3) use change from baseline as an outcome, and (4) evaluate and adjust for baseline imbalances.

4. Intention-to-treat (ITT) principle: Compare entire randomized arms, not only those who complied with treatment. Preserve randomized groups at all costs.

5. Regression to the mean: If entry criteria require large (resp., small) values of a variable, a subsequent measurement tends to be smaller (resp., larger) even with no intervention applied.

6. Concerning primary outcomes:

   (a) Limit the number (ideally to one).

   (b) Be wary of surrogate endpoints; they can sometimes mislead.

   (c) Make sure that the components of a composite outcome for a phase III trial are serious consequences of the disease under study.

   (d) Treatment should not have an effect on how the outcome is measured (see Examples 4.13 and 4.14).

7. Concerning variability:

   (a) **Variability ratio principle:** Many tests are based on the ratio of between- to within-arm variability; minimizing within-arm variability improves power.

   (b) Methods of reducing variability include replication (sources with greatest variability require the most replication), differencing, stratification, and regression modeling.

8. **Balanced block principle:** For blocks of positively correlated data:

   (a) The most efficient design assigns half to treatment and half to control (paired designs).

   (b) The least efficient design assigns all to treatment or all to control (cluster-randomized trials).

9. Multi-arm trials:

   (a) Comparisons with the same control: Multiplicity adjustment is common, and the optimal control-to-active arm ratio from power perspective is the square root of number of arms other than control.

   (b) Factorial trial: Like combining separate trials, and multiple comparison adjustment is often not done.

Chapter 5

Randomization/Allocation

We present a relatively brief review of randomization methods in clinical trials. Readers wishing to learn more are encouraged to read the comprehensive treatise by Rosenberger and Lachin (2016).

5.1 Sanctity and Placement of Randomization

Always remember that randomization is the key difference between a clinical trial and an observational study. Recall that randomization prevents selection bias in allocation of patients to different arms. As a result, arms tend to be balanced on both known and unknown prognostic factors. We will see in the next chapter that randomization allows valid inference with very few assumptions. For all of these reasons, it is imperative to get the randomization right and preserve the randomized arms at all costs.

Before getting into details of how to randomize, we note that where the randomization is placed dictates the question the trial will answer.

Example 5.1. Placement of randomization in CAST   Recall that in the Cardiac Arrhythmia Suppression Trial (CAST), the goal was to determine, in patients with cardiac arrhythmias and a prior heart attack, whether suppression of those arrhythmias reduces the risk of sudden arrhythmic death and cardiac arrest. This question cannot be answered in patients whose arrhythmias cannot be suppressed. Therefore, a drug titration period preceded randomization to find a drug suppressing at least 80% of the patient's arrhythmias. If no such drug was found, that patient was not randomized. If such a drug was found, the patient was randomized to that drug or a matching placebo. This placement of randomization allows the suppression hypothesis to be tested. A down side is that patients dying during the drug titration phase are not counted because such patients are not yet randomized.

A different question is whether **attempting** to suppress arryhthmias results in fewer sudden arrhythmic deaths and cardiac arrests. If this had been CAST's question, patients would have been randomized immediately (before finding out whether patients could be suppressed) to drug titration versus no drug titration. In this case, all deaths would count. If too many patients died in the attempt to find a suppressing drug, that would provide a negative answer to the question of whether one should attempt to suppress arrhythmias.

Once it was determined that two drugs, encainide and flecainide, resulted in increased event rates, CAST was modified into CAST II. The two offending drugs were eliminated and a placebo titration period was incorporated. Patients in CAST II were randomized immediately to drug or placebo titration. Early deaths **were** now counted. Excess mortality in the drug arm during the titration phase led to early stopping of CAST II.   □

DOI: 10.1201/9781315164090-5

5.2   Simple Randomization

Metaphorically, *simple randomization*, also called *complete randomization*, amounts to independent coin flips for different patients.   An advantage of simple randomization is that it is easy to explain and implement. If one wishes to assign a proportion p of patients to treatment, simply generate random numbers U_i uniformly on the interval $(0,1)$, and assign patient i to treatment if $U_i < p$ and control if $U_i > p$. Another advantage of simple randomization is that, regardless of treatment assignments of previous patients, the next patient's assignment is completely unpredictable. We will see in the next subsection why this may be important.

A disadvantage of simple randomization is that there may be an undesired imbalance in the number of patients assigned to the two arms at the end of the trial. Assume equal allocation (the same proportion assigned to treatment and control). On average, the same proportion of patients are assigned to each arm. However, in any given trial, those proportions may differ. One consequence is loss of efficiency. For example, suppose our trial compares arms A and B with respect to the difference $\hat{\delta} = \bar{Y}_A - \bar{Y}_B$ in sample means of a continuous outcome Y such as change in cholesterol or blood pressure. Suppose further that there are only 10 people in the entire trial (warning: never conduct such tiny trials!). The variance of the treatment effect estimate $\hat{\delta}$ is

$$\text{var}(\hat{\delta}) = \sigma^2(1/n_A + 1/n_B), \tag{5.1}$$

where n_A and n_B are the arm A and B sample sizes and σ^2 is the within-arm variance, assumed to be the same across arms. Equation (5.1) is smallest when exactly 5 people are assigned to each arm, and increases as the amount of imbalance between n_A and n_B increases. For example, if $(n_A, n_B) = (7,3)$ or $(3,7)$, the variance of $\hat{\delta}$ is about 19% larger than if $(n_A, n_B) = (5,5)$ because $(1/7 + 1/3)/(1/5 + 1/5) \approx 1.19$. Even worse would be $(n_A, n_B) = (10,0)$ or $(0,10)$, in which case $\hat{\delta}$ is not even defined!

Another consequence of imbalances in the proportion of patients assigned to the different arms is the potential for accidental imbalances in prognostic factors. For instance, suppose that diabetes is an important predictor of outcome, and there are two diabetics in our tiny trial of 10 people. It would be very unfortunate if both diabetics were assigned to the same arm. The probability that this happens is

$$P(\text{both A}) + P(\text{both B}) = \left(\frac{n_A}{n}\right)\left(\frac{n_A - 1}{n - 1}\right) + \left(\frac{n_B}{n}\right)\left(\frac{n_B - 1}{n - 1}\right), \tag{5.2}$$

where $n = n_A + n_B$. The probability (5.2) is lowest when $n_A = n_B = 5$, and increases as the imbalance between n_A and n_B increases.

5.3   Permuted Block Randomization

We have shown that balance in the proportions assigned to different arms increases efficiency and tends to equalize prognostic factors across arms. We would like balance not only at the end, but throughout a trial. After all, we monitor clinical trials repeatedly. The most common method of ensuring balance throughout is called *permuted block randomization* or just *blocked randomization*. Again assume equal allocation. We illustrate with blocks of size 4. Imagine placing 4 slips of paper, two of which have an "A" and two a "B", into a box. The next 4 patients of the trial are assigned by randomly drawing without replacement from the box. For instance, if the 4 draws are (A,A,B,B) then the first two patients are assigned to arm A and the next 2 to arm B. This is only one of $\binom{4}{2} = 6$ possible assignments for a block of size 4:

(A,A,B,B), (A,B,A,B), (A,B,B,A), (B,A,A,B), (B,A,B,A), (B,B,A,A).

Each of these blocks has exactly 2 people assigned to each arm. More generally, in a two-armed trial with equal allocation using blocks of size $2k$, k people are assigned to arm A and k to arm B in each block.

One way to program permuted block randomization first creates a list $L_1, \ldots, L_{2k}$ of As and Bs, where L_i is A if $i \leq k$ and B if $L_i > k$. Then generate $2k$ uniform numbers on $(0, 1)$, rank them $R_1, \ldots, R_{2k}$, and assign patient R_i to arm L_i (Table 5.1).

Table 5.1: Programming permuted blocks: create a list L_i of As and Bs, generate iid uniforms U_i, rank them (R_i), and assign patient R_i to arm L_i. For this example block of size 8, patients 2, 5, 7, and 8 are assigned to A, patients 1, 3, 4, and 6 to B.

L_i	A	A	A	A	B	B	B	B
U_i	0.25	0.92	0.80	0.48	0.33	0.44	0.06	0.60
R_i	2	8	7	5	3	4	1	6

Balance in the number of As and Bs is forced after every block. A small block size forces balance more frequently than a larger block size. A single large block comprising all trial patients is sometimes called *random allocation*. Among all permuted block designs, random allocation forces the least balance, whereas blocks of size 2 force the most balance. As we have seen, balance has the two advantages of precision and avoidance of accidental between-arm differences in prognostic factors.

There is a downside to forced balance of the numbers of patients assigned to the two arms. In an unblinded trial, some of the assignments will be known in advance. For instance, with equal allocation, if the first two patients in a block of size 4 are assigned to arm A, the next two are guaranteed to be assigned to arm B. The predictability of treatment assignments increases as the block size decreases. For instance, in an unblinded trial using blocks of size 2, the second assignment of each block is predictable in advance. Staff could keep track of previous treatment assignments and be certain about some future assignments. This can lead to *selection bias*, a nonrandom, between-arm imbalance in how sick patients are. For example, consider a trial randomizing patients to surgery or a pill using blocks of size 2. Once treatment is started, the patient and staff will know whether it was surgery or a pill (except for the rare trials using sham surgery to maintain the blind). If an investigator knows that the next patient will definitely receive surgery, the investigator may wait for a patient who is 'best suited' for surgery, and likewise if the next patient is guaranteed to receive a pill. The resulting groups may be systematically different, which could affect trial results. Trialists try to make treatment assignments more unpredictable by using different block sizes. For example, for the first block, flip a coin to decide whether to use a block size of 6 or 8. After the first block is complete, flip another coin to decide the size of the second block, etc. Nonetheless, in an unblinded trial, the amount of selection bias possible is unacceptable. Permuted block randomization should be avoided in unblinded trials.

Permuted block randomization can be applied with unequal allocation as well. For instance, we may want to assign twice as many patients to treatment as control. This may be more palatable to trial participants because they may prefer to be assigned to the experimental treatment. One could use blocks of size 3, with 2 Ts and 1 C, in random order. Likewise, one could use blocks of size 6, with 4 Ts and 2 Cs, in random order.

5.4   Biased Coin Randomization

One alternative that prevents complete knowledge of the next assignment is called *biased coin randomization* (Efron, 1971). Consider equal allocation. The first patient is assigned by simple randomization. Whenever there is an imbalance in the number of As and Bs, the next patient is assigned using a biased coin having fixed probability p, for the under-represented treatment, where $p > 1/2$ ($p = 2/3$ is recommended). For instance, suppose the first assignment is to A. Then patient 2 is assigned to arm B with probability 2/3. Suppose patient 2 is assigned to B. Then we revert to a fair coin when assigning patient 3. On the other hand, if patient 2 had also been assigned to A, then patient 3 is assigned to B with probability p, and so on. Like permuted block randomization, biased coin randomization tends to produce more balance than simple randomization in the proportion of assignments to A and B. Unlike permuted block randomization, biased coin randomization never results in the next assignment being perfectly predictable. Nonetheless, biased coin randomization is seldom used in clinical trials.

5.5   Stratified Randomization

Permuted block randomization does not ensure that the two treatment arms are balanced with respect to prognostic factors. For example, consider a clinical trial in patients at high risk of heart disease. Some patients have risk factors such as high cholesterol or family history of heart disease, while others have actually already survived a heart attack. The former and latter groups are known as *primary prevention* and *secondary prevention* patients, respectively. In a trial with permuted blocks of size 8 applied to the overall group, nothing precludes the block in Table 5.2 in which all primary prevention patients are assigned to arm A, while all secondary prevention patients are assigned to arm B.

Table 5.2: Example block of size 8 in a trial consisting of primary and secondary prevention patients. Inadvertently, all primary prevention patients are assigned to A, and all secondary prevention patients are assigned to B.

Primary (P) or Secondary (S) Prevention	P	S	S	S	P	S	P	P
Treatment Assignment	A	B	B	B	A	B	A	A

To prevent a scenario such as in Table 5.2, we need to use separate blocks within primary and secondary prevention subgroups. When a primary (resp., secondary) prevention patient arrives, we draw randomly from the primary (resp., secondary) prevention block. Had we done this, Table 5.2 might have been replaced by Table 5.3. Within both subgroups, there are exactly two patients assigned to arm A and two to arm B. This method of assignment is called *stratified randomization*.

Table 5.3: Stratified randomization uses separate blocks within subgroups, in this case, primary versus secondary prevention patients.

Primary (P) or Secondary (S) Prevention	P	S	S	S	P	S	P	P
Treatment Assignment	A	B	B	A	B	A	A	B

Stratified randomization is a wonderful tool to balance a few key prognostic factors across arms. When the number of combinations of subgroups is large compared to the number of patients, problems can result (Pocock and Simon, 1975; Thernau, 1993). For instance, consider a trial of 30 patients stratified by gender, race (4 categories), and age (4 categories). The total number of combinations of subgroups is $2 \times 4 \times 4 = 32$. On average, we expect only about one patient in each combination. If that turns out to be true, stratified randomization is equivalent to flipping a single coin in each subgroup combination (i.e., simple randomization). The problem is being caused by the fact that permuted block randomization attempts to balance the number of people in the different arms **within each combination of strata**, and some of these combinations may be very sparse.

5.6 Minimization and Covariate-Adaptive Randomization

As noted in the previous section, stratifying on more than a few baseline covariates can be counterproductive. In fact, in a small trial, one may be able to stratify on only one or two covariates. Consequently, an imbalance could mar the results of a small trial. *Covariate-adaptive randomization*, also called *dynamic allocation*, achieves better balance on multiple covariates simultaneously. Instead of trying to force balance within each **combination** of strata, covariate adaptive randomization computes the imbalance in the number of treatments and controls for each covariate **marginally** and sums imbalances over covariates to get a total imbalance score. When a new patient arrives, we compute the potential imbalance score for each possible treatment assignment for that patient. We then apportion higher probability to the arm that minimizes the total imbalance. The most extreme form of covariate-adaptive randomization assigns the patient deterministically to the arm that minimizes imbalance (if there is more than one choice leading to the minimum imbalance, we choose randomly). This extreme form of covariate-adaptive randomization is called *minimization.* (Taves, 1974). A less deterministic alternative is to assign the arm minimizing imbalance with high probability, say 0.75.

We illustrate the methodology using an example with two baseline covariates, gender and hypertension status. Suppose that at the time the next patient arrives, the marginal totals of patients in different genders and in different hypertension categories are as shown in Table 5.4. To date, 19 and 18 patients have been assigned to arms A and B, respectively. The next patient is female and hypertensive. We highlight this fact by boldfacing the female and hypertensive components of Table 5.4. These are the only portions of the table that change depending on the treatment assignment of this patient. If we assign her to arm A, the numbers assigned to arms A and B will be 9 versus 7 among females, and 7 versus 4 among hypertensives. The sum of imbalances among females and hypertensives will be $|9 - 7| + |7 - 4| = 2 + 3 = 5$. On the other hand, if she is assigned to arm B, the sum of imbalances among females and hypertensives will be $|8 - 8| + |6 - 5| = 0 + 1 = 1$. If we were using minimization, we would assign the patient to arm B because that assignment minimizes imbalance. If we were using a less extreme form of covariate-adaptive randomization, we might assign the patient to arm B with probability 0.75, for example.

Table 5.4: Marginal treatment totals within each of two covariates, gender and hypertension status.

	Male	**Female**		**Hypertensive**	Non-hypertensive
Arm A	11	**8**		**6**	13
Arm B	11	**7**		**4**	14

Note that in this example, if the patient had been a female, nonhypertensive, the imbalance would have been the same regardless of assignment: the imbalance would have been either $|9 - 7| + |14 - 14| = 2$ or $|8 - 8| + |13 - 15| = 2$ if she had been assigned to arm A or arm B, respectively. In this case, we would have assigned her with probability 0.5 to arm A or B.

5.7   Response-Adaptive Randomization

When the primary outcome of a trial is very short-term such as 24-hour mortality, we could update results after every new patient. Some have argued that we should change assignment probabilities to make the next patient more likely to be given the treatment with better results thus far. The technique was first proposed by Thompson (1933), and there has been controversy ever since. Proponents argue that this so-called *response-adaptive randomization* is more ethical than conventional randomization techniques. The claim is that fewer patients will be assigned to poorer treatments, especially in multi-armed trials. This claim has been disputed (Korn and Friedlin, 2011). We begin with a historical trial that ignited controversy over the procedure.

Example 5.2. (Remember the ECMO!)   The Extracorporeal Membrane Oxygenation (ECMO) trial was conducted in babies with primary pulmonary hypertension, a disease whose expected mortality under the standard treatment S was expected to be 80%. The new treatment N involved using an outside-the-body heart and lung machine to allow the baby's lungs to rest and recover. Because of the high expected mortality on S, Wei and Durham's (1978) response-adaptive urn randomization scheme was used that was conceptually equivalent to the following. Place one S ball and one N ball in an urn and randomly draw one out for the first baby. If the first baby is assigned to S and dies or N and lives, then the drawn ball is replaced and an N ball is added. Similarly, if the first baby is assigned to S and lives or N and dies, the original ball is replaced and an S ball is added. Either way, the second baby has a 2/3 probability of being assigned to the arm doing better so far. Likewise, for baby $i + 1$, if baby i receives S and dies or N and lives, ball i is replaced and an N ball is added, while if baby i receives N and dies or S and lives, ball i is replaced and an S ball is added.

As it turned out, baby 1 was assigned to N and survived, baby 2 was assigned to S and died, and the next 10 babies were all assigned to N and survived. At that point, randomization ended. Wei (1988) analyzed the results using a permutation test that will be described in much more detail in Chapter 6. Results of the trial did not convince the medical community. For one thing, the lone baby assigned to S was the sickest. Begg (1990) showed that different reasonable approaches lead to diametrically opposite conclusions. The controversy ended only after a much larger, definitive trial was conducted in the U.K. (UK Collaborative ECMO Group, 1996).   □

Many strides have been made in response-adaptive randomization since the ECMO trial. One improvement is the use of a 'burn-in' period of conventional randomization before beginning response-adaptive randomization. For example, one might begin with 50 patients per arm randomized with permuted blocks, and then begin the response-adaptive portion. That alleviates the problem of highly lopsided sample sizes seen in ECMO. A related improvement is that newer forms of response-adaptive randomization (RAR) are 'power oriented' as opposed to 'patient benefit oriented' (Villar, Bowden, and Wason, 2018). An improvement in multi-armed trials comparing arms to the same control is that if randomization probabilities are changed to favor one active treatment over the others, the control arm also gets higher weight. Asymptotic results now show that standard methods for constructing tests and confidence intervals can be applied to RAR (Melfi and Page, 2000; Hu and Rosenberger, 2006; Zhang et al. 2011). A vigorous defense of RAR is made in Robertson, Lee, López-

Kolkovska, and Villar (2020). Nonetheless, the potential for temporal trends to confound the estimate of treatment effect remains a concern. This issue is discussed in Section 5.8.

Incidentally, Bayesians have no problem analyzing data from a trial using RAR even if the sample size is small. After specifying a prior distribution for the treatment effect δ, they simply compute the posterior distribution of δ given the data and use it to make inference. ECMO showed that classical statisticians have more difficulty analyzing data from a small trial using RAR. One of very few valid analyses in that setting is discussed in Chapter 6.

5.8 Adaptive Randomization and Temporal Trends

One problem raised by the ECMO trial is that patients 3–12 were all assigned to the new treatment. What if a temporal trend caused earlier patients to be sicker than later patients? This could explain why results on the new treatment were better than on the standard treatment. In fact, the lone baby assigned to the standard treatment was objectively the sickest one, and may have died irrespective of treatment received. ECMO was extreme because only 1 patient was randomized to the new treatment, but whenever there are periods during which one treatment is under-represented, estimation of the treatment effect can be confounded by temporal trends.

Some implementations of response-adaptive randomization permit valid treatment effect estimation in the presence of temporal trends. Section 17.2 of Jennison and Turnbull (2000) describes such a scheme. The first block of B patients uses 1:1 randomization. Results of this first block are then used to modify the probability of assignment to T for the second block of B patients. Similarly, cumulative results on the first k blocks of size B are used to modify the probability of assignment to T for the $(k + 1)$st block of size B. At the end of the trial, a block-stratified analysis is used.

Korn and Friedlin (2012) evaluated response-adaptive randomization as described in the preceding paragraph and applied to an immediate response binary outcome. At the end of each block, they computed the posterior probability that T was better (i.e., had a higher response rate) than C, given the cumulative data thus far, and assuming a uniform prior distribution for $P(T$ better than $C)$. In the next block, they assigned T with probability

$$\frac{\sqrt{P(T \text{ better than C} \mid \text{data})}}{\sqrt{P(T \text{ better than C} \mid \text{data})} + \sqrt{1 - P(T \text{ better than C} \mid \text{data})}}.$$

At the end of the trial, they analyzed results using the Mantel-Haenszel statistic stratified by block. They found that this adaptive procedure required more patients to achieve the same power and generally resulted in a **greater** number of patients assigned to the inferior arm than would a fixed 1:1 randomization.

The reason that the response-adaptive trial led to poorer characteristics than the fixed 1:1 randomization is that the variance of the treatment effect estimator increases when there is an imbalance in the number of Ts and Cs. This phenomenon, discussed after Equation (5.1) in Section 5.2 for continuous outcomes, holds in the binary outcome setting as well. The resulting higher variability of within-block treatment effect estimates leads to higher variability for the stratified estimator than if fixed 1:1 randomization had been used.

Temporal trends can be problematic even with some implementations of covariate-adaptive randomization. Proschan, Brittain, and Kammerman (2011), motivated by the Late Onset Treatment Study (LOTS) in Pompé disease, gave a relatively simple hypothetical example of a 2:1 randomization of treatment to control in a clinical trial of a disease so rare that a very large number of centers is needed, each recruiting only 3 patients. The imbalance function is the squared difference between the actual and intended proportions of patients assigned to T and C at each center. Exercise 12 asks you to show that if strict minimization is followed at each center, the first patient will always be assigned to T, the second patient to C, and the third to T. In other words, there is no actual randomization! Because the disease is so rare, there may be a large time gap between patients. Any apparent treatment benefit might be explained by a temporal trend such that the earliest and latest patients are less sick than the middle patient. The problem is caused by unequal allocation.

Kuznetsova and Tymofyeyev (2012) pointed out that the problem caused by examples such as that of the preceding paragraph is that the marginal probability of being assigned to a given arm depends on patient order. They provided a very simple and elegant solution for unequal allocation. Instead of thinking of a trial with a 2:1 randomization to T versus C, imagine a trial with 2 active treatments, A and B, against a control, C, using 1:1:1 covariate-adaptive randomization. An assignment to arm A or B in the 1:1:1 trial is associated with an assignment to T in the 2:1 trial. The same idea applies for other randomization ratios. For instance, for 3:2 randomization, imagine a 5-armed trial with 1:1:1:1:1 randomization to D, E, F, G, and H. Arms D, E, and F (resp., G and H) of the five-armed trial correspond to T (resp., C) in the two-armed trial.

Section 6.4 will revisit temporal trends and LOTS in connection with a generalization of a permutation test.

Exercises

1. Why is it a good idea to try to achieve balance in the number of patients assigned to the two arms in a two-armed trial?

2. Evaluate expression (5.2) for a trial of size 10 when $n_A = 1$ and when $n_A = 5$. How much more likely is it that both diabetics will be assigned to the same arm when $n_A = 1$ than when $n_A = 5$?

3. Some trials use unequal allocation to treatment and control. Give a reason one might want to assign more patients to treatment than control. Is there ever a reason to make the control sample size larger? (See Section 4.7.5.)

4. In a trial of 100 patients using simple randomization, investigators notice that after 50 assignments, 27 patients are assigned to T. Do you think it is a good idea to change the randomization probability for the under-represented arm to 27/50 for the remaining 50 patients to try to fix the imbalance? Explain.

5. Consider a trial in which all patients are identified in advance, so that one could use a deterministic algorithm to assign treatments in a way that forces a lot of balance on known predictors of outcome. Compare and contrast that method with using simple randomization. Consider balance on both known and unknown prognostic factors in your answer.

6. Describe how to use permuted block randomization in a trial using a 3:2 ratio of treatment to control.

7. For the data in Table 5.4, what are the treatment assignments of the next 3 patients if strict minimization is used and the 3 patients are female hypertensive, female hypertensive, and male nonhypertensive, respectively.

8. Suppose the treatment assignments of the first 8 patients in a trial are (T, C, C, T, T, C, T, T).

   (a) If you know that either simple randomization or permuted block randomization with block size 4 was used, which was it? Explain.

    (b) If the assignments had been (T, C, C, T, T, C, T, C), would you have been able to tell for sure which randomization method was used? Explain.

9. Suppose one randomizes in blocks of size 8 by using simple randomization until 4 Ts or 4 Cs have been reached, assigning the remaining patients in the block to the remaining arm. This is called *truncated binomial randomization*. Show that the event that the first 4 patients are assigned to the same arm is more likely than with ordinary permuted block randomization.

10. Suppose that permuted block randomization is used with block sizes of 4 and 8 in an unblinded trial of size 16. As noted, the potential for selection bias exists.

    (a) List patient numbers of all **potential** starting points of blocks.

    (b) Suppose that the treatment assignments are (T, T, C, T, T, C, C, C, C, C, T, C, T, C, T, T). Which of the patients' treatment assignments could you have predicted with certainty?

11. Suppose that permuted blocks of sizes 4 and 6 are used in a trial with a large sample size.

    (a) List patient numbers of all **potential** starting points of blocks.

    (b) Do you get more information or less information about potential block starts with blocks of sizes 4 and 6 versus 4 and 8?

    (c) What does this say about whether it is wise, in terms of potential for selection bias, to make one block size a multiple of the other in an unblinded trial?

12. Consider a trial with 2:1 allocation conducted at a large number of centers, each with only 3 patients. Let $\hat{p}_T$ and $\hat{p}_C = 1 - \hat{p}_T$ denote the proportion of patients assigned to T and C so far at a given center, and define the imbalance function as $(\hat{p}_T - 2/3)^2 + (\hat{p}_C - 1/3)^2$. Show that if strict minimization is used, the first patient at each center is assigned to T, the second to C, and the third to T.

13. In Equation (5.1), fix the total sample size n and replace n_B by $n - n_A$. Let $f(n_A)$ be the resulting expression for $\mathrm{var}(\hat{\delta})$. Let $x = n_A$ and treat x as if it could take on any value (not just integers). Show that $f(x)$ decreases as x increases from 0 to $n/2$, and then increases as x increases from $n/2$ to n. Explain in words what this means and why it is important.

14. In Equation (5.2), fix the total sample size n and replace n_B by $n - n_A$. Let $f(n_A)$ be the resulting expression for $P(\text{both A}) + P(\text{both B})$. Let $x = n_A$ and treat x as if it could take on any value (not just integers). Show that $f(x)$ decreases as x increases from 0 to $n/2$, and then increases as x increases from $n/2$ to n. Explain in words what this means and why it is important.

15. If simple randomization is used in a trial of size $2n$:

    (a) Find an expression for the expected proportion of times there will be exact balance in numbers of Ts and Cs. Hint: The proportion of times of exact balance is $(2n)^{-1} \sum_{i=1}^{n} I(\text{balance after } 2i \text{ assignments})$. Now take the expectation.

    (b) Evaluate your expression for $n = 20$ (total sample size 40).

16. If permuted blocks of size 4 are used in a trial of size 40:

(a) Find an expression for the expected number of times there will be exact balance in numbers of Ts and Cs. Hint: The number of additional balances beyond those forced after every 4 is $\sum_{\text{blocks}} I(\text{balance in middle of block})$. Now take the expectation to get the expected number of balances and divide by $2n$.

(b) Compare your answer to part (a) to your answer to part (a) in Exercise 15.

17. In a trial randomizing patients to arm A, B, or C, how many different blocks of size 6, with 2As, 2Bs, and 2Cs, are there?

5.9   Summary

1. Randomization is the cornerstone of clinical trials, separating them from all other types of studies. Preserve the randomization at all costs:

    (a) Minimize the amount of missing data by emphasizing to patients the importance of continuing follow-up even if they stop taking their medication.

    (b) Never stop following noncompliant patients.

    (c) Do not condition on post-randomization covariates, such as compliance, in the primary analysis of a clinical trial.

2. Randomization methods attempt to achieve balance in the numbers of treatment and control assignments (and sometimes covariates) over time.

3. Such balance reduces accidental bias, but can lead to selection bias in unblinded trials.

4. Methods of achieving balance in the numbers of treatment and control assignments include:

    (a) Simple randomization (conceptually like coin flips). No selection bias is possible, but fairly large imbalances between the numbers of treatment and control assignments is possible.

    (b) Permuted block randomization (conceptually like drawing from a hat) achieves better balance of the numbers of treatment and control assignments over time, but is prone to selection bias in unblinded trials.

    (c) Efron's biased coin design, which is not commonly used.

5. Methods of randomization that balance covariates across arms include the following:

    (a) Stratified randomization (conceptually, drawing from a hat within combinations of covariates). This works well with large sample sizes and relatively few covariates.

    (b) Covariate-adaptive randomization, which can achieve better marginal balance when the sample size is small and there are several covariates.

6. Response-adaptive randomization changes assignment probabilities according to ongoing results in the trial. Although this option sounds attractive to patients, it is susceptible to bias from temporal trends. We believe that, currently, the risks outweigh the potential benefits of RAR.

Chapter 6

Randomization-Based Inference

6.1 Introduction

One of the beautiful features of randomization is that it provides a valid test of treatment effect under essentially no assumptions. Before introducing this test, we note that there are at least three possible explanations for a statistically significant treatment benefit in a clinical trial: (1) treatment works, (2) treatment does not work in the population of interest, but by luck we selected a group in which treatment does work, or (3) treatment does not work, but a chance imbalance caused patients randomized to treatment to be healthier than those randomized to control. Explanation 2 says that results do not generalize to our population of interest, whereas explanation 3 says that the arms are not comparable. We would like to exclude the latter two explanations and conclude that treatment really works. We can do that if the treatment and control groups are randomly sampled from the targeted population. In that case, it is unlikely that we happened to select a group that is uniquely susceptible to treatment and arms should be comparable. But how often do we actually take a random sample from the targeted population in a clinical trial? There is no list of all patients in the world with a given disease from which we can randomly sample. Even if there were, there is no guarantee that everyone selected would consent to be in the trial. Nonetheless, it seems reasonable to view the trial data as a random sample from **some** population, albeit not exactly the one originally intended. A statistically significant result implies that treatment works in at least some population.

Given that generalization is a matter of judgment, we focus on eliminating explanation 3 above. Regardless of whether these trial patients are representative of the population of interest, have we demonstrated that treatment works in them, or could a fluke of randomization have allocated healthier patients to treatment? We answer this question using a *re-randomization test*, also called a *randomization test*. This idea was first proposed by Fisher (1935) to test a woman's claim that she could discern whether milk or tea was added first to a cup. The experiment consisted of adding milk first to 4 cups selected randomly from 8, and tea first to the remaining 4. In a subsequent chapter of his book, Fisher employed the same analysis technique to an agricultural experiment involving growth rate of plants. The method goes by the name *permutation test* when simple randomization or random allocation is used, but it can be applied with any randomization method.

6.2   Paired Data

6.2.1   An Example

We begin with the setting of independent pairs of correlated observations, one member being assigned to treatment and the other to control. These pairs could be the same person under two different conditions in a crossover trial, or the same person with measurements in two ears, two eyes, etc. They could also result from pair matching of people or, as in the following example, communities.

Example 6.1. The Community Intervention Trial for Smoking Cessation (COMMIT) pair-matched communities on the basis of geographic location, size, and sociodemographic factors, and randomized one member of each pair to no intervention, and the other to a 4-year intervention to help smokers quit. The primary outcome in each community was the proportion of approximately 550 pre-selected heavy smokers in the age range 25-64 years who quit smoking, and the primary outcome in the ith pair of communities was the control minus intervention difference D_i in these quit rates. A one-tailed statistical test of $H_0 : \delta = 0$ versus $H_A : \delta < 0$ was conducted, where $\delta = \mathrm{E}(D)$.

Results are shown in Table 6.1. The mean control minus intervention difference of 0.0067 slightly favors the control group. A paired t-test yields a one-tailed p-value of 0.685, offering no evidence that the intervention has any benefit on smoking quit rates in the target population. However, a paired t-test assumes that paired differences are normally distributed. Our conclusion may be wrong if this assumption is violated. If the sample size were large, we could rely on the central limit theorem to ensure the validity of a t-test, but there are only 11 pairs.

An alternative method to analyze results of COMMIT can be used to test the null hypothesis:

$$H_0 : \quad \text{treatment has no effect in any of the 11 pairs versus} \tag{6.1}$$
$$H_1 : \quad \text{treatment has a beneficial effect in at least one of the 11 pairs.}$$

If intervention had no effect on smoking quit rates in any pair, then results observed in a given community would have happened regardless of treatment assignment. The within-pair quit rates would have been just as likely if we switched intervention and control labels. Such switching changes signs of paired differences. For example, consider the first pair in Table 6.1. The control minus intervention quit rate is $0.205 - 0.139 = 0.066$. If we switch the intervention and control labels, the difference becomes $0.139 - 0.205 = -0.066$. The absolute value of the difference remains constant (0.066), but the sign changes. The same argument can be used for other pairs. Different pairs are independent, so we can form a null distribution of the mean difference by considering each of the 2^{11} possible ways to either switch or retain the original intervention and control labels for the 11 pairs, and computing the mean difference for each. This collection of all possible values of the mean difference with their relative frequencies is called the *re-randomization distribution* of the mean difference. We can see whether the value of the mean difference actually observed in the trial is unusual by seeing where it lies in this re-randomization distribution.

Figure 6.1 is a histogram of the re-randomization distribution in COMMIT. It is symmetric about 0 because for each re-randomization yielding value $\bar{d}$, there is an 'equal and opposite' re-labeling (changing each treatment to control and vice versa) yielding mean difference $-\bar{d}$. The dot in Figure 6.1 is the value of the mean difference actually observed in the trial, 0.0067. It lies toward the middle of the re-randomization distribution, indicating that it is not at all unusual under null hypothesis (6.1). The one-tailed p-value is the proportion of mean differences in the re-randomization distribution less than or equal to 0.0067. The

Table 6.1: Smoking quit rates among approximately 550 pre-selected heavy smokers aged 25-64 in pair-matched intervention (I) and control (C) communities in the COMMIT trial.

Pair	1	2	3	4	5	6	7	8	9	10	11
I	.139	.163	.164	.204	.183	.164	.262	.193	.215	.136	.155
C	.205	.202	.163	.249	.160	.186	.230	.169	.127	.172	.189
C−I	+.066	+.039	-.002	+.045	-.022	+.022	-.032	-.024	-.088	+.036	+.034

resulting p-value of 0.686 is extremely close to the 0.685 figure from the t-test because the re-randomization distribution is closely approximated by a normal distribution with the same mean and variance (superimposed density in Figure 6.1). There is no evidence that intervention has an effect on smoking quit rates among the target group of heavy smokers aged 25 to 64 years.

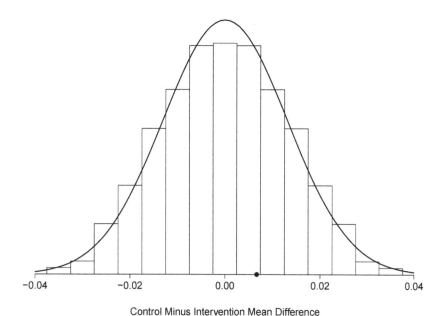

Control Minus Intervention Mean Difference

Figure 6.1: Re-randomization distribution of the mean control minus intervention paired difference of smoking quit rates in COMMIT. Superimposed is a normal density with the same mean and variance. The dot is the observed mean difference.

□

Because there were only 11 pairs in COMMIT, it was possible to enumerate all possible randomizations. If the number of pairs had been prohibitively large, the p-value could have been approximated by simulation by re-randomizing many thousands of times, calculating the control minus intervention sample mean difference for each, and using the proportion of re-randomized trials whose mean difference is at least as extreme as that of the actual trial. A slightly more accurate method when simulation, rather than exhaustive enumeration, is used is to always include in the numerator and denominator the result actually observed in the trial:

$$p = \frac{1 + \text{number of simulated re-randomized trials with at least as extreme result}}{1 + \text{number of re-randomized trials}}. \qquad (6.2)$$

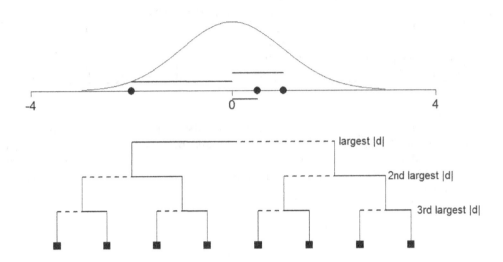

Figure 6.2: Generation of a null distribution: the t-test assumes random sampling from a normal distribution, whereas the re-randomization test fixes absolute values $|d_i|$ of paired differences and treats $\pm|d_i|$ as equally likely. The re-randomization distribution of the sum S of paired differences in this example consists of the 8 equally likely terminal nodes (filled squares) at the bottom of the figure.

Figure 6.2 contrasts the way a t-test and re-randomization test generate a null distribution for a very small example of 3 paired differences. For the t-test, we imagine repeatedly drawing 3 paired differences from a normal distribution with mean 0. For the re-randomization test, the 3 absolute values of differences, $|d_i|$, are fixed constants. The sign of the largest $|d_i|$ is negative. We form its mirror image on the other side of 0 using a dashed line. The actual and mirror images are treated as equally likely. From the two ends of that line segment, we attach actual and mirror images of the second largest $|d_i|$. To the actual and mirror images of the two new line segments, we attach actual and mirror images of the third largest $|d_i|$. The re-randomization distribution of the sum of the 3 paired differences consists of the 8 equally likely points shown at the bottom of Figure 6.2. Note that using the sum, rather than the mean, makes no difference, as the sum is just 3 times the mean.

The two key features of Example 6.1 that we will explore in greater detail are as follows:

1. The re-randomization distribution is the conditional distribution of the mean (or sum) of differences, given paired data $(y_1, y_1'), \ldots, (y_n, y_n')$, but no treatment labels. Equivalently, it is the conditional distribution of the mean difference given $|D_i| = |d_i|$, $i = 1, \ldots, n$, under null hypothesis (6.1). Therefore, a re-randomization test controls the conditional type I error rate given $|D_i| = |d_i|$, $i = 1, \ldots, n$.

2. A re-randomization test is asymptotically equivalent to a paired t-test if paired differences are iid with finite variance. This explains why the p-values using the re-randomization and t-test were so close in the COMMIT trial.

6.2.2   Control of Conditional Type I Error Rate

To see the first point at the end of the preceding section, think about how we would construct the conditional distribution of the mean difference given the pairs of data but not treatment labels under (6.1). The paired outcomes $(y_1, y_1'), \ldots, (y_n, y_n')$ become fixed constants, as do the absolute values $|d_i|$ of paired differences. The ith paired difference is $\pm|d_i|$ with probability $1/2$ each. If this sounds familiar, it should. This is exactly how we constructed the re-randomization distribution! Therefore, the re-randomization distribution of the mean difference is the conditional distribution of the mean difference given the paired outcomes, but not treatment labels. Rejecting (6.1) when the re-randomization p-value is $\leq \alpha$ is equivalent to rejecting (6.1) when the vector $\boldsymbol{D}$ of control minus treatment differences lies in some region R whose conditional probability given $|D_i| = |d_i|$, $i = 1, \ldots, n$ is $\leq \alpha$. In other words, by construction, the conditional type I error rate of the re-randomization test is controlled at level α. This applies to one-tailed, two-tailed, or any other test.

Theorem 6.2. *A re-randomization test with paired data controls the conditional type I error rate given the data, but not the treatment labels, under null hypothesis (6.1). Equivalently, a re-randomization test controls the conditional type I error given $|D_i| = |d_i|$, $i = 1, \ldots, n$.*

6.2.3   Asymptotic Equivalence to a T-test

The second point about a re-randomization test in a paired setting is that it is asymptotically equivalent to a t-test when pairs are iid and the variance of paired differences is finite. We offer a heuristic explanation for this fact and for the necessity of a finite variance. Given the vector $|\boldsymbol{D}| = |\boldsymbol{d}|$ of absolute values of paired differences, $S = \sum_{i=1}^{n} D_i$ is a sum of independent binary random variables, the ith of which takes values $\pm|d_i|$ with probability $1/2$ each. That is, conditionally,

$$S = \sum_{i=1}^{n} |d_i| \tau_i,$$

where τ_i, $i = 1, \ldots, n$, are iid variables taking values ± 1 with probability $1/2$ each. If the $|d_i|$ are all equal, then the re-randomization distribution is the distribution of a sum of iid random variables and is approximately normal by the central limit theorem. On the other hand, one can concoct $|d_i|$ such that the re-randomization distribution of S is far from normally distributed. For instance, suppose that one $|d_i|$ dominates all others. The resulting distribution for S can be bimodal (Figure 6.3).

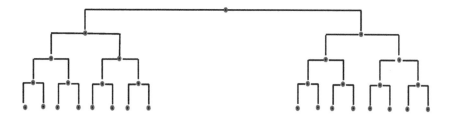

Figure 6.3: Depiction of the re-randomization distribution as in the bottom of Figure 6.2, but when the largest absolute paired difference dominates all others. The resulting re-randomization distribution is bimodal.

Fortunately, the probability that one $|d_i|$ dominates all others becomes negligible for large sample sizes if the D_i are a random sample from some distribution with finite variance.

In that case, the re-randomization distribution of S is approximately normal with mean 0 and variance

$$
\begin{aligned}
\text{var}(S) = \text{var}\left\{\sum_{i=1}^{n} |d_i| \tau_i\right\} &= \sum_{i=1}^{n} \text{var}(|d_i| \tau_i) \\
&= \sum_{i=1}^{n} d_i^2 \, \text{var}(\tau_i) = \sum_{i=1}^{n} d_i^2 \left[E(\tau_i^2) - \{E(\tau_i)\}^2 \right] \\
&= \sum_{i=1}^{n} d_i^2 \left\{ E(1) - 0^2 \right\} = \sum_{i=1}^{n} d_i^2.
\end{aligned}
\tag{6.3}
$$

Write the re-randomization variance of S as $n\tilde{\sigma}^2$, where

$$
\tilde{\sigma}^2 = (1/n) \sum_{i=1}^{n} d_i^2.
\tag{6.4}
$$

Note that $\tilde{\sigma}^2$ is closely related to the usual sample variance $\hat{\sigma}^2 = (n-1)^{-1} \sum_{i=1}^{n} (d_i - \bar{d})^2$. The two differences between $\tilde{\sigma}^2$ and $\hat{\sigma}^2$ are that (1) $\tilde{\sigma}^2$ uses a sum of squared deviations from its null mean of 0 instead of its estimated mean $\bar{d}$, and (2) $\tilde{\sigma}^2$ uses n instead of $n-1$ in the denominator. Not having to estimate the mean from the data saves one degree of freedom. $\tilde{\sigma}^2$ and $\hat{\sigma}^2$ can be quite different if the treatment effect is very large. In that case, paired differences will all tend to be on the same side of 0, so $\tilde{\sigma}^2$ will be very large compared to $\hat{\sigma}^2$. This explains why a re-randomization test is generally more conservative than a t-test. But very large treatment effects are unusual in clinical trials. If power is, say, 0.90, and the sample size is large, the true treatment effect cannot be huge (otherwise, power would be close to 1). Thus, in realistic clinical trial settings, $\tilde{\sigma}^2$ and $\hat{\sigma}^2$ will be very similar when the sample size is large.

In summary, the re-randomization and ordinary t-tests reject the null hypothesis for extreme values of the standardized statistics

$$
\frac{S}{\sqrt{n\tilde{\sigma}^2}} \quad \text{and} \quad \frac{S}{\sqrt{n\hat{\sigma}^2}},
\tag{6.5}
$$

respectively. In realistic settings, $\tilde{\sigma}^2$ and $\hat{\sigma}^2$ are nearly the same, and the two test statistics in (6.5) are nearly identical and asymptotically standard normal. A more precise statement of asymptotic equivalence of a re-randomization and t-test in a paired setting is as follows.

Theorem 6.3. *Consider a paired data setting in which paired differences are iid with finite variance. If power for the paired t-test approaches a constant in $(0,1)$ as $n \to \infty$, then the re-randomization and paired t-tests are asymptotically equivalent.*

Without the finite variance assumption, it is possible for one paired difference to dominate others, as in Figure 6.3. The resulting re-randomization distribution may not be asymptotically normal.

Equation (6.3) suggests that approximating a re-randomization p-value with one based on a t-statistic that uses $\tilde{\sigma}^2$ instead of $\hat{\sigma}^2$ might be even more accurate. To demonstrate the veracity of this conjecture, we simulated 100 paired differences as iid $N(\delta, 1)$ for different values of δ. The histograms in Figure 6.4 depict re-randomization distributions of $S_{100} = \sum_{i=1}^{100} |d_i| \tau_i$ when δ is such that power for a paired t-test is about 0.90 (left curve) and 0.99999 (right curve). The solid and dashed curves are densities of $\sqrt{100\tilde{\sigma}^2} T_{99}$ and $\sqrt{100\hat{\sigma}^2} T_{99}$, respectively, where T_{99} is t with 99 degrees of freedom. When the treatment effect δ is typical, such that power is about 0.90, the two approximations nearly coincide and approximate the re-randomization distribution extremely well. In very unusual circumstances, when δ is so large that the paired t-test has power approximately 0.99999, the solid curve better approximates the re-randomization distribution of $\sum_{i=1}^{100} |d_i| \tau_i$. Thus, even though the standard t-test closely approximates a re-randomization test when n is large, replacing $\hat{\sigma}^2$ by $\tilde{\sigma}^2$ in the t-statistic approximates a re-randomization test even more closely.

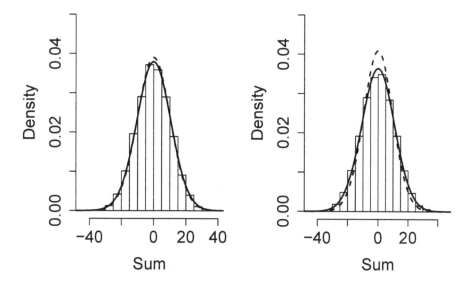

Figure 6.4: The re-randomization distributions of S_{100} when the true mean is such that power for a t-test is 0.90 (left) and 0.99999 (right). The solid and dashed curves are densities of $\sqrt{100\tilde{\sigma}^2} T_{99}$ and $\sqrt{100\hat{\sigma}^2} T_{99}$, respectively, where T_{99} is t with 99 degrees of freedom.

6.2.4 Null Hypothesis and Generalizing

Null hypothesis (6.1) and the fact that a re-randomization test conditions on observed data suggest that conclusions apply to the specific pairs in the trial. Can we make a statement about more than just the specific pairs in our study? Actually, rejection of null hypothesis (6.1) should make us confident that the following null hypothesis is also false:

$$H_0 : \text{treatment has no effect on any pair in the population} \qquad (6.6)$$

After all, if we reject (6.1) in favor of a one-sided alternative hypothesis, we conclude that treatment has a beneficial effect on at least one pair in the trial, which implies that it has a beneficial effect on at least one pair in the population.

But (6.1) and (6.6) are strong null hypotheses because they say that no pair was affected by treatment. What if treatment helps some pairs and hurts others? If a one-tailed test is statistically significant, can we conclude that the average effect of treatment over all pairs in the population is beneficial? Rejection of (6.1) or (6.6) does not allow this conclusion. Critics of re-randomization tests argue that the ability to generalize to a population is a major advantage of t-tests over re-randomization tests. This creates a conundrum. Section 6.2.3 shows that the re-randomization and t-tests coincide as the number of pairs becomes large. The two tests usually yield similar results even with moderate n. In Example 6.1, p-values for the two tests were nearly identical with only 11 pairs. Can the t-test, but not the re-randomization test, permit generalization when they give nearly the same answers for moderate sample sizes? Something seems awry. The truth is that generalization for either test requires an implicit assumption that the trial data can be viewed as being a random sample from some meaningful population, albeit not necessarily the one we originally intended. If we did not believe this assumption, we would never have undertaken the trial. The ability to generalize depends on this assumption, **not** on whether a re-randomization test or t-test was used.

We can formulate null and alternative hypotheses to permit generalization by assuming that the D_i are iid with density or mass function $f(d - \delta)$, where $f(d)$ is symmetric about 0. Then $f(d - \delta)$ is symmetric about δ. We test

$$H_0 : \delta = 0 \tag{6.7}$$

against a one-sided (e.g., $\delta > 0$) or two-sided alternative ($\delta \neq 0$). Hypothesis (6.7) says that treatment is just as likely to have a detrimental versus a beneficial effect of a given size. Under (6.7), the conditional density of D_i given $|D_i| = |d_i|$ still places probability $1/2$ on each of $\pm |d_i|$. Therefore, the re-randomization test controls the conditional type I error rate given $|\boldsymbol{D}| = |\boldsymbol{d}|$, so remains valid for testing null hypothesis (6.7).

Null hypothesis (6.7) also does not require data to be continuous. A re-randomization test can be applied with paired binary data as well. For example, a new treatment might be applied to one eye and a control treatment to the other. A re-randomization test in the paired data setting is an exact version of *McNemar's test* (McNemar, 1947; see also page 349 of Pagano and Gauvreau, 2000). This exact version looks only at *discordant pairs*, pairs for which one member is 1 and the other is 0. Among the m discordant pairs, the number for which the control member is 1 has a binomial distribution with m trials and probability parameter

$$p = P(\text{control} = 1 \,|\, \text{discordant pair}).$$

We can test the null hypothesis that $p = 1/2$ using the procedure described in Section 1.2.1.
‘

6.2.5   Does a Re-randomization Test Assume Independence?

If we do not want to make the assumption that the D_i are iid from some population, and are willing to settle for a conclusion about only the pairs in the trial, a re-randomization test is valid even without the assumption that the D_i are independent. Let $\boldsymbol{Z}$ be the sequence of treatment indicators. Consider the following null hypothesis.

$$H_0 : \ D_1, \ldots, D_n \text{ and } \boldsymbol{Z} \text{ are independent.} \tag{6.8}$$

Null hypothesis (6.8) makes **no** assumption about the joint distribution of $D_1, \ldots, D_n$. In particular, they need not be independent. Assume that (6.8) holds. Then $\boldsymbol{Z}$ is also independent of $|D_1|, \ldots, |D_n|$. Conditioned on $|\boldsymbol{D}| = |\boldsymbol{d}|$, the $|d_i|$ are fixed constants and the distribution of $\boldsymbol{Z}$ is unchanged. The re-randomization distribution continues to be the conditional distribution of $\bar{D}$ given $|\boldsymbol{D}| = |\boldsymbol{d}|$, so the re-randomization test continues to control the conditional error rate given $|\boldsymbol{D}| = |\boldsymbol{d}|$. Accordingly, the re-randomization test is a valid test of null hypothesis (6.8) without assuming that the D_i are independent or identically distributed.

The only caveat to the preceding paragraph is that, without the assumption that the D_i are iid from some population, generalization is not possible. This is especially problematic when the sample size is very small because the sample may be quite different from the intended population, so observed results may apply only to a small subset of the population. The re-randomization test has a built-in protection in this circumstance: rejection of the null hypothesis is literally impossible for tiny sample sizes. For instance, with 4 pairs, there are only $2^4 = 16$ re-randomizations. The smallest possible one-tailed p-value is $1/16$. By contrast, the paired t-test can be statistically significant even with only 2 paired differences! We consider it an advantage of a re-randomization test that a very small sample size cannot result in a statistically significant difference. One should never be confident with a tiny sample size. For one thing, there is no way to verify the assumptions underlying a t-test. Even if one were confident about the assumptions, observed differences between arms could easily be explained by imbalances in important prognostic variables if sample sizes are very small.

6.3 Unpaired Data: Traditional Randomization

6.3.1 Introduction

A re-randomization test can be applied in an unpaired data setting as well. There is no conceptual difference between re-randomization tests in an unpaired versus paired setting, but the variety of randomization methods is broader in the unpaired setting. With paired data, the designation of members of the pair, (A,B), is usually arbitrary. There is often no need to think about balancing the numbers of pairs in which member A, versus member B, was assigned to treatment. In contrast, in an unpaired setting, there is concern about the potential for temporal trends to create bias. For instance, if many consecutive patients are assigned to the same arm, then any between-arm difference could be explained by the fact that patients recruited during that period were sicker or less sick than patients recruited at other times. Therefore, randomization methods in an unpaired setting tend to try to force balance between numbers of treatments and controls throughout the study and within different subgroups.

We find it useful to distinguish between two types of randomization.

Definition 6.4. We use *traditional randomization* to mean either simple or permuted block randomization, and *adaptive randomization* to mean either covariate- or response-adaptive randomization.

Some features of re-randomization tests apply to all forms of randomization, while others are guaranteed to hold for traditional randomization, but not necessarily for adaptive randomization. We will see that for both classes, re-randomization tests control the conditional type I error rate given the data. This is completely analogous to the paired data setting of Section 6.2. The other feature of re-randomization tests in the paired data setting was asymptotic equivalence to a t-test. We will see that this property carries over to unpaired data when traditional randomization is used, but not necessarily when adaptive-randomization is used. This section focuses on traditional randomization.

Let $T(\boldsymbol{Y}, \boldsymbol{Z})$ be a test statistic, where $\boldsymbol{Y} = (Y_1, \ldots, Y_n)^T$, Y_i is the outcome for patient i, and $\boldsymbol{Z} = (Z_1, \ldots, Z_n)^T$, $Z_i = 0$ or 1 denoting that patient i was assigned to control or treatment, respectively. For a trial with a continuous, binary, or survival outcome, T might be the t-statistic, z-statistic for proportions, or logrank statistic, respectively. Alternatively, T might be an estimator like a difference in means or proportions. Fix the outcome vector $\boldsymbol{Y}$ at its observed value $\boldsymbol{y}$ and create a null distribution by re-randomizing patients according to the original randomization scheme. We begin with a relatively straightforward example.

Example 6.5. Pretend that the data in Table 6.1 resulted from an unpaired, rather than paired, setting. Suppose that the 22 communities were assigned to intervention or control using simple randomization. Let $\boldsymbol{Y}$ be the vector of 22 smoking quit rates in the different communities, and $\boldsymbol{Z}$ be the vector of treatment indicators. We would like to test the null hypothesis that the intervention has no effect on any community versus a one-tailed alternative that it results in greater quit rates.

The test statistic is

$$T(\boldsymbol{Y}, \boldsymbol{Z}) = \frac{\sum_{i=1}^{22} Y_i(1 - Z_i)}{\sum_{i=1}^{22}(1 - Z_i)} - \frac{\sum_{i=1}^{22} Y_i Z_i}{\sum_{i=1}^{22} Z_i} = \bar{Y}_C - \bar{Y}_T.$$

Because this difference in sample means is identical to the mean of the pairwise differences computed in Example 6.1, the observed value T_{obs} of T is 0.0067. To compute the exact p-value using a re-randomization test, perform the following steps:

1. Enumerate all possible re-randomization vectors $\boldsymbol{z}_{\text{re}}$.

2. For each $\boldsymbol{z}_{\text{re}}$, compute $T_{\text{re}} = T(\boldsymbol{y}, \boldsymbol{z}_{\text{re}})$ as if the re-randomization assignments were actual assignments. For example, compute the mean difference in ys between the group with $z_{\text{re}} = 0$ and the group with $z_{\text{re}} = 1$.

3. Compute the p-value as the proportion of T_{re}s that are at least as extreme, in the direction of the alternative hypothesis, as the observed value $T_{\text{obs}} = 0.0067$. For example, for a one-sided test rejecting H_0 for small values of T, use the proportion of T_{re}s that are less than or equal to $T_{\text{obs}} = 0.0067$; for a two-sided test, use the proportion of $|T_{\text{re}}|$s that are greater than or equal to $|T_{\text{obs}}| = 0.0067$.

If the number of possible re-randomization vectors is prohibitively large, we can replace enumeration by simulation of thousands of re-randomization vectors.

An interesting nuance arises: two potential re-randomizations are $\boldsymbol{z} = (0, 0, \ldots, 0)^T$ and $\boldsymbol{z} = (1, 1, \ldots, 1)^T$. Under either of these extreme re-randomizations, the test statistic is not even well defined because one of the arms contains no observations. The probability of seeing one of these extreme re-randomizations is exceedingly small, but it could still happen. One solution is to discard either of these re-randomization vectors and generate a new one. Effectively, this means that the re-randomization probability that $\boldsymbol{Z} = \boldsymbol{z}$ is $1/\{2^{22} - 2\}$ for each of the $2^{22} - 2$ $\boldsymbol{z}$s other than $\boldsymbol{z} = (0, 0, \ldots, 0)^T$ or $\boldsymbol{z} = (1, 1, \ldots, 1)^T$.

Restricting the set of randomization vectors to those yielding a well-defined test statistic does not seem to go far enough. For example, it includes randomization vectors with only one person assigned to one of the arms. For the observed randomization vector, $\sum z_i = 11$. That is, exactly 11 communities are assigned to each arm. The difference in sample means is much less variable with the observed $\boldsymbol{z}$ than with a more extreme $\boldsymbol{z}$ with $\sum z_i = 1$ or $\sum z_i = 21$, for example. For this reason, we condition additionally on the observed sample sizes per arm with simple randomization. That is, we consider only those re-randomization vectors yielding the same per-arm sample sizes as the observed randomization vector. Such re-randomization vectors may be viewed as concatenating 11 zeros and 11 ones, and permuting these 22 numbers. That is why a re-randomization test with simple randomization is called a *permutation test* when we condition on sample sizes. The $\binom{22}{11} = 705{,}432$ possible permutation vectors are equally likely; of these, 473,264 yield a control minus intervention mean difference of 0.0067 or smaller. Therefore, if COMMIT had not been pair-matched, and simple randomization had been used to assign communities to intervention or control, the one-tailed p-value using a permutation test would have been 473,264/705,432=0.667. Note that this p-value is close to the p-value of 0.686 computed using the actual randomization of pairs in Example 6.1.   □

Conditioning on sample sizes to obtain the re-randomization p-value in Example 6.5 is consistent with how we usually treat sample sizes. For instance, the p-value for a t-test treats sample sizes as fixed constants rather than as random variables whose distribution must be estimated. This is because sample sizes give us no information about the parameter of interest, namely the intervention effect. We call a quantity whose distribution does not depend on the parameter an *ancillary statistic*. Conditioning on ancillary statistics is a widely accepted principle called the *conditionality principle* (see page 293 of Casella and Berger, 2002). The principle applies when permuted block randomization is used as well. The following example is an illustration.

Example 6.6. Consider again the COMMIT trial of Example 6.1, but pretend that instead of pair matching communities, the trial randomly assigned the 22 communities to intervention or control using blocks of size 2 and 4. Assume that each time a new block was to start, a fair coin was used to choose between block sizes 2 and 4. Pretend that the first 5 blocks turned out to be of size 4, while the last block was of size 2, as shown in Table 6.2.

Table 6.2: Smoking quit rates within the embellished version of COMMIT with five blocks of size 4 and one block of size 2. The first and second rows of numbers show control and intervention quit rates, respectively, in different communities of the blocks.

	Block 1		Block 2		Block 3		Block 4		Block 5		Block 6
I	.139	.163	.164	.204	.183	.164	.262	.193	.215	.136	.155
C	.205	.202	.163	.249	.160	.186	.230	.169	.127	.172	.189

If we re-randomized using the blocked randomization scheme, we might not get five blocks of size 4 and one block of size 2. Instead, we might get eleven blocks of size 2 or six blocks of size 4. In the latter case, we would take only the first two assignments of the last block. The distribution of the intervention effect estimate is different depending on the number of blocks of different sizes and whether the total sample size was accrued in the middle or end of the last block. Therefore, with permuted block randomization, we condition not only on the sample sizes per arm, but also on the specific set of block sizes, in their observed order. In our re-randomizations in this example, the first five blocks are of size 4, and the last is of size 2. We simply permute intervention and control labels within each block. Within each block of size 4, there are $\binom{4}{2} = 6$ different ways to assign exactly 2 communities to intervention. This yields 6 possible values, not necessarily unique, for $\hat{\delta}_i$, the difference between the mean of the two control communities and the mean of the two intervention communities in block i, $i = 1, \ldots, 5$. There are two possible values for $\hat{\delta}_6$, the control minus intervention difference in the final block of size 2. Table 6.3 shows the set of possible $\hat{\delta}_i$ for blocks $1, \ldots, 6$. The difference between the control and intervention means of all 11 communities per arm is $(2\sum_{i=1}^{5} \hat{\delta}_i + \hat{\delta}_6)/11$. Therefore, the re-randomization distribution of the intervention effect estimate is the distribution of $(2\sum_{i=1}^{5} \hat{\delta}_i + \hat{\delta}_6)/11$, where $\hat{\delta}_i$ is the difference in means within pair i when the two control observations are randomly selected from the numbers in block i of Table 6.3. Of the $6^5 \cdot 2 = 15{,}552$ ways to pick 2 numbers from each of the first 5 blocks of Table 6.3 and one number from the last block, 10,450 yielded a control minus intervention mean less than or equal to the observed difference, 0.0067. Therefore, the one-tailed re-randomization p-value for the embellished version of the COMMIT trial is 10,450/15,552= 0.672. This is very similar to the p-value of 0.686 obtained in Example 6.1 using the actual randomization method, namely eleven blocks of size 2.

Again if the number of possible re-randomizations had been huge, we would have approximated the re-randomization p-value by simulation. We draw a huge number of re-randomization vectors z, compute $T(y, z)$ for each, and compute the p-value using (6.2). □

Table 6.3: All possible values of the control mean minus intervention mean within each of the five blocks of size 4 and the last block of size 2 for the embellished version of the randomization in COMMIT.

Block 1	Block 2	Block 3	Block 4	Block 5	Block 6
-.0525	-.0630	-.0225	-.0650	-.0620	-.0340
-.0135	-.0230	-.0035	-.0280	-.0260	.0340
-.0105	-.0220	-.0005	-.0040	-.0170	
.0105	.0220	.0005	.0040	.0170	
.0135	.0230	.0035	.0280	.0260	
.0525	.0630	.0225	.0650	.0620	

6.3.2   Control of Conditional type I Error Rate

As mentioned in Section 6.3.1, two key features of a re-randomization test in the paired setting carry over to the unpaired setting with traditional randomization: (1) a re-randomization test conditions on outcome data, thereby controlling the conditional type I error rate and (2) a re-randomization test is asymptotically equivalent to a t-test when the common variance is finite. This section considers the first fact, conditional error rate control.

To see fact 1 above, let I denote additional information we intend to condition on, in the form of ancillary statistics such as per-arm sample sizes or block sizes. We will show that the re-randomization distribution of the test statistic $T(Y, Z)$ is the conditional distribution of $T(Y, Z)$ given $Y = y$ and $I = i$ under a certain null hypothesis. To see this, note that the conditional distribution of $T(Y, Z)$, given $Y = y$ and $I = i$, is

$$F(t \mid y, i) \overset{\text{Def}}{=} P\{T(Y, Z) \leq t \mid Y = y, I = i\}$$
$$= P\{T(y, Z) \leq t \mid Y = y, I = i\}$$
$$= \sum_{z : T(y, z) \leq t} P(Z = z \mid Y = y, I = i) \qquad (6.9)$$

Now suppose the following null hypothesis is true:

$$H_0 : Y \text{ and } Z \text{ are conditionally independent, given } I = i. \qquad (6.10)$$

Then once we condition on $I = i$, the distribution of Z does not change if we condition additionally on $Y = y$. That is, $P(Z = z \mid Y = y, I = i) = P(Z = z \mid I = i)$. In that case, (6.9) becomes

$$\sum_{z : T(y, z) \leq t} P(Z = z \mid I = i). \qquad (6.11)$$

Notice that (6.11) is obtained by fixing Y at its observed value y and using the distribution of T induced by the randomization distribution of Z given $I = i$. But that is exactly how we compute the re-randomization distribution of T given $I = i$. This shows that the conditional distribution of $T(Y, Z)$ given $Y = y$ and $I = i$, computed under null hypothesis (6.10), is the re-randomization distribution of $T(Y, Z)$ given $I = i$. Accordingly, the re-randomization test controls the conditional type I error rate given $Y = y$ and $I = i$.

The same reasoning is used in the slightly simpler setting when we do not condition on additional information I. In that case, the null hypothesis being tested is

$$H_0 : Y \text{ and } Z \text{ are independent.} \qquad (6.12)$$

We summarize these results as follows.

Theorem 6.7. (Control of conditional type I error rate)

1. *A re-randomization test that conditions on $I = i$ controls the conditional type I error rate given $Y = y$ and $I = i$, under null hypothesis 6.10.*

2. *A re-randomization that does not condition on ancillary information I controls the conditional type I error rate given $Y = y$, under null hypothesis 6.12.*

6.3.3 The Null Hypothesis and Generalizing

Let us explore more deeply the null hypothesis being tested by a re-randomization test when traditional randomization is used. Consider the simpler setting in which we do not condition on ancillary information I. Null hypothesis (6.12) says that treatment has no effect on the distribution of the observations Y. A slightly stronger null hypothesis is often assumed, namely,

$$H_0 : \text{The same values } Y = y \text{ would have occurred regardless of } z. \qquad (6.13)$$

In fact, we can restate this by thinking of the data generating mechanism as follows:

$$H_0 : Y \text{ was generated first, then } Z \text{ according to the randomization method.} \qquad (6.14)$$

Null hypothesis (6.14) seems strange because we know it is false, but the real question is whether the data provide compelling evidence that it is false. If treatment truly had no effect on anyone, we should not be able to rule out (6.14). On the other hand, if treatment worked, we should have strong evidence that (6.14) is false. Null (6.13) implies null (6.12), but not vice versa. For example, suppose we generate data Y as follows. We consider, in advance, every possible randomization vector z. For each possible z, we draw a new observation Y from the same distribution F. Then hypothesis (6.13) is false because we could get a different value Y for each z. Nonetheless, the distribution of Y is the same regardless of z. Therefore, (6.12) still holds. A re-randomization test is valid for testing any of null hypotheses (6.12), (6.13), or (6.14). Likewise, when we condition on ancillary information I, the re-randomization test can be viewed as testing any of null hypotheses (6.10), (6.13), or (6.14). The reason we bring up null hypothesis (6.13) is that it is used to construct confidence intervals for re-randomization tests, a topic we defer to Section 6.7.

All of the above null hypotheses are strong in the sense that they imply that treatment had no effect on anyone. As in the paired data setting, if the truth is that treatment helps some people and hurts others, technically, rejection of the null hypothesis does not permit a conclusion that treatment is helpful on average. Some people argue that a t-test is preferable because it does allow the conclusion that treatment helps on average. They claim that a permutation test applies only to participants in the trial, but a t-test allows generalization to a population. This argument is as lame as it was in Section 6.2.4. A re-randomization test is asymptotically equivalent to a t-test under mild assumptions; it must be testing nearly the same null hypothesis as the t-test for large sample sizes. The truth is that the ability to generalize depends not on what test is used, but whether data can be regarded as a random sample from some population of interest.

6.3.4 Does a Re-randomization Test Require Independence?

If we are willing to abandon the idea of generalizing, then we do not have to make the assumption that the Y_i are independent of each other. None of hypotheses (6.10), (6.12), (6.13), and (6.14) require that assumption. The fact that re-randomization tests do not require an independence assumption has been known for a long time (see, for example,

Fisher, 1935, section 2; Welch, 1937; Wilk, 1955; and Cox and Reid, 2000, page 24-27). Nonetheless, when this topic arose in the following trial, it led to controversy.

Example 6.8. Vaccine trial with lack of independence   VAX004 (Flynn, Forthal, Harro et al., 2005) was an HIV vaccine trial in which the primary outcome Y_i was 1 if participant i became HIV-positive and 0 otherwise. The trial was designed under the assumption of independent Y_i. During the course of the trial, nearly identical genetic HIV viruses were found. This is extremely strong evidence that participants within the trial were having sex with either each other or a common partner. This casts serious doubt on the independence assumption. For instance, if trial participant i becomes HIV-infected and has sex with trial participant j, then participant j has a higher probability of becoming HIV-infected. Y_i and Y_j are likely to be positively correlated. The comments preceding this example imply that a re-randomization test remains a valid test of the strong null hypothesis that the vaccine has no effect in anyone. But exactly what does this statement mean? One way for the strong null hypothesis to be false is as follows. Suppose that the vaccine has no other effect than to increase libido compared to receiving a placebo. This might cause more sexual sharing and more HIV among vaccine participants than among placebo participants. The probability that a two-tailed re-randomization test declares a difference between arms might exceed α even though the vaccine might have no **direct** effect on HIV. This seems to contradict our statement that a re-randomization test remains valid. In fact, this is not a contradiction. The strong null hypothesis is false: the vaccine does have an effect on HIV through its **indirect** effect on libido. Given that the null hypothesis is false, no type I error can be made. Rejection of the null hypothesis allows us to say only that there is **some** effect of vaccine, but not necessarily the one we were hoping for (Proschan and Follmann, 2008).   □

6.3.5   Asymptotic Equivalence to a t-Test

The other feature of a re-randomization test in a traditional randomization setting is asymptotic equivalence to a t-test. This is often proven using a permutation central limit theorem that treats data as fixed constants and gives conditions on those constants that ensure that the permutation distribution is asymptotically standard normal (Wald and Wolfowitz, 1944; Noether, 1949; Hoeffding, 1951). These conditions concern infinite sequences of constants, and essentially prevent any single observation or a few observations from dominating all others in terms of variability. Given that we have a fixed sample of size n, how would we know whether such a condition on an infinite sequence holds? We could only be confident by assuming some other condition such as that observations are random samples from some populations with finite variance. We make that assumption in what follows.

Consider simple randomization to the two arms, and suppose we condition on sample sizes, so our re-randomization test is a permutation test. The difference in sample means can be written as

$$\bar{y}_C - \bar{y}_T = \frac{\sum_{i=1}^n y_i(1 - Z_i)}{n_C} - \frac{\sum_{i=1}^n y_i Z_i}{n_T}$$

$$= \frac{\sum_{i=1}^n y_i}{n_C} - \left(\sum_{i=1}^n y_i Z_i\right)(1/n_T + 1/n_C). \tag{6.15}$$

We use lower case letters for the y_i and upper case letters for the Z_i to emphasize that only the Z_i are random variables when it comes to re-randomization inference. The appendix shows that the re-randomization variance of $\bar{y}_T - \bar{y}_C$ is

$$s_L^2(1/n_T + 1/n_C), \text{ where } s_L^2 = (n - 1)^{-1}\sum_{i=1}^n (y_i - \bar{y})^2$$

is the lumped variance of all $n = n_T + n_C$ observations. Note that the estimated variance of $\bar{Y}_T - \bar{Y}_C$ used by the t-test is very similar:

$$s_P^2(1/n_T + 1/n_C), \text{ where } s_p^2 = \frac{(n_T - 1)s_T^2 + (n_C - 1)s_C^2}{n_T + n_C - 1}$$

is the pooled variance estimate. The difference between the two variance estimators s_L^2 and s_P^2 is that s_L^2 assumes the null hypothesis, so the common mean in the two arms is estimated by the overall mean $\bar{y}$. This is analogous to what happens in the paired setting of Section 6.2.3, where the re-randomization variance of paired differences assumed the null mean of 0. If the treatment effect is huge, the separation between treatment and control observations makes the lumped variance much larger than the pooled variance. This explains why a permutation test tends to be more conservative than a t-test. However, if sample sizes are large and power for the t-test is, say, 0.90, the two variances will be very similar. Moreover, the re-randomization distribution of $\bar{y}_T - \bar{y}_C$ is approximately normal. A similar derivation can be used with permuted block randomization. We summarize as follows. Readers with an advanced probability background can find the details in Proschan and Shaw (2016).

Theorem 6.9. *Consider a clinical trial with either simple or permuted block randomization. Under regularity conditions, the re-randomization test is asymptotically equivalent to:*

1. *a t-test if simple randomization is used and one conditions on sample sizes (i.e., a permutation test is used),*

2. *a stratified t-test (stratified by permuted blocks) if permuted block randomization is used and one conditions on block sizes.*

The regularity conditions are that the common population variance in the two arms is finite and that power of the respective t-test approaches a fixed number in $(0, 1)$ as n_T and n_C approach ∞ in such a way that n_T/n_C approaches a constant.

As in the paired setting, a slightly better approximation for the re-randomization test is to use a t-test based on the null variance estimator s_L^2 rather than the pooled variance estimator s_P^2. Understanding the asymptotic connection between re-randomization and t-tests is very helpful, especially in adaptive settings (Proschan, Glimm, and Posch, 2014).

6.3.6 Protection Against Temporal Trends

One very important feature of a re-randomization test is that it protects against possible temporal trends, even with a very poor randomization scheme that is prone to bias from temporal trends. The following example illustrates the point.

Example 6.10. Protection against temporal trends Consider a trial of 20 patients in which a permuted block with 9 Cs and 1 T is used for the first 10 patients, and a permuted block with 9 Ts and 1 C is used for the last 10 patients. This randomization method is prone to confounding by temporal trends because almost all control patients are among the first 10, while almost all treatment patients are among the second 10. Suppose that treatment has no effect, but there is a temporal trend such that the second 10 patients have higher values than the first 10. Then the ordinary treatment effect estimator $\bar{Y}_T - \bar{Y}_C$ will be positive, and the type I error rate of an unstratified, one-tailed t-test will be inflated.

If a re-randomization test is used, each re-randomization will also have nearly all Cs from the first half and Ts from the second half. Therefore, any temporal trend will be reflected in each re-randomization, causing the mean of the re-randomization distribution to have the same sign as the observed test statistic (see Exercise 11). The treatment effect estimate for the actual randomization will not look unusual in the re-randomization distribution. In this way, a re-randomization test automatically protects the type I error rate in the presence of temporal trends.   □

6.3.7   Fisher's Exact Test as a Re-Randomization Test

Note that a re-randomization test can be used even when the outcome is not continuous. Consider a binary outcome setting with simple randomization and test statistic

$$T(\boldsymbol{Y}, \boldsymbol{Z}) = \sum_{i=1}^{n} Z_i Y_i = \# \text{ treatment events.}$$

Condition on $\boldsymbol{Y} = \boldsymbol{y}$, and suppose that there are $\sum_{i=1}^{n} y_i = s$ events combined across both arms. We get the same answer whether we fix $\boldsymbol{y}$ and permute $\boldsymbol{z}$ or fix $\boldsymbol{z}$ and permute $\boldsymbol{y}$. The first way can be viewed as assigning n_T Ts and n_C Cs to the data vector $\boldsymbol{y}$, while the second assigns s ones and $n_T + n_C - s$ zeroes to the randomization vector $\boldsymbol{z}$. Consider the second way.

1. The number of ways to assign k ones among the n_T treatment participants is the number of ways of choosing a subset of size k from n_T people, namely $\binom{n_T}{k}$. The other $n_T - k$ treatment patients are all assigned zeroes (in only one way).

2. The remaining $s - k$ ones can be assigned among the n_C control patients in $\binom{n_C}{s-k}$ ways. The other $n_C - (s-k)$ control patients are all assigned zeroes (in only one way).

3. The total number of ways of assigning s ones to the $n_T + n_C$ people is $\binom{n_T+n_C}{s}$.

Therefore, the re-randomization probability of exactly k treatment events is

$$\frac{\binom{n_T}{k}\binom{n_C}{s-k}}{\binom{n_T+n_C}{s}}. \tag{6.16}$$

Consider a one-tailed test of whether $H_0 : p_T = p_C$ versus $H_1 : p_T < p_C$, where p_T and p_C are the event probabilities in the treatment and control arms. To compute the p-value, sum the probabilities (6.16) over all k less than or equal to the observed number of treatment events. But this is exactly how we compute a p-value for Fisher's exact test (see Section 2.2.1). We have established the following result.

Proposition 6.11. *When the outcome Y is binary, a permutation test is equivalent to Fisher's exact test.*

6.4   Unpaired Data: Covariate-Adaptive Randomization

6.4.1   Introduction

For the remainder of the chapter, we consider adaptive randomization strategies (covariate- and response-adaptive). Before getting into the details, we must point out one crucial difference between traditional and adaptive randomization strategies:

Remark 6.12. *For adaptive randomization strategies, the per-arm sample sizes may no longer be ancillary statistics. Consequently, it may **not** be advisable to condition on them when generating the null distribution of the test statistic. See Example 6.21.*

Simon and Simon (2011) prove, in one fell swoop, the validity of re-randomization tests with covariate- or response-adaptive randomization. We prefer to separate these two, as they are conceptually quite different. This section considers covariate-adaptive randomization. For simplicity of presentation, assume there is a single covariate x, and let $\boldsymbol{x}_i = (x_1, \ldots, x_i)$ denote the covariate values for patients $1, \ldots, i$, and similarly define $\boldsymbol{y}_i$ and $\boldsymbol{z}_i$. With covariate-adaptive randomization, the probability that patient i is assigned to treatment depends on $\boldsymbol{x}_i$ and $\boldsymbol{z}_{i-1}$:

$$P(Z_i = 1 \mid \boldsymbol{x}_i, \boldsymbol{z}_{i-1}) = p_i = p_i(\boldsymbol{x}_i, \boldsymbol{z}_{i-1}).$$

We begin with null hypothesis (6.14) modified for covariate-adaptive randomization:

$H_0 : (\boldsymbol{X}, \boldsymbol{Y})$ were generated **first**, then $\boldsymbol{Z}$ was generated using
the covariate $-$ adaptive algorithm. $\hfill (6.17)$

In reality, $(\boldsymbol{X}, \boldsymbol{Y})$ were not generated first, but again the question is whether the data provide strong evidence against (6.17). Null hypothesis (6.17) is a reasonable way to express the fact that treatment has no effect. After all, if outcomes were generated before treatment was assigned, then treatment could not possibly affect outcome. On the other hand, if treatment works, then $Z_i = 1$ should be a good predictor of a favorable Y_i even after adjusting for covariates, in which case we ought to be able to reject null hypothesis (6.17).

6.4.2 Control of Conditional type I Error Rate

Under null hypothesis (6.17), $(\boldsymbol{x}, \boldsymbol{y})$ are fixed constants by the time $\boldsymbol{Z}$ is generated. We can write the re-randomization probability that $Z_1 = z_1$ in the canonical way as $p_1^{z_1}(1 - p_1)^{1-z_1}$, which is p_1 if $z_1 = 1$ and $1 - p_1$ if $z_1 = 0$. Similarly, the re-randomization probability that $\boldsymbol{Z} = \boldsymbol{z}$ is

$$\prod_{i=1}^{n} \{p_i(\boldsymbol{x}_i, \boldsymbol{z}_{i-1})\}^{z_i} \{1 - p_i(\boldsymbol{x}_i, \boldsymbol{z}_{i-1})\}^{1-z_i}. \hfill (6.18)$$

This is also the conditional probability that $\boldsymbol{Z} = \boldsymbol{z}$ given $\boldsymbol{X} = \boldsymbol{x}, \boldsymbol{Y} = \boldsymbol{y}$ under (6.17) because the randomization algorithm for Z_i looks only at $\boldsymbol{x}_i$ and $\boldsymbol{z}_{i-1}$. The re-randomization distribution of the test statistic $T(\boldsymbol{Y}, \boldsymbol{Z})$, namely

$$H_{\boldsymbol{x},\boldsymbol{y}}(t) \overset{\text{Def}}{=} P\{T(\boldsymbol{Y}, \boldsymbol{Z}) \le t \mid \boldsymbol{X} = \boldsymbol{x}, \boldsymbol{Y} = \boldsymbol{y})$$
$$= \sum_{\boldsymbol{z}:T(\boldsymbol{y},\boldsymbol{z})\le t} \prod_{i=1}^{n} \{p_i(\boldsymbol{x}_i, \boldsymbol{z}_{i-1})\}^{z_i} \{1 - p_i(\boldsymbol{x}_i, \boldsymbol{z}_{i-1})\}^{1-z_i}, \hfill (6.19)$$

is the conditional distribution function of $T(\boldsymbol{Y}, \boldsymbol{Z})$ given $(\boldsymbol{x}, \boldsymbol{y})$ when null hypothesis (6.17) is true. This means that by construction, the re-randomization test controls the conditional type I error rate given $\boldsymbol{X} = \boldsymbol{x}, \boldsymbol{Y} = \boldsymbol{y}$ under hypothesis (6.17).

Theorem 6.13. (Control of conditional error rate) *Under null hypothesis (6.17), a re-randomization test controls the conditional type I error rate given $\boldsymbol{X} = \boldsymbol{x}, \boldsymbol{Y} = \boldsymbol{y}$.*

6.4.3 Protection Against Temporal Trends

Example 6.10 illustrated the protective effect of re-randomization tests against temporal trends in the context of permuted block randomization. The same phenomenon occurred in a more subtle way in the following trial that used what turned out to be a sub-optimal covariate-adaptive randomization scheme with unequal allocation. The problems caused by this trial led to improved methods of covariate-adaptive randomization with unequal allocation.

Example 6.14. In October 2008, the FDA's Endocrinologic and Metabolic Drugs Advisory Committee discussed safety and efficacy of algucosidase alpha for the treatment of Pompé disease, a very rare neuromuscular disorder. The sponsor, Genzyme Corporation, conducted the Late Onset Treatment Study (LOTS), a double-blind trial randomizing patients with late onset Pompé disease to algucosidase alpha or placebo in a 2:1 ratio. The primary outcome used the 6-minute walk test (6MWT), the distance a patient could walk in 6 minutes. Covariate-adaptive randomization was used with covariates study site (8 sites), baseline 6MWT stratum (≤ 300 meters versus > 300 meters), and forced vital capacity stratum ($\le 55\%$ versus $> 55\%$ of predicted), a measure of lung function.

The FDA requested that a re-randomization test be conducted to support the statistically significant result ($p = 0.035$) of a parametric analysis of covariance. The p-value from the re-randomization test was 0.06, narrowly missing the 0.05 level required. The sponsor argued that the re-randomization test should not be used because the mean of the re-randomization distribution was not 0 (Figure 6.5).

Two questions immediately come to mind: (1) why was the mean of the re-randomization distribution not 0 and (2) what are the consequences of this nonzero mean?

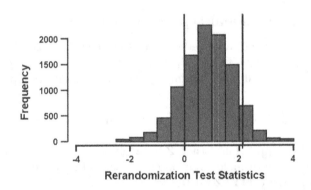

Distribution of 6MWT ANCOVA test statistics

Rerandomization Test Statistics

Figure 6.5: Plot presented at the October 2008 Endocrinologic and Metabolic Drugs Advisory Committee showing the re-randomization distribution of the ANCOVA z-statistic in the Late Onset Treatment Study. The vertical line slightly larger than 2 represents the observed z-score.

To see why the mean of the re-randomization distribution was nonzero, note that the difference in sample means is

$$\bar{y}_T(\boldsymbol{Z}) - \bar{y}_C(\boldsymbol{Z}) = \frac{\sum Z_i y_i}{\sum Z_i} - \frac{\sum (1 - Z_i) y_i}{\sum (1 - Z_i)}. \tag{6.20}$$

The 2:1 randomization scheme ensured that $\sum Z_i$ would be very close to the intended target of $(2/3)n$, where n is the total sample size. Replace $\sum Z_i$ by $(2/3)n$ and $\sum (1 - Z_i)$ by $(1/3)n$ in the denominators of (6.20). Then

$$\mathrm{E}\{\bar{y}_T(\boldsymbol{Z}) - \bar{y}_C(\boldsymbol{Z})\} \approx \frac{\sum \{\mathrm{E}(Z_i)\} y_i}{(2/3)n} - \frac{\sum \{\mathrm{E}(1 - Z_i)\} y_i}{(1/3)n}. \tag{6.21}$$

If the expected value of Z_i, namely $P(Z_i = 1)$, were 2/3 for each i, then the right side of (6.21) would be

$$\frac{\sum (2/3) y_i}{(2/3)n} - \frac{\sum (1/3) y_i}{(1/3)n} = \bar{y} - \bar{y} = 0.$$

In other words, the mean of the re-randomization distribution can differ appreciably from 0 only if $P(Z_i = 1)$ differs across i. A suboptimal application of response-adaptive randomization caused the probability of assignment to algucosidase alpha in LOTS to differ by patient order, resulting in a nonzero mean of the re-randomization distribution.

A serious consequence of having a nonzero mean of the re-randomization distribution is that power can be substantially lower than for a parametric analysis. Proschan, Brittain, and Kammerman (2011) gave a hypothetical example in which power of the re-randomization test remained lower than that of a t-test, even asymptotically. This is in contrast to what happens when more traditional randomization methods (e.g., simple or permuted block) are used (see Theorem 6.9).

The fact that power is lost when the re-randomization distribution has nonzero mean is arguably an appropriate punishment. As noted above, the nonzero mean occurs because $P(Z_i = 1)$ is not constant. Suppose there is a temporal trend such that patients tend to be healthier on days for which $P(X_i = 1)$ is high. We could not easily disentangle a treatment effect from a time effect. A re-randomization test delivers an appropriate punishment by tending to make the mean of the re-randomization distribution have the same sign as the observed treatment effect. We saw this in Example 6.10, and the same thing happened in the algucosidase trial. The 'punished' p-value from the re-randomization test was 0.06.

The problem of nonzero mean of a re-randomization distribution with $k : 1$ randomization can be avoided by ensuring that $P(Z_i = 1)$ is approximately constant over i. The method of Kuznetsova and Tymofyeyev (2012), described in Section 5.8, is a good way to do this. □

Extra Protection: Adjusting for Covariates

Using a treatment effect estimate that adjusts for at least the covariates used in the randomization process gives an added layer of protection in covariate-adaptive trials. After all, if we used the correct model and our estimates of the parameters were precise enough, the covariate-adjusted residuals should be close to iid observations under the null hypothesis. If they really were iid, then our allocation method should not matter. Even if we used a completely deterministic algorithm to allocate patients to arms, parametric and nonparametric tests should perform well.

Some people worry about adjusting for covariates on the grounds that models require more assumptions. However, one can get the best of both worlds by applying a re-randomization test to a covariate-adjusted outcome. The most pristine way to do this is to first fit a model that does not include the treatment variable. One may even rummage through a host of different models and use any method for choosing the best one (e.g., the Akaike information criterion or Bayesian information criterion). The key requirements are that only baseline variables are used and treatment assignments are not included. Once the model is fit, apply a re-randomization test to the residuals $Y_i' = Y_i - \hat{\beta}_0 - \hat{\beta}_1 x_1 - \ldots - \hat{\beta}_k x_k$, $i = 1, \ldots, n$. We can view this as a re-randomization test on the part of the outcome that is not explained by baseline covariates. In this way, one obtains the benefit of covariate adjustment and the robustness of a re-randomization test. Even if the model is wrong, the type I error rate of a re-randomization test is guaranteed to be α or less under a strong null hypothesis of no treatment effect on anyone.

6.4.4 More Rigorous Null Hypothesis

Null hypothesis (6.17) sidesteps some technical difficulties with formulating a more rigorous null hypothesis. Still, (6.17) is not very statistical. We would prefer a null hypothesis like (6.10), but (6.10) is false with covariate-adaptive randomization because Z depends on X, which is correlated with Y. Therefore, Z and Y are not independent. Since the dependence between Z and Y is mediated through X, it seems that conditioning on X should make Y and Z independent. Therefore, it is natural to specify the following null hypothesis:

$$H_0 : Z \text{ and } Y \text{ are conditionally independent given } X. \tag{6.22}$$

It is tempting to assert that the re-randomization distribution of T is the conditional distribution of $T(Y, Z)$ given $X = x, Y = y$ under null hypothesis (6.22). If true, that would show that Theorem 6.13 holds when we replace null hypothesis (6.17) by (6.22). However, there is a technical difficulty requiring the following additional assumption (Simon and Simon, 2011).

$$Z_i \text{ and } (X_{i+1}, \ldots, X_n) \text{ are conditionally independent given } X_i, Z_{i-1}. \tag{6.23}$$

Remark 6.15. *One way of viewing (6.23) is that, given the information used in the randomization of Z_i, namely X_i and Z_{i-1}, covariate values of future patients give no additional information about Z_i. This seems like a given: at the time patient i is assigned, covariate values of future patients are not even available. But another way to view (6.23) is that, given the information used in the randomization of Z_i, Z_i gives no additional information about $X_{i+1}, \ldots, X_n$. This can be violated if we change the covariate composition of future patients depending on the value of Z_i, as in the following example.*

Example 6.16. Consider a tiny trial of 12 people. First recruit 6 women and use simple randomization. If all 6 are assigned to T or all to C, recruit 6 more women and assign them all to the opposite arm. On the other hand, if the first 6 women are not all assigned to the same arm, recruit 6 men and use simple randomization. Let covariate X_i be the indicator that patient i is a man. Suppose the information available just prior to assignment of patient 6 is $X_1 = 0, \ldots, X_6 = 0$ and $Z_1 = 0, \ldots, Z_5 = 0$. Then $X_7, \ldots, X_{12}$ will all be 0 if $Z_6 = 0$ and 1 if $Z_6 = 1$. Therefore, (6.23) does not hold.

To see the consequence of the fact that (6.23) does not hold, suppose there is a temporal effect such that the last 6 patients have astronomically larger values than the first 6. Conditioned on $X_{12} = (0, \ldots, 0)$, the first and last 6 patients were assigned to opposite arms, so the observed difference in means is the most extreme possible for a two-tailed test. The p-value for a two-tailed re-randomization test is the re-randomization probability that $Z_1 = 0, \ldots, Z_6 = 0$ or $Z_1 = 1, \ldots, Z_6 = 1$, namely $2(1/2)^6 = 0.031$. As this p-value is ≤ 0.05, the re-randomization test will be statistically significant. This says that, given $X_{12} = (0, \ldots, 0)$ and the observed y (which is such that $|y_i - y_j|$ is huge for any $i \leq 6$ and $j \geq 7$), the type I error rate of the re-randomization test is 1. This example shows that null hypothesis (6.22) is not sufficient to ensure control of the conditional type I error rate for a re-randomization test.   □

We must fix the loophole that allows counterexamples such as Example 6.16. Condition (6.23) is needed to prevent an indirect effect of Z_i on future Y values through Z_i's effect on future X values.

Theorem 6.17. *Under the additional condition (6.23), Theorem 6.13 holds with null hypothesis (6.17) replaced by null hypothesis (6.22).*

6.5   Unpaired Data: Response-Adaptive Randomization

6.5.1   Introduction

With response-adaptive randomization, the probability that patient i is assigned to treatment depends on outcomes y_{i-1} and treatment assignments z_{i-1} of patients $1, \ldots, i-1$:

$$P(Z_i = 1 \mid y_{i-1}, z_{i-1}) = p_i = p_i(y_{i-1}, z_{i-1}).$$

We are convinced by the arguments of Korn and Friedlin (2012), which we review in Chapter 5, Section 5.8, that response-adaptive randomization should be avoided in two-armed trials. It may be more appealing in multi-armed trials. Nonetheless, to understand how a re-randomization test works with response-adaptive randomization, we focus on two-armed trials. The development that follows is very similar to that of covariate-adaptive randomization covered in Section 6.4. Therefore, we will be brief.

Null hypothesis (6.14) applied to response-adaptive randomization is as follows:

$$H_0 : \boldsymbol{Y} \text{ was generated } \textbf{first}, \text{ then } \boldsymbol{Z} \text{ was generated using}$$
$$\text{the response} - \text{adaptive algorithm.} \tag{6.24}$$

The re-randomization probability that $\boldsymbol{Z} = \boldsymbol{z}$ under null hypothesis (6.24) is

$$\prod_{i=1}^{n} \{p_i(\boldsymbol{y}_{i-1}, \boldsymbol{z}_{i-1})\}^{z_i} \{1 - p_i(\boldsymbol{y}_{i-1}, \boldsymbol{z}_{i-1})\}^{1-z_i}, \tag{6.25}$$

and the re-randomization distribution of the test statistic T under (6.24) is

$$H_{\boldsymbol{y}}(t) \overset{\text{Def}}{=} P\{T(\boldsymbol{Y}, \boldsymbol{Z}) \leq t \mid \boldsymbol{Y} = \boldsymbol{y}\}$$
$$= \sum_{\boldsymbol{z}:T(\boldsymbol{y},\boldsymbol{z})\leq t} \prod_{i=1}^{n} \{p_i(\boldsymbol{y}_{i-1}, \boldsymbol{z}_{i-1})\}^{z_i} \{1 - p_i(\boldsymbol{y}_{i-1}, \boldsymbol{z}_{i-1})\}^{1-z_i}. \tag{6.26}$$

This can be shown to be the conditional distribution function of $T(\boldsymbol{Y}, \boldsymbol{Z})$ given $\boldsymbol{Y} = \boldsymbol{y}$ under null hypothesis (6.24). This implies:

Theorem 6.18. *Under null hypothesis (6.24), a re-randomization test controls the conditional type I error rate given* $\boldsymbol{Y} = \boldsymbol{y}$.

As in the preceding section, we can formulate the null hypothesis more mathematically. Under null hypothesis (6.24), the conditional distribution of Z_i given $\boldsymbol{y}_n, \boldsymbol{z}_{i-1}$ depends on $\boldsymbol{y}_n$ only through $\boldsymbol{y}_{i-1}$. That is, the conditional distribution of Z_i given $(\boldsymbol{y}_{i-1}, (y_i, \ldots, y_n), \boldsymbol{z}_{i-1})$ does not depend on $(y_i, \ldots, y_n)$. Therefore,

$$H_0 : Z_i \text{ and } (Y_i, \ldots, Y_n) \text{ are conditionally independent given } \boldsymbol{Y}_{i-1},$$
$$\boldsymbol{Z}_{i-1}, \ i = 1, \ldots, n. \tag{6.27}$$

Remark 6.19. *Null (6.27) says that once we include data used in the randomization algorithm for* Z_i, *we get no additional information about* Z_i *by looking at current or future outcome data. Of course, if treatment did have an effect on outcome, then a favorable value of* Y_i *should be correlated with* $Z_i = 1$, *and null hypothesis (6.27) should be easy to reject.*

Theorem 6.20. *Theorem 6.18 holds with null hypothesis (6.24) replaced by null hypothesis (6.27).*

The following is an historical example that caused a firestorm of controversy. Methods of response-adaptive randomization have improved, but this trial remains very instructive, both to illustrate calculations and highlight potential pitfalls of response-adaptive randomization.

Example 6.21. (ECMO Trial) The Extracorporeal Membrane Oxygenation (ECMO) trial in infants with primary pulmonary hypertension was described in Example 5.2. Briefly, babies with primary pulmonary hypertension were randomized to a standard treatment S (putting the baby on a ventilator) or a new treatment N (an outside the body heart and lung machine). Because of the very high expected mortality on S, a response-adaptive urn randomization scheme was used. The urn initially had 1 N ball and 1 S ball, so the first baby had probability 1/2 of being assigned to N (resp., S). If the ith baby was assigned to N and lived or S and died, the selected ball would be replaced and an N ball would be added, while if baby i was assigned to N and died or S and lived, the selected ball would be replaced and an S ball would be added. The actual results were as follows. The first baby was assigned to N and survived, the second was assigned to S and died, and the next 10 were all assigned to N and survived. Randomization ceased at that point with the results shown in Table 6.4.

Table 6.4: Results of the ECMO trial.

	Dead	Alive	
New Treatment	0	11	11
Standard Treatment	1	0	1
	1	11	12

Begg (1990) and commentary thereafter delineate several potential problems with attempts to analyze ECMO data. First, the trial was stopped not because results surpassed a pre-specified boundary, but because of a perception that the totality of evidence supported a beneficial effect of the new treatment. Second, the total sample size was small and the imbalance in numbers of babies assigned to the two treatments was huge. The only more lopsided sample size would be 12-0, in which case the difference in mortality proportions would not even be defined! Moreover, the sample sizes themselves give information about the treatment effect: the reason so many babies were assigned to the new treatment was that it appeared to be working. This dependence between sample size and treatment effect is problematic for standard analysis methods.

Table 6.5: Outcome vector y (0 for survival, 1 for death) and the 12 possible treatment assignment vectors $z^{(1)}, \ldots, z^{(12)}$ yielding 11 babies assigned to N ($z_i = 1$) and 1 baby assigned to S ($z_i = 0$) in ECMO.

Baby	1	2	3	4	5	6	7	8	9	10	11	12
y	0	1	0	0	0	0	0	0	0	0	0	0
$z^{(1)}$	0	1	1	1	1	1	1	1	1	1	1	1
$z^{(2)}$	1	0	1	1	1	1	1	1	1	1	1	1
$\vdots$												
$z^{(12)}$	1	1	1	1	1	1	1	1	1	1	1	0

One common method that is not valid for analyzing the ECMO trial is Fisher's exact test. It considers each possible randomization vector that produces the same numbers, 11 and 1, of babies assigned to N and S. The 12 such randomization vectors shown in Table 6.5 are then assumed to be equally likely. Because the actual randomization vector z_{act} yields the most extreme value, 0, for the upper left cell of Table 6.4, the one-tailed p-value using Fisher's exact test is $1/12 = 0.083$. Equivalently, we can perform the usual Fisher exact calculation:

$$p = \binom{11}{0}\binom{1}{1} / \binom{12}{1} = 1/12 = 0.083. \tag{6.28}$$

However, we will see below that the different randomizations leading to 11 Ns and 1 S are not equally likely, so Fisher's exact test is **not** appropriate.

A re-randomization test is one of very few valid frequentist analyses of ECMO data, as asymptotic methods are inappropriate with such small sample sizes. To perform a re-randomization test, fix y shown in Table 6.5, and compute the conditional distribution of Z given $Y = y$. For example, consider the treatment assignment vector actually observed, $z_{act} = (1, 0, 1, 1, 1, 1, 1, 1, 1, 1, 1, 1)$. The first baby's assignment is Bernoulli $(1/2)$. Because that baby was assigned to N and survived, there are 2 N balls and 1 S ball in the urn at the time baby 2 is assigned. Therefore, the probability that baby 2 is assigned to S is $1/3$. Because baby 2 was assigned to S and died, there are 3 N balls and 1 S ball at the time baby 3 is assigned: baby 3 has probability $3/4$ of being assigned to N, and so on. Table 6.6 shows, for each baby, the composition of the urn just prior to that baby's treatment assignment.

Table 6.6: Actual treatment assignment vector (row 2) and numbers of new therapy (N) and standard therapy (S) balls in the urn just prior to each assignment (row 3) in the ECMO trial.

Baby	1	2	3	4	5	6	7	8	9	10	11	12
z_{act}	1	0	1	1	1	1	1	1	1	1	1	1
# N,	1 N	2 N	3 N	4 N	5 N	6 N	7 N	8 N	9 N	10 N	11 N	12 N
# S	1 S	1 S	1 S	1 S	1 S	1 S	1 S	1 S	1 S	1 S	1 S	1 S

The probability of the actual randomization z_{act} is

$$P(Z = z_{act}) = \left(\frac{1}{2}\right)\left(\frac{1}{3}\right)\left(\frac{3}{4}\right)\left(\frac{4}{5}\right)\left(\frac{5}{6}\right)\left(\frac{6}{7}\right)\left(\frac{7}{8}\right)$$
$$\times \left(\frac{8}{9}\right)\left(\frac{9}{10}\right)\left(\frac{10}{11}\right)\left(\frac{11}{12}\right)\left(\frac{12}{13}\right) = \frac{1}{26}.$$

Similar calculations show that $P\{Z = (0, 1, \ldots, 1)\} = 1/1716$ (exercise) and $P(Z = z) = 1/429$ for each z with a single 0, where that 0 occurs in one of positions 3–12. There are 10 such zs. This shows that if we condition on row and column totals of Table 6.4, as in Fisher's exact test, the one-tailed p-value is actually

$$\frac{1/26}{1/26 + 1/1716 + 10/429} = 66/107 = 0.617. \tag{6.29}$$

What a stark difference between (6.29) and (6.28)! The much larger p-value (6.29) results from the fact that z_{act} is the most likely by far among randomizations yielding the row and column totals of Table 6.4. But we should **not** condition on row and column totals because they are very informative about the treatment effect. With simple randomization, the row and column totals give very little information about the treatment effect, so it is appropriate to condition on them. However, conditioning on them when response-adaptive randomization is used actually conditions away a large part of the treatment effect.

If we do not condition on row and column totals, we have a different problem: all 12 babies could be assigned to the same treatment. If we continue to use as test statistic the upper left cell of Table 6.4, then the same test statistic value is obtained for the actual randomization vector as for the one randomizing all babies to the new treatment. It seems odd to consider these two cases comparable when the latter offers no data about the mortality on the standard treatment! If we instead try to use the difference in proportions, this test statistic is not even defined when $z = (0, \ldots, 0)$ or $(1, \ldots, 1)$. One possible solution is to use the difference in proportions but compute a p-value by excluding these two extreme randomization vectors. In short, not conditioning on row and column totals is far preferable to conditioning on them, but has its own problems.

The bottom line is that analysis of ECMO data was very problematic for classical statisticians. Bayesians, on the other hand, have no problems analyzing ECMO data. Their inferences depend only on the prior distribution and the observed data, not the method of randomization. This may explain the perception that a higher proportion of Bayesians than classical statisticians support response-adaptive randomization.   □

6.6   Re-randomization Tests and Strength of Randomized Evidence

Re-randomization tests properly express the strength of evidence in a clinical trial by focusing on randomization as the basis for inference. For example, consider a community-randomized trial with a continuous outcome. Suppose there are 1,000 people in each community, and 20 communities. Once a community is randomized, all 1,000 people receive T or all 1,000 receive C. A re-randomization corresponds to either keeping all 1,000 on the assigned condition or switching all 1,000 to the opposite condition (permuting en masse). The re-randomization test is approximately equivalent to an unpaired t-test on 20 community-specific sample means (i.e., 18 degrees of freedom). The re-randomization test automatically equates the strength of evidence to roughly an unpaired t-test on 20 observations, recognizing that the data for the 1,000 people within a community are correlated.

A statistical novice might erroneously use a t-test based on 20x1,000=20,000 observations, not realizing that data within the same community are correlated. This erroneous test is asymptotically equivalent to a re-randomization test in which **individuals** are re-randomized rather than communities. One who carefully follows the original randomization scheme when conducting a re-randomization test will not make this mistake.

You may think that the above error is too obvious for any real statistician to commit, but it can occur in a more subtle form. For example, people sometimes argue that differences between patients can be modeled and removed using covariates, resulting in data that can be treated as independent. This would again be like having virtually 20x1,000=20,000 independent pieces of data. A proper adjusted analysis could be performed using a re-randomization test. Without knowledge of community-specific treatment labels, fit a model with covariates and a community-specific intercept. Now do a re-randomization test on these intercepts. The level of evidence would properly reflect roughly 20 independent pieces of information instead of 20,000.

Another illustration of how re-randomization tests gauge the level of actual randomized evidence is provided by the following example.

Example 6.22. Very Poor Allocation Scheme   Imagine a very poorly designed trial in which the following allocation scheme is used. The first patient is assigned randomly to one of the arms. The same treatment continues to be given until a failure occurs, at which time the opposite treatment is given until a failure occurs, and so on. For example, suppose that the randomization vector is (T,T,C,C,C,T,C...). The first failure occurred at patient number 2, causing the third patient to be assigned to C. The next failure occurred at patient number 5, causing a switch to T, and so on. With this allocation scheme, the only patient actually **randomized** is the first one. Therefore, given the outcomes, there are only 2 possible treatment sequences, (T,T,C,C,C,T,C,...) and (C,C,T,T,T,C,T...). The conditional probability of each of these sequences, given the data, is 1/2. A two-tailed re-randomization test will have p-value 1, even if the sample size is 10,000. The re-randomization test is reflecting the amount of actual **randomized** trial evidence.   □

Example 6.22 seems silly, but a similar phenomenon can occur when the assignment probabilities become close to 0 or 1. This happened in the ECMO trial (see Examples 5.2 and 6.21); the urn became stacked so heavily in favor of the new treatment that assignment to the new treatment became almost deterministic. One should avoid allocation schemes with such extreme probabilities.

6.7   Confidence Intervals

Thus far we have focused exclusively on re-randomization tests, but confidence intervals are also an important component of the analysis of a clinical trial. Associated with a re-randomization test is a confidence interval that assumes a common treatment effect across participants (Branson and Bind, 2019). The first step in constructing a confidence interval is constructing a test of a nonzero null hypothesis using the notion of *potential outcomes.*
 Potential outcomes are the outcome the patient would have if assigned to control and the outcome the patient would have if assigned to treatment. We see the outcome for the treatment actually assigned, but we do not see the *counterfactual outcome,* the outcome that would have occurred if the patient had been assigned to the opposite treatment.

We illustrate how to use potential outcomes to construct a test of a nonzero null hypothesis using a clinical trial of patients coinfected with HIV and hepatitis C virus (HCV). Hepatitis C treatment is less effective if the patient also has HIV. We hope that the new treatment N lowers viral load, the amount of virus in the blood, better than the standard treatment S. The primary outcome is change in log viral load from baseline to 7 days. The first two columns of Table 6.7 are the 1-week change in log viral load (y) and treatment assignment (z), where $z = 0$ (resp., $z = 1$) denotes the standard (resp., new) treatment.

Table 6.7: y =change in hepatitis C log viral load from baseline to 1 week, z =treatment assignment (0 for standard treatment, 1 for new treatment), and y_{cf} =counterfactual outcome had the opposite randomization occurred, computed under the assumption that the new treatment reduces log viral load by 0.5 more than the standard treatment.

y	z	y_{cf} for assignment $1 - z$
-1.11	0	-1.61
-0.57	0	-1.07
-0.01	0	-0.51
-1.02	0	-1.52
0.00	0	-0.50
-0.13	0	-0.63
-0.77	0	-1.27
-0.38	0	-0.88
0.08	0	-0.42
-0.09	0	-0.59
-1.01	1	-0.51
0.07	1	0.57
-2.15	1	-1.65
-0.24	1	0.26
-0.23	1	0.27
-1.59	1	-1.09
-2.31	1	-1.81
-1.47	1	-0.97

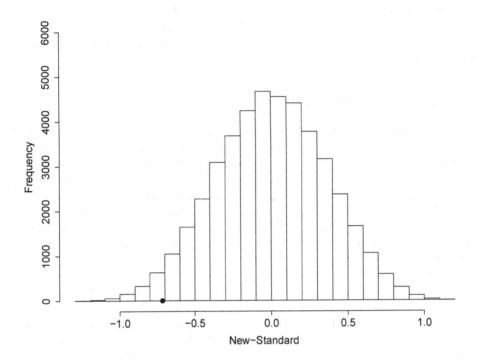

Figure 6.6: Re-randomization distribution for the difference in means, new minus standard, in change in log HCV viral load from baseline to 1 week in the HIV/HCV trial. The dot shows the observed difference in means.

The new minus standard mean log viral load was -0.716, which lies in the left tail of the re-randomization distribution shown in Figure 6.6. Assume that the true effect of the new treatment **in every patient** is a lowering of log viral load by the same amount, δ, relative to the standard treatment. The one-tailed p-value for the null hypothesis $H_0 : \delta = 0$ versus alternative hypothesis $H_1 : \delta < 0$ is 0.022. Because this p-value is less than 0.025, we have good evidence that $\delta < 0$, but can we rule out other values of δ? For example, can we be confident that the benefit of the new treatment relative to the standard treatment is at least 0.5 (i.e., that $\delta < -0.5$)? Column 3 of Table 6.7 shows the counterfactual outcome if the patient had been assigned to the opposite arm under the assumption that $\delta = -0.5$. For example, the first patient was actually assigned to the standard treatment and had a 1.11 reduction in log viral load at 1 week (i.e., $y = -1.11$). Assume that if the patient had been assigned to the new treatment, he/she would have had a benefit 0.5 better than under the standard treatment. That is, the change in log viral load would have been $-1.11 - 0.5 = -1.61$. Similarly, for every patient assigned to the standard treatment, that patient's counterfactual outcome would have been $y_{\mathrm{cf}} = y - 0.5$ if assigned to the new treatment. Every patient assigned to the new treatment would have had a 0.5 worse change in log viral load if the treatment assignment had instead been to the standard treatment. Thus, the counterfactual outcome for a patient actually assigned to the new treatment would have been $y_{\mathrm{cf}} = y + 0.5$ if he/she had instead been assigned to the standard treatment.

Construct a re-randomization p-value for the test of $H_0 : \delta = -0.5$ versus $H_1 : \delta < -0.5$ as follows:

1. Re-randomize according to the original randomization scheme.

2. For a patient whose re-randomization assignment z_{re} was the same as the actual assignment z of that patient, use y from column 1 of Table 6.7, but for patients whose re-randomization assignment z_{re} was $1 - z$, the opposite of what was actually assigned, use counterfactual outcome y_{cf} from column 3 of Table 6.7.

3. Compute $\bar{y}_{N,re} - \bar{y}_{S,re}$ for the re-randomized assignments.

4. Repeat the above steps for every possible re-randomization vector (or, if that is too computationally intensive, simulate a large number of re-randomization vectors) and compute the proportion of re-randomized results with a new minus standard mean log viral load of -0.716 or less (i.e., a difference at least as strong, in favor of the new treatment, as the observed difference, -0.716).

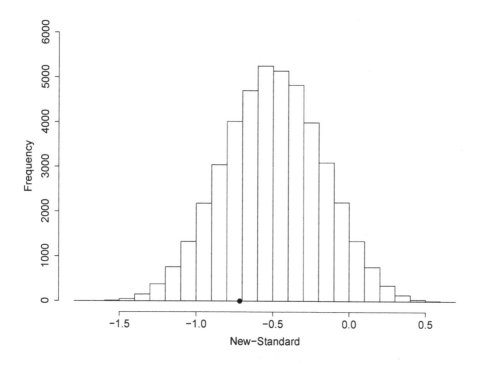

Figure 6.7: Re-randomization distribution of the difference in means, new minus standard, for the test of $H_0 : \delta = -0.5$ versus $H_1 : \delta < -0.5$ in the HIV/HCV trial. The dot shows the observed difference in means.

Figure 6.7 shows the reference distribution constructed using the counterfactual method assuming that $\delta = -0.5$. Now the observed result does not look unusually small as it did in Figure 6.6. The one-tailed p-value for testing $H_0 : \delta = -0.5$ versus $H_1 : \delta < -0.5$, namely the proportion of re-randomized trials with $\bar{y}_{N,re} - \bar{y}_{S,re} \leq -0.716$, is 0.26. Therefore, we do not have strong evidence that $\delta < -0.5$. We can successively test $H_0 : \delta = \delta_0$ versus $H_1 : \delta < \delta_0$ for different values of δ_0 until we find δ_0 such that the re-randomization p-value is 0.025. We denote that value of δ_0 by δ_U because it will become the upper limit of the 95% confidence interval for δ. In this example, $\delta_U = -0.01$. Similarly, we can test $H_0 : \delta = \delta_0$ versus $H_1 : \delta > \delta_0$ for different values of δ_0 and find the value δ_L for δ_0 such that the re-randomization p-value is 0.025; δ_L is the lower limit of the 95% confidence interval for δ. In this example, $\delta_L = -1.424$ (see Figure 6.8). The errors associated with the lower and upper endpoint are each 2.5%, so the error associated with the statement that both $\delta < -0.01$ and $\delta > -1.424$ is $2.5\% + 2.5\% = 5\%$. In other words, we are $(100 - 5)\% = 95\%$ confident that

$$-1.424 < \delta < -0.01.$$

The same technique works for different randomization methods, and can be generalized to allow different patients to have different responses to treatment (Branson and Bind, 2019).

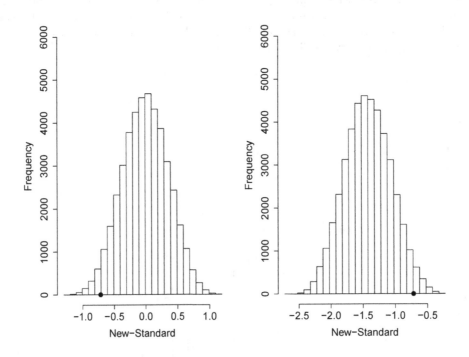

Figure 6.8: Re-randomization distributions of the difference in means, new minus standard, for the test of $H_0 : \delta = -0.01$ versus $H_1 : \delta < -0.01$ (left) and of $H_0 : \delta = -1.424$ versus $H_1 : \delta > -1.424$ (right) in the HIV/HCV trial. The dot shows the observed difference in means. The p-value for each test is 0.025.

6.8   Philosophical Criticism of Re-randomization Tests

Basu (1980) criticizes re-randomization tests on the grounds that they incorporate information from random experiments that should not influence decision-making. Consider the ECMO response-adaptive trial of Example 6.21. Suppose you know nothing about the trial, and someone tells you that none of the eleven babies randomized to the new treatment died, while the lone baby assigned to the standard treatment died. Then you are told that additional experiments were performed in which certain numbers of balls of two different colors were placed in an urn and drawn randomly. Once you know the numbers of babies who died under the two different treatments, should results of the random urn experiments have any bearing on your inferences? Intuitively, the answer is no. The only relevant information is that 0 out of 11 babies given the new treatment died and 1 out of 1 baby given the standard treatment died. While we understand this criticism, we are more persuaded by performance of procedures than by philosophical arguments. Re-randomization tests are very flexible; they can be used with any randomization method. They are often asymptotically equivalent to t-tests that are known to have optimal properties. Re-randomization tests protect against temporal trends and control the conditional type I error rate given the outcome data, which is advantageous with adaptive methods. For instance, we have seen that one can rummage through different models, pick the baseline covariates most correlated with outcome, and use a re-randomization test on residuals without paying a penalty for multiple comparisons. We do not believe that there is an alternative method that achieves all of the advantages of re-randomization tests and avoids the philosophical concern raised above. Bayesian methodology has some advantages, including avoiding the philosophical issue, but also has the disadvantage that results depend on the prior distribution selected. Re-randomization tests and Bayesian approaches both have attractive features, and should be part of the armamentarium of any clinical trialist.

Exercises

1. Name an advantage of a re-randomization test over a parametric test in a clinical trial.

2. Suppose that in the COMMIT example (Example 6.1), within each pair, the quit rate had been higher in the intervention community than in the control community. What would the one-tailed p-value have been for the re-randomization test?

3. In a paired data setting with a re-randomization test, what is the minimum number of pairs required to be able to achieve a one-tailed p-value of 0.05 or less?

4. Consider a re-randomization test in a paired setting using the treatment minus control mean difference $\bar{D}$ as test statistic. Suppose that the paired differences are $5, 2, 0, -1$.

    (a) What is the p-value if we reject the null hypothesis for large values of $\bar{D}$?

    (b) Now eliminate the 0 and recompute the p-value. Does the p-value change?

5. Consider an unpaired setting with n patients per arm using statistic $\bar{Y}_T - \bar{Y}_C$, the difference in sample means. If all of the treatment observations exceed all of the control observations, what will be the p-value for a one-tailed re-randomization test with alternative hypothesis that treatment tends to produce larger values?

6. In an unpaired setting with n patients per arm using $\bar{Y}_T - \bar{Y}_C$ as test statistic, what is the smallest n for which a one-tailed re-randomization test can be statistically significant at level $\alpha = 0.05$?

7. In an unpaired setting using $\bar{Y}_T - \bar{Y}_C$ as test statistic, the data are shown in Table 6.8. What is the two-tailed p-value when you condition on sample sizes of 3 per arm? If $\alpha = 0.05$, is there enough evidence to conclude that treatment has any effect?

Table 6.8: Data from a very small trial.

Control	0.52	1.67	1.00
Treatment	2.18	3.15	1.45

8. The following data were generated by simulation from a $N(0, 1)$ distribution in the control arm and a $N(\delta, 1)$ distribution in the treatment arm, where δ is such that power for a two-tailed, unpaired t-test is approximately 0.85. Compute the lumped and pooled variances, s_L^2 and S_P^2. Are they similar?

Table 6.9: Data from a an unpaired trial.

C	.13	-.24	.10	.49	.84	-.55	-.72	.01	1.68	1.02
T	1.59	2.09	-.38	.73	-.53	1.77	-.08	.26	-.77	-.14

9. Consider the setting of problem 12 of Chapter 5, where at each center, the first and third patients are assigned to T and the second is assigned to C. If there is a temporal trend such that the first patient at each center tends to have larger values than subsequent patients, will a t-test control the type I error rate? What about a re-randomization test?

10. Do you think that the sample sizes in the ECMO trial would have been as lopsided as they were if they had started with 10 N balls and 10 S balls in the urn instead of 1 and 1? What is the tradeoff of starting with a larger number of balls of each type?

11. Suppose that the data in Example 6.10 are $y = (120, 111, 116, 133, 100, 110, 127, 140, 95, 122, 135, 147, 155, 130, 160, 150, 139, 125, 165, 102)$. What is the mean of the re-randomization distribution of $\bar{Y}_T - \bar{Y}_C = (1/10) \sum_{i=1}^{20} (2Z_i - 1)y_i$?

12. Consider a trial of two different eyedrops, A or B, to eliminate redness. One trial design randomizes participants to eyedrop A or B, and the participant applies that eyedrop to both eyes. The second design randomizes eyes within each participant, one eye receiving eyedrop A, the other eyedrop B.

   (a) Describe how you would you conduct the re-randomization test for each trial.

   (b) If the number of participants is large, what type of t-test (paired or unpaired) will the re-randomization test be close to for each design?

   (c) If the correlation between the degree of redness in the two eyes is high, which of the two trial designs is more efficient?

13. For the ECMO trial, given the observed outcome vector:

   (a) Show that the probability that $Z = (0, 1, 1, \ldots, 1)$ is 1/1716 by constructing a table similar to Table 6.6 and mimicking the calculations that follow the table.

   (b) What is the probability that $Z = (1, 1, \ldots, 1)$?

14. An 'n of 1' trial was conducted to see whether ritalin improved concentration in a specific student diagnosed with attention deficit disorder. Ritalin can be given episodically because it is excreted from the body within hours. Each week, a coin flip determined whether ritalin would be given on Monday and placebo on Tuesday, or placebo on Monday and ritalin on Tuesday. The primary outcome was the teacher's rating of the student's performance using a 5-point scale similar to the grades A,B,C,D, and F. Suppose that a paired re-randomization test is used whereby treatment and placebo labels for each (Monday, Tuesday) pair are switched or not.

   (a) Is this re-randomization test 'valid' for drawing conclusions about this individual student?

   (b) Would you be confident that the results of this n-of-1 study apply to other students? Would your answer to this question be different if you used a paired t-test instead of a re-randomization test to analyze the data?

(c) If the number of weeks is large and the weeks can be regarded as a random sample from this student, will the re-randomization test give approximately the same results as a paired t-test?

15. In a trial of a very rare disease with an extremely promising treatment, 6 people are randomized to treatment or control in a block of size 6, but in such a way that simple randomization is used until there are 3 Ts or 3 Cs, with the remaining patients assigned to the remaining arm (this is called *truncated binomial randomization*). All 3 patients on treatment have a successful outcome, while none in the control arm have a successful outcome.

    (a) If a p-value is computed by erroneously assuming ordinary permuted block randomization in which each block is equally likely, what is the one-tailed p-value?

    (b) Conditioned on the outcome vector $y = (1, 0, 0, 1, 1, 0)$ but not z, what is the actual type I error rate if we reject H_0 when the erroneously computed one-tailed p-value in part (a) is ≤ 0.05?

16. One big difference between patient-randomized and community-randomized trials is that communities are identified in advance, whereas patients usually arrive sequentially. This makes it possible in a community-randomized trial to evaluate, before randomization, the between-arm covariate balance for each possible randomization vector z. Suppose that one identifies the k randomization vectors $z_1, \ldots, z_k$ that produce the most balance, and then randomly picks one of these z_i.

    (a) Describe how a re-randomization test could be conducted.

    (b) Suppose that $k = 1$ (i.e., we always select the randomization vector that produces the greatest balance). What is the re-randomization p-value?

    (c) What are the tradeoffs of picking a small versus large value of k?

17. In a *stepped wedge* community-randomized vaccine trial with 2 periods, each community will receive vaccine eventually and will continue receiving it until the end of the trial. Randomization of communities is to time of start of the vaccine; half will start in period 1 and half in period 2. Suppose that the outcome for each community is the difference in rates of infection between the first and second periods. Describe how you could conduct a re-randomization test.

18. For simplicity, we have focused on re-randomization tests when there is a single primary outcome variable, but re-randomization tests can be used with multiple primary outcomes as well. Consider a trial with three primary outcome variables, Y_1, Y_2, Y_3, and let P_1, P_2, P_3 be the p-values for comparing treatment and control with respect to Y_1, Y_2, Y_3. Describe how to conduct a re-randomization test for the statistic $\min(P_1, P_2, P_3)$. Does the re-randomization test work regardless of the correlation between the Ys?

6.9 Appendix: The Permutation Variance of $\bar{Y}_C - \bar{Y}_T$

The permutation variance of $\bar{y}_T - \bar{y}_C$, from (6.15), is

$\text{var}_{\mathbf{Z}}(\bar{y}_C - \bar{y}_T)$

$$= \text{var}\left\{ \frac{\sum_{i=1}^{n} y_i}{n_C} - \left(\sum_{i=1}^{n} y_i Z_i\right)(1/n_T + 1/n_C) \right\}$$

$$= 0 + (1/n_T + 1/n_C)^2 \text{var}\left(\sum_{i=1}^{n} y_i Z_i\right)$$

$$= \frac{n^2}{n_T^2 n_C^2} \text{cov}\left(\sum_{i=1}^{n} y_i Z_i, \sum_{j=1}^{n} y_j Z_j\right) \quad \text{where } n = n_T + n_C$$

$$= \frac{n^2}{n_T^2 n_C^2} \sum_{i=1}^{n}\sum_{j=1}^{n} y_i y_j \text{cov}(Z_i, Z_j). \tag{6.30}$$

When $i = j$, the covariance between Z_i and Z_j is the variance of Z_i. The marginal distribution of Z_i is Bernoulli with parameter $p = n_T/n$, so its variance is $p(1-p) = n_T n_C/n^2$.

When $i \neq j$,

$$\text{cov}(Z_i, Z_j) = \text{E}(Z_i Z_j) - \text{E}(Z_i)\text{E}(Z_j)$$

$$= P(Z_i = 1, Z_j = 1) - p^2$$

$$= P(Z_i = 1)P(Z_j = 1 \mid Z_i = 1) - \left(\frac{n_T}{n}\right)^2$$

$$= \left(\frac{n_T}{n}\right)\left(\frac{n_T - 1}{n - 1}\right) - \left(\frac{n_T}{n}\right)^2$$

$$= \left(\frac{n_T}{n}\right)\left\{\frac{n_T - 1}{n - 1} - \frac{n_T}{n}\right\}$$

$$= -\frac{n_T n_C}{n^2(n - 1)} \tag{6.31}$$

Putting everything together, we find that the re-randomization variance of $\bar{y}_T - \bar{y}_C$ is

$$\frac{n^2}{n_T^2 n_C^2}\left[\sum_{i=1}^{n} y_i^2\left(\frac{n_T n_C}{n^2}\right) + \sum\sum_{i \neq j} y_i y_j\left\{-\frac{n_T n_C}{n^2(n - 1)}\right\}\right]$$

$$= \frac{\sum_{i=1}^{n} y_i^2}{n_T n_C} - \frac{\sum\sum_{i \neq j} y_i y_j}{n_T n_C(n - 1)}$$

$$= \frac{1}{n_T n_C}\left\{\sum_{i=1}^{n} y_i^2 - \frac{(\sum_{i=1}^{n} y_i)^2 - \sum_{i=1}^{n} y_i^2}{(n - 1)}\right\}$$

$$= \frac{1}{n_T n_C}\left\{\left(1 + \frac{1}{n - 1}\right)\sum_{i=1}^{n} y_i^2 - \frac{(\sum_{i=1}^{n} y_i)^2}{n - 1}\right\}$$

$$= \left(\frac{1}{n_T n_C}\right)\left(\frac{n}{n - 1}\right)\left\{\sum_{i=1}^{n} y_i^2 - \frac{(\sum_{i=1}^{n} y_i)^2}{n}\right\}$$

$$= \left(\frac{1}{n_T n_C}\right)\left(\frac{n}{n - 1}\right)\sum_{i=1}^{n}(y_i - \bar{y})^2$$

$$= s_L^2(1/n_T + 1/n_C), \tag{6.32}$$

where $s_L^2 = (n - 1)^{-1}\sum_{i=1}^{n}(y_i - \bar{y})^2$ is the lumped variance of all $n = n_T + n_C$ observations.

6.10 Summary

Re-randomization tests have the following properties:

1. They condition on outcome data (randomness stems solely from the treatment labels), so they control the conditional type I error rate given outcome data.

2. They can condition on ancillary statistics like sample sizes, but not with adaptive randomization because sample sizes may not be ancillary.

3. They are valid tests of the (strong) null hypothesis that treatment has no effect on anyone. We can view the null hypothesis as H_0 : data were generated first, then treatment labels according to the given randomization method.

4. They protect against temporal trends.

5. They are asymptotically equivalent to t-tests when traditional randomization is used.

6. They can be used on adjusted treatment effect estimators to attain an added layer of protection.

7. They can be inverted to produce confidence intervals.

We recommend following the 'analyze as you randomize principle':

Principle 6.23. Analyze as you randomize principle *Always analyze data the same way they were randomized. A re-randomization test is the strictest form of this principle. A weaker form asserts that a stratified analysis should be performed whenever stratified randomization is used.*

Chapter 7

Survival Analysis

7.1 Introduction to Survival Methods

In this chapter, we summarize the most common methods of dealing with time-to-event data. These methods constitute *survival analysis*, although the event need not be death. It is often a composite event such as either heart attack or death. The clock usually begins at the time of randomization, and ends at the first event of the composite. For instance, if a patient experiences a heart attack 1 year following randomization and dies 6 months later, the time to event is 1 year. In some cases the event is beneficial. For example, in trials of infectious diseases, interest may be on time to clearance of the disease.

How is time to an event different from other continuous outcomes such as cholesterol, blood pressure, or amount of virus in the body? Many people may not have the event of interest over the course of the study. If a patient amasses 3 years of follow-up without having the event, what is his/her time to event? Likewise, if a patient leaves the trial after 1 year of follow-up and has not yet had the event, what do we do? In either case, we do not actually know the time to event because the event has not yet occurred. All we know is that the time to event was at least 3 years for patient 1 and at least 1 year for patient 2. Their actual time to event is said to be *censored*. We call the data *right-censored* because the event occurred at some point to the 'right' of (i.e., after) the censoring time. *Left censoring*, on the other hand, indicates that the event occurred to the 'left' of (i.e., before) the censoring time. For example, we may know only that the patient had the disease at the end of the trial, but the time the patient actually acquired it is not known. *Interval censoring* results when the event of interest is known to have occurred some point between time A and time B. For example, the disease status was known to be negative at time A, and positive at time B. We focus on the most common and straightforward type of censoring in clinical trials, namely right censoring.

How do we handle right-censored observations? Treating them as times to event underestimates the actual times to event. On the other hand, omitting patients with censored observations fails to credit them for the time they amassed without experiencing the event. Either way, we get a biased estimate of the actual time to event. To make any progress, we usually make the assumption that the censoring mechanism does not give us any information about the remaining time to event. This is called *noninformative censoring*. A patient who leaves the study because her job forces her to relocate to another country probably constitutes a case of noninformative censoring. On the other hand, in a clinical trial of substance abusers, someone who stops showing up for his drug tests because he is arrested for possession of drugs undoubtedly constitutes a case of *informative censoring*, meaning that the censoring gives us additional information about the time to event.

DOI: 10.1201/9781315164090-7

7.2   Kaplan-Meier Survival Curve

The first step in survival analysis is to construct a *survival curve*, namely the probability of surviving t years, for different values of t. The most popular survival curve is the *Kaplan-Meier survival curve*. Table 7.1 shows results from a small, 2-year study with only 11 patients. Six patients died at times 0.8, 1.2, 1.2, 1.3, 1.4, and 1.8 years. The other times are followed by a plus sign, indicating right-censored observations. One patient left the study after 1 year, while 4 patients survived to the end of their follow-up at 2 years.

Table 7.1: Data from a survival study with 11 patients.

t	0.8	1.0+	1.2	1.2	1.3	1.4	1.8	2+	2+	2+	2+

Consider the probability of surviving past the first observed time, 0.8 years. Because 10 of 11 patients survived 0.8 years, we estimate $S(0.8)$, the probability of surviving 0.8 years, as $\hat{S}(0.8) = 10/11$. Now consider the second time, 1 year. To survive 1 year, one must first survive 0.8 years, then survive 1 year given survival to 0.8 years. All 10 people who survived 0.8 years, including the one who was censored at 1 year, survived 1 year. Therefore, we estimate the conditional probability $S(1\,|\,T > 0.8) = P(T > 1\,|\,T > 0.8)$ as $10/10$. We estimate $S(1)$ by

$$\hat{S}(1) = \hat{S}(0.8)\hat{S}(1\,|\,T > 0.8) = (10/11)(10/10) = 10/11.$$

Similarly, to compute the probability of surviving 1.2 years, we multiply the estimated probability of surviving 1 year by an estimate of the conditional probability of surviving 1.2 years, given survival to 1 year. The censored observation at 1 year cannot be used to calculate this conditional probability because we have no information on that patient after 1 year. Of the 9 other patients who have not died or been censored by 1 year, 7 survived 1.2 years. Therefore, we estimate $S(1.2\,|\,T > 1)$ by $7/9$. Our estimate of $S(1.2)$ is

$$\hat{S}(1.2) = \hat{S}(1)\hat{S}(1.2\,|\,T > 1) = (10/11)(7/9) = 70/99.$$

We continue this process at all censoring and death times.

The computation of the survival curve is depicted in Figure 7.2. The arrows show the zigzagging process of multiplying the estimated survival probability $\hat{S}(t_{i-1})$ at the preceding time point by the estimate $\hat{S}(t_i\,|\,T > t_{i-1})$ of the conditional probability of surviving the current time point, given survival to the previous time point. Note that the Kaplan-Meier curve changes only at death times. We can express the Kaplan-Meier estimator in compact form as follows. Let n_i be the *number at risk* at time t_i, meaning the number of people who, immediately prior to time t_i, have not yet died or been censored. Let d_i denote the number of people who die at time t_i. Then the Kaplan-Meier estimator of the probability of surviving time t is

$$\hat{S}(t) = \prod_{i:t_i \leq t} \left(1 - \frac{d_i}{n_i}\right).$$

Note that if there is no censoring, the Kaplan-Meier estimate reduces to $1 - \hat{F}(t)$, where $\hat{F}(t) = (1/n)\sum_{i=1}^{n} d_i I(d_i \leq t)$ is the sample distribution function.

Plotting the survival probabilities against time produces the Kaplan-Meier curve in Figure 7.2.

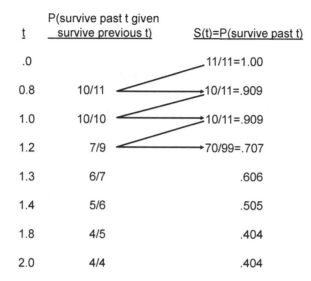

Figure 7.1: Process of computing the Kaplan-Meier survival curve.

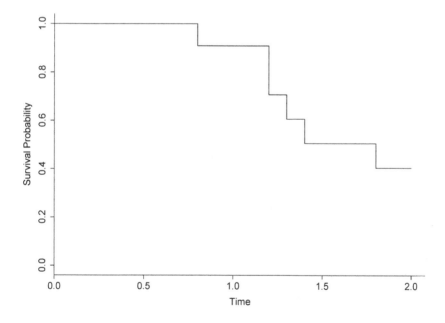

Figure 7.2: Kaplan-Meier survival curve.

In small trials, sizes of drops in the survival curve are large and the curve is unstable (Figure 7.2). In large trials, sizes of drops are small and the survival curve appears nearly continuous (Figure 7.3).

The Kaplan-Meier estimate $\hat{S}(t)$ is approximately normally distributed if the sample size is large and the true survival probability $S(t)$ is not too close to 0 or 1. One method of constructing a confidence interval or test for the probability of surviving a given time point

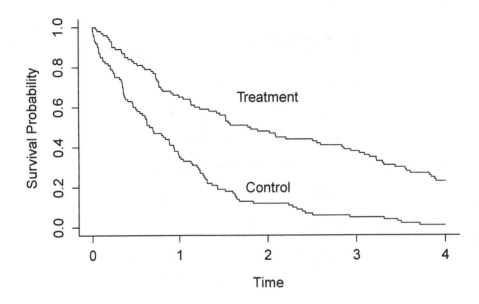

Figure 7.3: Kaplan-Meier survival curve in a more typical clinical trial with more than 100 events.

uses *Greenwood's variance formula*:

$$\widehat{V}_{GW} = \widehat{\mathrm{var}}\{\widehat{S}(t)\} = \{\widehat{S}(t)\}^2 \sum_{i:t_i \leq t}^{n} \frac{d_i}{n_i(n_i - d_i)}. \tag{7.1}$$

An approximate $100(1 - \alpha)\%$ confidence interval for $S(t)$ is therefore

$$\widehat{S}(t) \pm z_{\alpha/2}\sqrt{\widehat{V}_{GW}}. \tag{7.2}$$

A problem with confidence interval (7.2) is that the endpoints of the interval can be outside the range $[0, 1]$, whereas $S(t)$ must lie in $[0, 1]$. When an estimator is nonnegative such as $\widehat{S}(t)$, a logarithmic transformation often reduces skew and improves accuracy. Using the delta method, we see that $\ln\{\widehat{S}(t)\}$ is approximately normally distributed with mean $\ln\{S(t)\}$ and variance estimated by $= \sum_{i:t_i \leq t} \frac{d_i}{n_i(n_i - d_i)}$. But because $\widehat{S}(t) \leq 1$, $\ln\{\widehat{S}(t)\} \leq 0$. That is, $-\ln\{\widehat{S}(t)\} \geq 0$. A second logarithmic transformation $\ln[-\ln\{\widehat{S}(t)\}]$ seems in order. Again using the delta method, we find that $\ln[-\ln\{\widehat{S}(t)\}]$ is asymptotically normal with mean $\ln[-\ln\{\widehat{S}(t)\}]$ and variance

$$\widehat{V}_{LL} = \widehat{\mathrm{var}}\left(\ln[-\ln\{\widehat{S}(t)\}]\right) = \frac{1}{[\ln\{\widehat{S}(t)\}]^2} \sum_{i:t_i \leq t} \frac{d_i}{n_i(n_i - d_i)}. \tag{7.3}$$

The subscript LL denotes the "log log" method. The idea is to first use (7.3) to get a confidence interval for $\ln[-\ln\{S(t)\}]$, then transform back to get the following $100(1 - \alpha)\%$ confidence interval for $S(t)$:

$$\left(\widehat{S}(t)^{\exp\{z_{\alpha/2}\sqrt{\widehat{V}_{LL}}\}}, \ \widehat{S}(t)^{\exp\{-z_{\alpha/2}\sqrt{\widehat{V}_{LL}}\}}\right). \tag{7.4}$$

Interval (7.4) is guaranteed to lie in $[0, 1]$ because its lower and upper limits are both $\widehat{S}(t)$ raised to nonnegative powers.

Table 7.2: Small dataset solely to illustrate the calculation of confidence intervals for a survival trial.

t_i	d_i	n_i	$\frac{d_i}{n_i(n_i-d_i)}$
0.8	1	11	$1/110$
1.2	2	9	$2/63$
1.3	1	7	$1/42$
1.4	1	6	$1/30$
1.8	1	5	$1/20$

Solely to demonstrate the calculations, we compute confidence intervals for $S(1.35)$ for the data of Table 7.1 using the Greenwood and log-log methods. The number of events is not large enough to be confident that such intervals will have approximately the correct coverage probabilities.

The first 3 columns of Table 7.1 show times t_i of events, numbers d_i of events at each time, and numbers n_i of patients at risk just prior to each event. The fourth columns shows $d_i/\{n_i(n_i - d_i)\}$. The Kaplan-Meier estimate of survival at time 1.35 is $\hat{S}(1.35) = 60/99 = 0.606$. Therefore, the Greenwood (GW) and log-log (LL) standard deviations are

$$\sqrt{V_{\text{GW}}} = \sqrt{(60/99)^2(1/110 + 2/63 + 1/42)} = 0.154 \text{ and}$$

$$\sqrt{V_{\text{LL}}} = \sqrt{\left[\frac{1}{\{\ln(60/99)\}^2}\right](1/110 + 2/63 + 1/42)} = 0.508, \tag{7.5}$$

respectively. Therefore, the GW and LL confidence intervals for $S(1.35)$ are

$$\left(60/99 - 1.96(0.154), 60/99 + 1.96(0.154)\right) = (0.304, 0.908) \text{ and}$$

$$\left((60/99)^{\exp\{1.96\cdot0.508\}}, (60/99)^{\exp\{-1.96\cdot0.508\}}\right) = (0.258, 0.831). \tag{7.6}$$

If the numbers of events were much larger, GW's method and the LL method would produce very similar intervals, and coverage probabilities would be close to 0.95.

7.3 Comparing Survival Across Arms

7.3.1 Comparing Survival at a Specific Time

In clinical trials, we are usually interested in comparing two or more groups. To compare the survival probability at a fixed time t in the control and treatment arms, we compute the z-score

$$Z = \frac{\hat{E}_C - \hat{E}_T}{\sqrt{\hat{V}_C + \hat{V}_T}}, \tag{7.7}$$

where T and C denote treatment and control, $\hat{E}$ denotes an estimator of either $S(t)$ or $\ln[-\ln\{S(t)\}]$, and $\hat{V}$ denotes an estimator of var$(\hat{E})$. Large z-scores indicate that treatment is effective. If the number of deaths is large and the survival probabilities are not very close to 0 or 1, the z-score (7.7) has an approximate standard normal distribution under the null hypothesis that the two survival probabilities $S_T(t)$ and $S_C(t)$ are equal. Accordingly, the two-tailed p-value after observing $Z = z$ is $2\{1 - \Phi(|z|)\}$.

For example, if the Kaplan-Meier estimate of 28-day mortality and its standard error are $\hat{S}_C(28) = 0.20$ and $SE_C = 0.014$ in the control arm and $\hat{S}_T(28) = 0.15$ and $SE_T = 0.019$ in the treatment arm, the z-statistic comparing the two arms is

$$Z = \frac{0.20 - 0.15}{\sqrt{(0.014)^2 + (0.019)^2}} = 2.119,$$

so the two-tailed p-value is $2\{1 - \Phi(2.119)\} = 0.034$. A 95% confidence interval for the difference in survival probabilities is

$$0.20 - 0.15 \pm 1.96\sqrt{(0.014)^2 + (0.019)^2} = (0.004, 0.096).$$

The treatment improves survival by between 0.4 and 9.6 percentage points.

7.3.2 Logrank Test

We are often interested in comparing entire survival curves rather than survival probabilities at a single time point. When there is wide separation between curves relative to sizes of jumps within each curve, we can be confident that survival curves differ. The situation is analogous to t- or F-tests with continuous outcomes: when between-arm variability dwarfs within-arm variability, the difference between arms will be highly statistically significant (see the variability ratio principle, Principle 4.15).

A very common method to compare survival curves in treatment and control arms is the *logrank test*. The idea was first described by Mantel (1966) in a medical journal, but Peto and Peto (1972) fully developed its statistical properties. The test begins by ordering times to death, $t_1, \ldots, t_d$. Assume first that there is only one death at any given time, so that $t_1 < \ldots < t_d$. Let n_T and n_C be the numbers of patients at risk in the treatment and control arms immediately prior to the first death at time t_1. Let O_1 be 1 or 0 according to whether the first death came from the control or treatment arm, respectively. We could equally well define O_i to be the indicator of a treatment event, but we parameterize such that large values of the test statistic indicate a treatment benefit. If treatment has no effect on survival, the death is equally likely to have been any of the $n_{T1} + n_{C1}$ patients at risk. Therefore, conditioned on n_{T1} and n_{C1} and the fact that there is a single death at t_1, O_1 is a Bernoulli random variable with probability parameter $E_1 = n_{C1}/(n_{C1} + n_{T1})$; its null mean and variance are E_1 and $V_1 = E_1(1 - E_1)$. Note that we treat E_1 and V_1 as fixed constants.

Table 7.3: Typical 2×2 table.

	Dead	Alive	
Control	O_i		n_{Ci}
Treatment			n_{Ti}
	1	$n_i - 1$	n_i

$$E_i = \frac{n_{Ci} \times 1}{n_{Ci} + n_{Ti}} = \frac{n_{Ci}}{n_i} \text{ and } V_i = E_i(1 - E_i). \qquad (7.8)$$

Continuing in this way, we construct a 2×2 table at death i. Combine data across all death times: $\sum_{i=1}^{d} O_i$ and $\sum_{i=1}^{d} E_i$ are the observed and expected numbers of deaths in the control arm if treatment has no effect. The difference $\sum_{i=1}^{d}(O_i - E_i)$ is the number of excess control deaths from what would be expected by chance. If $\sum_{i=1}^{d}(O_i - E_i)$ is large enough, we conclude that treatment is effective. To determine whether the number of excess deaths is too large to have occurred by chance, we create a z-score by dividing by the null standard deviation of $\sum_{i=1}^{d}(O_i - E_i)$. Although the $(O_i - E_i)$ are not independent, they are uncorrelated under the null hypothesis of no treatment effect. Therefore, $\text{var}\{\sum_{i=1}^{d}(O_i - E_i)\} = \sum_{i=1}^{d} V_i$. The z-score is

$$Z = \frac{\sum_{i=1}^{d}(O_i - E_i)}{\sqrt{\sum_{i=1}^{d} V_i}}. \tag{7.9}$$

If the number of deaths is large, Z is approximately standard normal under the null hypothesis. Therefore, an approximate two-tailed test rejects the null hypothesis of no treatment effect if $|Z| > z_{\alpha/2}$, where $z_{\alpha/2}$ is the $(1 - \alpha/2)$th quantile of the standard normal distribution. Equivalently, we could refer Z^2 to a chi-squared distribution with 1 degree of freedom for a two-tailed test.

Table 7.4: d_i deaths at time t_i.

	Dead	Alive	
Control	O_i		n_{Ci}
Treatment			n_{Ti}
	d_i	$n_i - d_i$	n_i

If d_i events occur at the same time, as in Table 7.4, then E_i and V_i become:

$$E_i = \frac{n_{Ci} \times d_i}{n_{Ci} + n_{Ti}} = \frac{n_{Ci} d_i}{n_i} \text{ and } V_i = \frac{(n_{Ci})(n_{Ti})(d_i)(n_i - d_i)}{n_i^2(n_i - 1)}.$$

These are the mean and variance of a (central) hypergeometric distribution corresponding to drawing d_i labels without replacement from an urn containing n_{Ti} and n_{Ci} treatment and control labels. The z-score is computed as in (7.9). Note that the value of the logrank statistic does not depend on the actual times of deaths as long as the treatment labels at the first event, second event, etc., remain the same.

Table 7.5: Data to illustrate the logrank statistic. Plus signs indicate censored observations.

C	1.5	2.0+	2.2	2.3	2.5	2.5	2.6
T	0.3	0.3	0.4	0.7+	0.9	1.1	1.8

We illustrate the logrank test for the data in Table 7.5, which seem to show longer times to event in the treatment arm relative to the control arm. Combine and order data from smallest to largest and imagine placing an arrow immediately preceding deaths, as shown in Figure 7.4. We construct the 2×2 table at death time i using the numbers per arm to the right of the ith arrow as the row totals. Note that we can stop as soon as there are no more observations to the right in one arm because $O_i - E_i = 0$ and $V_i = 0$ for those event times.

Table 7.6 shows O_i, E_i, and V_i (until there are no more observations in the control arm), together with their sums. The logrank z-score is

$$Z = \frac{\sum(O_i - E_i)}{\sqrt{\sum V_i}} = \frac{6 - 2.2067}{\sqrt{1.3193}} = 3.3025.$$

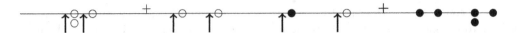

Figure 7.4: Logrank test applied to the data in Table 7.5. Open and filled circles are control and treatment events, respectively. Light and dark pluses are censored observations in the respective arms. Arrows immediately precede events; populate row totals in 2 × 2 table 7.4 by the numbers per-arm to the right of the ith arrow. Arrows stop when no more observations are to the right in one arm because, in that case, $O_i = E_i$ and $V_i = 0$.

The large sample approximation for the p-value is $2\{1 - \Phi(3.3025)\} \approx 0.001$, although this approximation should not be trusted with only 12 events.

Table 7.6: Summary data of O, E, V, and their sums for the data of Table 7.5. Only deaths for which both arms have at least one patient at risk are shown.

Time	0.3	0.4	0.9	1.1	1.5	1.8	Total
O	2	1	1	1	0	1	6
E	1	5/12	3/10	2/9	1/8	1/7	2.2067
V	6/13	(5/12)(7/12)	(3/10)(7/10)	(2/9)(7/9)	(1/8)(7/8)	(1/7)(6/7)	1.3193

A re-randomization test is useful in examples such as this where the number of events is small. Re-randomize according to the original randomization scheme, re-compute the logrank z-score for the re-randomized treatment labels, repeat until all (or a very large number of) re-randomizations are generated, and compute the proportion of re-randomized z-statistics at least as extreme as the observed z-statistic. This re-randomization approach tests the strong null hypothesis that the survival and censoring distributions are the same in treatment and control arms. In a carefully designed and conducted clinical trial, staff emphasize to the patients the importance of continuing to be followed up even if they stop taking their medicine. Most of the censoring should be *administrative*, meaning that the patient completed the study without having the event. In that case, a statistically significant re-randomization test is evidence of a treatment effect, not a difference in censoring distributions. A permutation test applied to the above data results in a two-tailed p-value of 0.002. This p-value is qualitatively similar to the asymptotic p-value of 0.001 found above.

7.4   Hazard Rate and Cox Model

What is the conditional probability of dying within the next year, given that you have survived to now? How old do you have to be before this conditional probability is at least 50%? Questions like this are of great interest. More generally, consider the conditional probability of dying within the next interval of time $(t, t + \Delta t]$, given that you have survived to time t. If $F(t)$ is the distribution function for time to death, this conditional probability is

$$
\begin{aligned}
P\{T \in (t, t + \Delta t] \mid T > t\} &= \frac{P\{T \in (t, t + \Delta t] \cap T > t\}}{P(T > t)} \\
&= \frac{P\{T \in (t, t + \Delta t]\}}{S(t)} \\
&= \frac{F(t + \Delta t) - F(t)}{S(t)}.
\end{aligned}
\tag{7.10}
$$

We can turn this conditional probability into a rate by dividing by Δt:

$$\frac{P(T \in (t, t+\Delta t] \mid T > t)}{\Delta t} = \left(\frac{F(t+\Delta t) - F(t)}{\Delta t}\right)\left(\frac{1}{S(t)}\right) \qquad (7.11)$$

As $\Delta t \to 0$, $\{F(t+\Delta t) - F(t)\}/\Delta t$ converges to the density function $f(t)$ for $F(t)$, and (7.11) converges to $f(t)/S(t)$. This instantaneous death rate at time t, $r(t) = f(t)/S(t)$, is called the *hazard rate* or *hazard function*.

In simple cases, the hazard rate may be a constant function of t. A classic example in engineering is 'death' of an airplane engine caused by ingestion of a bird. This so-called *foreign object damage (FOD)* is what forced Captain "Sully" Sullenberger to land U.S Airways flight 1549 onto the Hudson River on January 15, 2009. FOD is a very rare, completely random event. A bird must happen to be flying directly in front of the engine when the airplane is flying at a low altitude. The probability of such an occurrence is the same regardless of the age t of the engine. Therefore, the hazard rate $r(t)$ for FOD is constant. In biostatistics, the hazard rate for death among 30-year-olds might be relatively constant over time for the same reason. Many such deaths result from car accidents and other unintentional injuries that would be expected to be random.

In other settings, the hazard rate may be increasing or decreasing over time. For example, in older persons, the hazard rate for death increases with each additional year. On the other hand, consider the hazard rate $r(t)$ for rejection of an organ t months following a transplant. The probability of a rejection is highest early after the transplant. Therefore, $r(t)$ decreases over time in this setting. More generally, the hazard function for an event can increase over some periods, stay the same over others, and decrease over others. The sample size needed to accurately estimate the hazard rate is very large.

One popular model for the hazard rate $r(t)$ is called the *Cox proportional hazards model*. Let $x_1, \ldots, x_k$ denote baseline covariates like randomization assignment (1 for treatment, 0 for control), age, sex, hypertension status, and so on. Instead of modeling $r(t)$ in an absolute sense, the Cox model specifies the relative effect of covariates on the hazard function. Let $r_0(t)$ denote the *baseline hazard function* corresponding to $x_i = 0$, $i = 1, \ldots, k$. The Cox model specifies that the ratio $r(t)/r_0(t)$ of the hazard function for the given covariate values to the baseline hazard function is of the form

$$\ln\left\{\frac{r(t)}{r_0(t)}\right\} = \beta_1 x_1 + \ldots + \beta_k x_k. \qquad (7.12)$$

Equivalently,

$$r(t) = r_0(t)\exp(\beta_1 x_1 + \ldots + \beta_k x_k).. \qquad (7.13)$$

This so-called *proportional hazards* assumption implies that the hazard ratio is the same for all t. A major advantage is that the parameters $\beta_1, \ldots, \beta_k$ can be estimated without the need to estimate the unknown baseline hazard function. By imposing this proportional hazards assumption, the Cox model avoids a much stronger assumption such as that the survival curve follows an exponential, Weibull, or other family of survival functions.

The hazard ratio for a 1 unit increase in a covariate x_i, when other covariates are held constant, is

$$\frac{r_0(t)\exp\{\sum_{j\neq i}\beta_j x_j\}\exp\{\beta_i(x_i + 1)\}}{r_0(t)\exp\{\sum_{j\neq i}\beta_j x_j\}\exp\{\beta_i x_i\}} = \exp(\beta_i).$$

Note the similarity between the Cox model in a survival setting and logistic regression in a binary outcome setting. The Cox (resp., logistic regression) model specifies that the logarithm of the hazard (resp., odds) ratio is a linear function of baseline covariates. Exponentiating the regression coefficient yields the hazard (resp., odds) ratio for a 1 unit change in x_i when other covariates are fixed.

The simplest Cox model in a clinical trial contains a single covariate x_1, the treatment indicator. In that case, $\exp(\beta_1)$ is the treatment to control hazard ratio. The p-value from this simplest Cox model is nearly the same as that of the logrank test. Yusuf et al. (1985) used an extension of the O minus E except after V principle (Principle 2.2) to estimate the log of the treatment-to-control hazard ratio.

Principle 7.1. O minus E except after V *(Yusuf et al. 1985) In a survival setting in which 2 tables are updated at each event, $(O_i - E_i)/V_i$ estimates the log hazard ratio with variance $1/V_i$. The common log odds ratio over all events is estimated by*

$$\ln\left(\widehat{\text{HR}}\right) = \frac{\sum_{i:d_i \geq 1}(O_i - E_i)}{\sum V_i},$$
(7.14)

which has estimated variance $1/\sum_{i:d_i \geq 1} V_i$.

Details of the derivation are in the appendix to this chapter.

If the Cox model includes other baseline covariates besides the treatment indicator x_1, $\exp(\beta_1)$ is the treatment to control hazard ratio after adjusting for the between-arm difference in baseline values of covariates.

7.5 Competing Risk Analysis

Up to now we have considered settings with noninformative censoring. The most obvious example of noninformative censoring is *administrative censoring*, meaning that the patient reached the end of the trial without experiencing the event. One could imagine continuing follow-up until the event of interest occurs. A slightly more complicated scenario is when the patient has a freak accident such as being struck by lightning or hit by a train. One could still ponder what would have happened had the accident been prevented. The accident probably gives no information about when the participant would have had the event of interest. In other words, the accident is not informative about the time to event.

Now consider an even more complicated scenario in which the event of interest is coronary heart disease death, which consists primarily of fatal heart attacks, and the patient dies of an ischemic stroke. An ischemic stroke is like a heart attack, but in the brain. Even if we could imagine magically reviving the fatal stroke victim, the stroke is likely to portend an earlier time to coronary heart disease death. In other words, the stroke is informative about the time to fatal heart attack. Tools like the Kaplan-Meier estimate or log-rank test, which assume that censoring is independent of time to event, are inappropriate. When one type of event (e.g., fatal stroke) prevents us from being able to observe the event of interest (e.g., coronary heart disease death), we say there are *competing risks*. In this example, fatal stroke is a competing risk for fatal coronary heart disease. We present a very brief introduction to the issues of competing risks.

Instead of focusing on what the time to an event of interest would have been if we could magically eliminate competing risks, the *cumulative incidence function* approach (Fine and Gray, 1999) considers something much easier to conceptualize, namely the probability of experiencing the event of interest by time t in the presence of competing risks. In other words, the cumulative incidence function is the probability of being able to observe the event of interest by time t (i.e., the event of interest occurs by t and no competing risk precedes it). In the above example, fatal events could result from any of three possible causes: (1) coronary heart disease (CHD), (2) other cardiovascular disease, or (3) non-cardiovascular causes. To calculate the cumulative incidence function for CHD, we first consider the probability of not dying of any cause by time t, and then dying of CHD between time t and $t + dt$, where dt is an infinitesimally small amount of time:

$$P(\{\text{survive to } t\} \cap \{\text{die of CHD in } (t, t + dt]\})$$
$$= S(t)P(\text{die of CHD in } (t, t + dt] \,|\, \text{survive to } t)$$
$$= S(t)\lambda_{\text{CHD}}(t)dt, \tag{7.15}$$

where $S(t)$ is the probability of surviving to time t and $\lambda_{\text{CHD}}(t)$ is the *cause-specific hazard function* for CHD death at time t, defined as

$$\lim_{\Delta t \to 0} \frac{P(\text{die of CHD in } (t, t + \Delta t] \,|\, \text{survive to } t)}{\Delta t}. \tag{7.16}$$

The *cumulative incidence function* $F(t)$ is obtained by integrating (7.15):

$$F(t) = \int_0^t S(u)\lambda_{\text{CHD}}(u)du. \tag{7.17}$$

Notice that $F(t)$ is a *subdistribution function*, meaning that it is a distribution function in every sense except that $\lim_{t \to \infty} F(t)$ is strictly less than 1 because the patient has nonzero probability of dying of something else. In fact, we can think of (7.15), (7.16), and (7.17) as the density function, hazard function, and distribution function for an improper random variable that has nonzero probability of equaling ∞. More specifically, let X be the time to the event of interest among people who do not die of a competing risk. Then X has some proper distribution function G. The time to **observing** a CHD death is X with probability $1 - \epsilon$ and ∞ with probability ϵ, where $\epsilon > 0$ is the probability of death by a competing risk before the event of interest occurs.

The sample analog to Formula (7.17) is the Aalen-Johansen estimator:

$$\hat{F}(t_i) = \sum \hat{S}(t_{i-1})\frac{n_{\text{CHD},i}}{R(t_{i-1})},$$

where $n_{\text{CHD},i}$ is the number of people who die of CHD at time t_i and $R(t_{i-1})$ is the number of people in the risk set, namely the number of people who are still alive just prior to the ith CHD death.

More generally, suppose there are k competing risks including the one of primary interest (CHD death in the above example), which we arbitrarily denote as cause 1. Let $S(t)$ be the probability of survival past time t. Thus, $S(t)$ is the probability of not experiencing any of the k competing risks by time t. Let $\hat{S}(t)$ be the Kaplan-Meier estimate of $S(t)$. Then the cumulative incidence function at time t and its Aalen-Johansen estimator are

$$F(t) = P(\text{event 1 by time } t) = \int_0^t S(u)\lambda_1(u)du \tag{7.18}$$

and

$$\hat{F}(t_i) = \sum \hat{S}(t_{i-1})\frac{n_{1,i}}{R(t_{i-1})}. \tag{7.19}$$

We can compare treatment arms with respect to the cumulative incidence function of CHD death by different times. One issue is that the cumulative incidence function for CHD depends on more than just CHD because the survival function $S(t)$ depends on the hazard functions for other types of mortality. For example, a very large hazard rate for other cardiovascular mortality (or for non-cardiovascular mortality, for that matter) will decrease overall survival, which affects (7.17) and (7.19). For this reason, one must compare the cumulative incidence function for each of the three types of death to get a full picture.

Fine and Gray (1999) also showed how to do proportional hazards regression modeling in the presence of competing risks. Patients who have had a competing risk remain in the risk set for the primary outcome. The method is very similar to using ordinary Cox regression on the primary outcome, ignoring the competing risk. In other words, patients who have had a competing risk remain in the risk set when estimating the parameters of the Cox model. Although this feels unnatural, it yields valid estimates.

An example in which competing risk methodology could be used is the ACTT-1 clinical trial in coronavirus disease (COVID-19). COVID-19, which can lead to severe pneumonia and serious consequences in other organs, became a pandemic in 2020. ACTT-1 compared the antiviral drug Remdesivir plus standard care to placebo plus standard care with respect to time to recovery up to 28 days. Death is a competing risk, but the special feature of this example is that all such deaths are presumably due to COVID-19. Therefore, a treatment that reduces the probability of death is effective against COVID-19. The approach taken in ACTT-1 and in some other trials was to count any death prior to day 28 as a censored observation at 28 days (the end of follow-up) and use the Cox model to estimate the treatment to control 'hazard' ratio. They called this hazard ratio the *recovery rate ratio* to emphasize that a large hazard ratio means that treatment is beneficial. Censoring deaths at any time after the end of follow-up would have given the same answer. Thus, the approach taken in ACTT-1 is effectively the same thing as treating a death as an infinite recovery time. Interestingly, the Fine-Gray method yields virtually the same answer as censoring deaths at 28 days. In fact, it can be shown that with complete follow-up, the Fine-Gray method gives the same answer as the method adopted in ACTT-1.

7.6 Parametric Approaches

We have emphasized survival methods that make no assumptions about the distribution of time to an event. Before these methods were developed, it was common to assume that time to an event follows an exponential distribution with probability density, distribution, and survival functions $f(y)$, $F(y)$, and $S(y)$ given by

$$f(y) = \lambda \exp(-\lambda y), \ F(y) = 1 - \exp(-\lambda y) \text{ and } S(y) = \exp(-\lambda y).$$

There are several advantages to assuming an exponential. First, the exponential has constant hazard rate λ because

$$\frac{f(y)}{S(y)} = \frac{\lambda \exp(-\lambda y)}{\exp(-\lambda y)} = \lambda.$$

Second, the exponential distribution has the *lack of memory property*, which is that the conditional probability of surviving an additional time u, given survival to time t, is also exponential with parameter λ:

$$
\begin{aligned}
P(Y > t + u \mid Y > t) &= \frac{P(Y > t + u, Y > t)}{P(Y > t)} = \frac{P(Y > t + u)}{P(Y > t)} \\
&= \frac{\exp\{-\lambda(t + u)\}}{\exp(-\lambda t)} = \exp(-\lambda u). \quad (7.20)
\end{aligned}
$$

Another convenient property of the exponential distribution is that the maximum likelihood estimator of λ for a sample of iid exponential random variables is $1/\bar{Y} = n/\sum_{i=1}^{n} Y_i$, the number of failures divided by the total time. With censored data, the MLE is also the number of failures divided by the total amount of time.

The problem is that the exponential distribution may not be realistic because the true hazard function may be increasing or decreasing over time. A more realistic class of distribution functions is the family of Weibull distributions with density, distribution, and survival functions given by

$$\exp\{-(y/\eta)^\beta\}$$

The Weibull has decreasing, constant, or increasing hazard rate depending on whether $\beta < 1$, $\beta = 1$, or $\beta > 1$.

One way to view a Weibull distribution is that we can transform to an exponential distribution using the power transformation Y^β. Although the Weibull distribution is flexible in that it can accommodate an increasing, decreasing, or constant hazard rate, the robustness principle suggests that the logrank test or proportional hazards model is preferable because it makes fewer assumptions.

7.6.1 Conditional Binomial Procedure

One parametric method for dealing with time-to-event data is often used in vaccine trials whose primary endpoint is occurrence of a relatively rare disease. Consider first the data in a given arm. If everyone is followed for the same amount of time, t, the number of people who get the disease has a binomial distribution with n trials and probability parameter p, where n is the sample size and p is the probability of disease by fixed time t. By what is sometimes called the *law of small numbers*, a binomial distribution with large n and small p is well approximated by a Poisson distribution with parameter $\lambda = np$. More precisely, if $n \to \infty$ and $p_n \to 0$ at such a rate that $np_n \to \lambda > 0$, then the binomial (n, p_n) probability mass function (pmf) converges to the Poisson pmf with parameter λ (see, for example, Parzen, 1960 or Proschan and Shaw, 2016).

Now consider the comparison of vaccine and control arms. For simplicity, assume common sample size n in the two arms. By the law of small numbers, the numbers of vaccine and control events, Y_V and Y_C, are approximately Poisson with parameters $\lambda_V = np_V$ and $\lambda_C = np_C$. The null hypothesis that $p_V = p_C$ is equivalent to $\lambda_V = \lambda_C$. We can test this latter hypothesis by taking advantage of the following theorem.

Theorem 7.2. *If Y_V and Y_C are independent Poisson random variables with parameters λ_V and λ_C and $S = Y_C + Y_V$, then the conditional distribution of Y_C given $S = s$ is binomial (s, p), where $p = \lambda_C/(\lambda_C + \lambda_V)$.*

The theorem suggests a *conditional binomial procedure* to test $H_0 : \lambda_V = \lambda_C$. Conditioned on the total number of events s, the number of control events has a binomial distribution with s trials and probability parameter

$$p = \frac{\lambda_C}{\lambda_C + \lambda_V} = \frac{np_C}{np_C + np_V} = \frac{p_C}{p_C + p_V}.$$

Under the null hypothesis that $\lambda_V = \lambda_C$ (equivalently, $p_V = p_C$), the binomial probability parameter p is $1/2$. We can now conduct an exact binomial test of $H_0 : p = 1/2$, as in Section 1.2.1

In reality, sample sizes may differ by arm, and staggered entry, dropout, and loss to follow-up cause people to have different amounts of follow-up. Exclusion of those who have not had full follow-up is unappealing and potentially misleading. Theorem 7.2 can be used in a way that includes everyone with any amount of follow-up. Let t_i be the follow-up time of patient i, and assume that the number of disease events for patient i has an approximate Poisson distribution with parameter λt_i. Even though the primary endpoint in vaccine trials is binary (disease/no disease) and a Poisson distribution allows more than 1 event per person, the Poisson approximation works well because the Poisson probability of more than one event for a given patient is very close to 0 if λ is very small. The sum of independent Poisson random variables has a Poisson distribution with parameter equal to the sum of the individual parameters. Accordingly, the total numbers of events in the control (C) and vaccine (V) arms are independent Poissons with parameters $\lambda_C t_C$ and $\lambda_V t_V$, where $t_C = \sum_{i=1}^{n_C} t_{Ci}$ and $t_V = \sum_{i=1}^{n_V} t_{Vi}$ are the total follow-up times in the control and vaccine arms, respectively. Let $\theta = \lambda_V / \lambda_C$. By Theorem 7.2, the conditional distribution of X_C given $X_C + X_V = s$ is binomial (s, p), where

$$p = \frac{\lambda_C t_C}{\lambda_C t_C + \lambda_V t_V} = \frac{t_C}{t_C + (\lambda_V/\lambda_C) t_V} = \frac{t_C}{t_C + \theta t_V}. \tag{7.21}$$

We can test the null hypothesis

$$H_0 : \theta = \theta_0$$

by testing

$$H_0 : p = \frac{t_C}{t_C + \theta_0 t_V}.$$

Likewise, we can obtain a $100(1 - \alpha)\%$ confidence interval (L, U) for $\theta = \lambda_V / \lambda_C$ by first computing a $100(1 - \alpha)\%$ Clopper-Pearson confidence interval (l, u) for p and then solving the inequality

$$l \le \frac{t_C}{t_C + \theta t_V} \le u$$

for θ. This yields the following $100(1 - \alpha)\%$ confidence interval for $\theta = \lambda_V / \lambda_C$:

$$\frac{t_c(1 - u)}{t_v u} \le \theta \le \frac{t_c(1 - l)}{t_v l}. \tag{7.22}$$

Example 7.3. In the COVID-19 pandemic beginning at the end of 2019, efficacious vaccines were desperately needed. On December 10, 2020 and December 17, 2020, the FDA's Vaccines and Related Biological Products Advisory Committee (VRBPAC) recommended Emergency Use Authorization for two messenger RNA vaccines with estimated efficacy exceeding 90%. We illustrate the conditional binomial procedure by estimating and testing the efficacy of the mRNA-1273 vaccine developed by ModernaTX, Inc. and presented to the FDA's VRBPAC on December 17, 2020.

Table 7.7: Results of Moderna's Study 301.

	Vaccine	Control (Placebo)
Sample size	14,134	14,073
Person years	3,304.9	3,273.7
Events	11	185

Data from the manufacturer's pivotal, Phase III, placebo controlled trial 301 are shown in Table 7.7. The primary endpoint is COVID-19. The numbers of participants with COVID-19 are 11 of 14, 134 over 3, 304.9 person years of follow-up and 185 of 14, 073 over 3, 273.7 years of follow-up in the vaccine and control arms, respectively. Let λ_V and λ_C be the yearly rates of acquiring COVID-19 in the vaccine and control arms and assume that the numbers of vaccine and control COVID-19 events are approximately Poisson with respective parameters $3, 304.9 \lambda_V$ and $3, 273.7 \lambda_C$. We are interested in making inferences about λ_V / λ_C. Equation (7.21) shows that, conditioned on the $11 + 185 = 196$ total events and total follow-up times of $3, 304.9$ and $3, 273.7$, the number of placebo participants with COVID-19 is binomial with 196 trials and probability parameter $p = 3, 273.7/(3, 273.7 + 3, 304.9\,\theta)$, where $\theta = \lambda_V / \lambda_C$. The FDA guidance called for demonstration that the true efficacy, defined by

$100(1 - \lambda_V/\lambda_C)$, exceeds 30%. This is equivalent to showing that $\theta \leq 1 - 0.30 = 0.70$. One way to do this is to conduct an exact binomial test of $H_0 : \theta = 0.70$ versus the alternative hypothesis $H_1 : \theta < 0.70$. Equivalently, we test the following hypothesis for the binomial probability parameter p:

$$H_0 : p = \frac{3,273.7}{3,273.7 + 3,304.9(0.70)} = 0.586 \text{ versus } H_1 : p > 0.586. \qquad (7.23)$$

The one-tailed p-value for an exact binomial test of (7.23) with 185 events out of 196 trials is

$$\text{p-value} = \sum_{i=185}^{196} \binom{196}{i} (0.586)^i (1 - 0.586)^{196-i} < 0.0001.$$

The manufacturer also obtained a p-value < 0.0001 using a different method of analysis, the stratified Cox model.

Also of interest is a 95% confidence interval for vaccine efficacy. The Clopper-Pearson confidence interval for p for a binomial with 185 events out of 196 trials is $(0.9018, 0.9717)$. From (7.22), the 95% confidence interval for $\theta = \lambda_V/\lambda_C$ is

$$\left(\frac{3,273.7(1 - 0.9717)}{3,304.9(0.9717)}, \frac{3,273.7(1 - 0.9018)}{3,304.9(0.9018)} \right) = (0.029, 0.108).$$

The confidence interval for vaccine efficacy is $100(1 - 0.108, 1 - 0.029) = (89.2\%, 97.1\%)$. This is in close agreement with the confidence interval of $(89.3\%, 96.8\%)$ reported by the manufacturer using a stratified Cox model. □

Exercises

1. What is the advantage of using survival methods over using the proportion of patients who survive a fixed amount of time such as 1 year?

2. In a clinical trial of a drug to reduce the risk of heart attacks, some patients receive a heart transplant. Receiving a new heart profoundly changes the time to heart attack, so investigators propose censoring the time to heart attack at the time of receipt of a heart transplant.

   (a) Do you think that this represents non-informative censoring? Explain your answer.

   (b) Does your answer to part (a) change if you are told that everyone in the trial is sick enough to receive a heart transplant, and the only reason that some did was that a matching heart happened to be available for them.

   (c) What is an alternative method of handling a heart transplant?

3. Find the Kaplan-Meier survival estimate of $S(t)$ for the following data that contains no censored data: 1.4, 2.1, 3.0, 0.8, 1.9, and 3.3.

4. ↑ Show that in problem 3, the Kaplan-Meier estimate $\hat{S}(t)$ is $1 - \hat{F}(t)$, where $\hat{F}$ is the sample distribution function $F(t) = \sum_{i=1}^{n} I(Y_i \leq t)$.

5. True or false: the logrank test is invalid when the proportional hazards assumption is not satisfied. Explain your answer.

6. Describe how the competing risk approach differs from the approach of the Cox proportional hazards model.

7. Show that when there are no censored observations, the Kaplan-Meier estimator simplifies to the sample distribution function $F(t) = \sum_{i=1}^{n} I(Y_i \leq t)$.

7.7   Appendix: Partial Likelihood

Estimation using the proportional hazards model simplifies tremendously using a clever conditioning argument of Cox. Condition on the fact that a death occurred in the interval $(t - dt, t]$ and calculate the probability that it was participant i. Consider the risk set $R(t)$, namely the people who are alive and have not been censored by time $t - dt$, where dt is an infinitesimally small number. Let $D_{t,i}$ be the event that participant i in $R(t)$ dies by time t. Then

$$P(D_{t,i}) = P(\text{participant } i \text{ dies by } t \mid \text{alive at } t - dt) \approx \lambda_0(t) \exp(\boldsymbol{\beta} \cdot \boldsymbol{x}_i) dt.$$

Let $D_t = \cup_{i \in R(t)} D_{t,i}$ be the event that at least one person in the risk set $R(t)$ dies by time t. The probability of more than one death or a censoring and a death occurring in $(t - dt, t]$ is ignorably small for tiny t. Therefore, given that a death occurred in $(t - dt, t]$, the probability that the decedent is participant i is

$$
\begin{aligned}
P(D_{t,i} \mid D_t) &= \frac{P(D_t \cap D_{t,i})}{P(D_t)} = \frac{P(D_t \cap D_{t,i})}{\sum_{j \in R(t)} P(D_t \cap D_{t,j})} \\
&\approx \frac{P(D_{t,i})}{\sum_{j \in R(t)} P(D_{t,j})} = \frac{\lambda_0(t) \exp(\boldsymbol{\beta} \cdot \boldsymbol{x}_i) dt}{\sum_{j \in R(t)} \lambda_0(t) \exp(\boldsymbol{\beta} \cdot \boldsymbol{x}_j) dt} \\
&= \frac{\exp(\boldsymbol{\beta} \cdot \boldsymbol{x}_i)}{\sum_{j \in R(t)} \exp(\boldsymbol{\beta} \cdot \boldsymbol{x}_j)}.
\end{aligned}
\tag{7.24}
$$

The baseline hazard function $\lambda_0(t)$ cancels out in the numerator and denominator, so we never need to deal with it! Cox argued that the data at different death times can be treated as independent Bernoullis with probabilities given by (7.24), which results in the *partial likelihood*

$$\mathcal{L}(\boldsymbol{\beta}) = \prod_{i \in \text{deaths}} \frac{\exp(\boldsymbol{\beta} \cdot \boldsymbol{x}_i)}{\sum_{j \in R(t_i)} \exp(\boldsymbol{\beta} \cdot \boldsymbol{x}_j)}. \tag{7.25}$$

We can maximize the partial likelihood by differentiating the logarithm of (7.25) with respect to each β_i, equate to 0, and solve numerically.

We illustrate how to use the partial likelihood to get a surprisingly accurate estimate of the log odds ratio in a clinical trial. Use the Cox model with a single predictor $\boldsymbol{x}$, the treatment indicator vector whose ith component is 1 or 0 depending on whether patient i is assigned to treatment or control. The logarithm of the partial likelihood and its derivative are

$$
\begin{aligned}
L(\beta) &= \sum_i \ln\left\{ \frac{\exp(\beta x_i)}{\sum_{j \in R(t_i)} \exp(\beta x_j)} \right\} \\
&= \sum_i \left[\beta x_i - \ln\left\{ \sum_{j \in R(t_i)} \exp(\beta x_j) \right\} \right] \\
L'(\beta) &= \sum_i \left[x_i - \frac{\sum_{j \in R(t_i)} x_j \exp(\beta x_j)}{\sum_{j \in R(t_i)} \exp(\beta x_j)} \right]
\end{aligned}
\tag{7.26}
$$

We could equate $L'(\beta)$ to 0 and solve for β numerically using Newton's method. Recall that Newton's method of finding a root of a function $f(\beta)$ begins with an initial guess β_{init} and uses the first-order Taylor series approximation

$$f(\beta_{\text{init}}) + f'(\beta_{\text{init}})(\beta - \beta_{\text{init}}) \tag{7.27}$$

or $f(\beta)$. Equating (7.27) to 0 and solving for β yields the new estimate

$$\beta_{\text{new}} = \beta_{\text{init}} - \frac{f(\beta_{\text{init}})}{f'(\beta_{\text{init}})}.$$

In our setting, $f(\beta) = L'(\beta)$. Our initial estimate of β is 0, so

$$\beta_{\text{new}} = -\frac{L'(0)}{L''(0)}. \tag{7.28}$$

We get

$$L'(0) = \sum_i \left[x_i - \frac{\sum_{j \in R(t_i)} x_j}{\sum_{j \in R(t_i)} 1} \right] = \sum_i \left[x_i - \frac{\sum_{j \in R(t_i)} x_j}{n_i} \right],$$

the difference between the observed number and expected number of treatment deaths. Also, from (7.26),

$$L''(\beta) = -\sum_i \left[\frac{\sum_{j \in R(t_i)} \exp(\beta x_j) \sum_{j \in R(t_i)} x_j^2 \exp(\beta x_j) - \left\{ \sum_{j \in R(t_i)} x_j \exp(\beta x_j) \right\}^2}{\left(\sum_{j \in R(t_i)} \exp(\beta x_j) \right)^2} \right], \tag{7.29}$$

so

$$L''(0) = -\sum_i \left[\frac{n_i \sum_{j \in R(t_i)} x_j^2 - \left\{ \sum_{j \in R(t_i)} x_j \right\}^2}{n_i^2} \right]$$

$$= -\sum_i \left[\frac{n_i \sum_{j \in R(t_i)} x_j - \left\{ \sum_{j \in R(t_i)} x_j \right\}^2}{n_i^2} \right] \quad \text{(because } x_i = 0 \text{ or } 1)$$

$$= -\sum_i p_i(1 - p_i), \tag{7.30}$$

where $p_i = (1/n_i) \sum_{j \in R(t_i)} x_j$ is the Bernoulli parameter of the conditional distribution of X_i given the numbers at risk at time t_i in the two arms. Accordingly, $\sum_i p_i(1 - p_i)$ is the conditional variance of X_i. In other words, the first step of Newton's method reproduces the approximate log hazard ratio estimator

$$\frac{\sum_i (O_i - E_i)}{\sum V_i}.$$

This is the basis for the survival version of the O minus E except after V principle (Principle 7.1).

7.8   Summary

1. Survival analysis accounts for censored observations when dealing with time to an event.

2. Most methods assume that censoring is noninformative, meaning that it is independent of the time to event.

3. The most common way to estimate the survival distribution $S(t)$ is the Kaplan-Meier method.

4. Survival distributions are often compared across arms using the log-rank test.

5. The hazard function $\lambda(t)$ is the instantaneous event rate given that the event has not yet occurred in an individual.

6. The Cox proportional hazards model can be used to compare arms while accounting for baseline differences in covariates

   (a) $\lambda(t) = \lambda_0(t) \exp(\beta_1 x_1 + \ldots + \beta_k x_k$, where $\lambda_0(t)$ is the baseline hazard function.

Chapter 8

Sample Size/Power

8.1 Introduction

A hypothesis test in a clinical trial is designed to require a strong burden of proof to declare the treatment beneficial. Consequently, a statistically significant result makes us confident that the treatment is effective. Should we be confident that the treatment is ineffective if the result is not statistically significant? That depends on the *type II error rate* β of the test, namely the probability of 'accepting' the null hypothesis when it is false. If β is a small number like 0.10, then a non statistically significant result would be a rare event if the true treatment effect is as specified in the protocol. Therefore, a non statistically significant result should make us confident that the true treatment effect is not large. We can frame this argument in an equivalent way in terms of statistical *power* $1 - \beta$, the probability of rejecting the null hypothesis when it is false. If power is high and we fail to reject the null hypothesis, we should be confident that the treatment does not have a large effect.

What power level is acceptable? Typical levels in clinical trials are between 0.80 and 0.90. Even though 0.80 is considered acceptable (values lower than 0.80 are not), we advise against using power 0.80. Should it really be acceptable to have a 1 in 5 chance of missing a truly effective treatment? Using 80% power is like playing Russian roulette with a 5-shooter. In certain situations, it might actually be preferable to make the type II error probability smaller than the type I error probability. In a phase I or II trial, making a type II error means abandoning an effective treatment for any future testing. This is an especially grave error if the disease is serious and there are no effective treatments. But usually there is at least one known effective treatment. In that case, a type I error on a new treatment might cause patients to erroneously eschew the known effective treatment in favor of the ineffective new treatment. Given the serious consequences of such a mistake, the type I error rate is usually set lower than the type II error rate. Using type I and II error rates of 0.05 and 0.10, respectively, strikes a good balance.

We begin this chapter with calculation of approximate power and sample size using a simple equation that can be applied to continuous, binary, or survival outcomes. Then we discuss practical aspects of sample size calculations, and end with exact power calculations and computer programs. The reader who is tempted to skip to the exact programs is advised not to. The approximate technique at the beginning of the chapter is extremely useful for quickly checking the accuracy of, and developing intuition about, sample size and power.

8.2   EZ Principle Illustrated through the 2-Sample t-Test

Consider a trial with a continuous primary endpoint Y like blood pressure, and suppose that large values of Y indicate worse outcomes. Let $\delta = \mu_C - \mu_T$ be the between-arm difference in means. The two-sample t-statistic with n patients per arm for testing $H_0 : \delta = 0$ versus the one-tailed alternative $H_1 : \delta > 0$ is

$$t = \frac{\bar{Y}_C - \bar{Y}_T}{\sqrt{2s^2/n}}.$$

If n is large, the distribution of the t-statistic can be approximated by replacing s by the true standard deviation σ. We denote this large sample version of t by Z. By the central limit theorem, $\bar{Y}_T$ and $\bar{Y}_C$ are asymptotically normally distributed, so Z is approximately normal with mean $\theta = \delta/\{2\sigma^2/n\}^{1/2}$ and variance 1. Under the null hypothesis, $\theta = 0$.

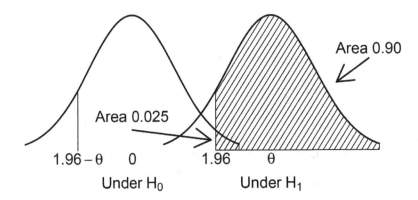

Figure 8.1: The null (left curve) and alternative (right curve) normal densities for the z-statistic. Power is the area to the right of 1.96 under the right curve, which equals the area to the right of $1.96 - \theta$ under the left curve. This area is $1 - \Phi(1.96 - \theta)$.

Figure 8.1 shows the large sample normal density for Z under the null and alternative hypotheses. The rejection region for a one-tailed test with alternative $H_1 : \delta > 0$ at $\alpha = 0.025$ is $Z > 1.96$. The shaded area depicted in the left (resp., right) curve is the type I error rate (resp., power when $E(Z) = \theta$). Because the two normal curves have the same variance 1, the right curve is simply the left curve shifted θ units to the right. Therefore, the shaded area in the right curve equals the area to the right of $1.96 - \theta$ under the standard normal curve on the left. The 0.10th quantile of the standard normal density is -1.28, so the area to the right of -1.28 for the standard normal density is $1 - 0.10 = 0.90$. Consequently, to achieve power 0.90, equate $1.96 - \theta$ to -1.28 and solve for θ: $\theta = 1.96 + 1.28$. That is,

$$E(Z) = 1.96 + 1.28 = 3.24. \tag{8.1}$$

We have considered a one-tailed test at $\alpha = 0.025$, but the same equation applies approximately to a two-tailed test at level 0.05 for the following reason. If power for a one-tailed test at level 0.025 is 0.90, then power for a two-tailed test at level 0.05 is higher than 0.90 because rejection of the null hypothesis could occur in either the correct or incorrect tail. But it is extremely unlikely that a two-tailed test would produce a z-score in the incorrect tail. Therefore, power for a two-tailed test at level α is nearly identical to power for a one-tailed test at level $\alpha/2$ whenever the latter is a typical level like 0.80 or 0.90.

The same reasoning can be applied to other values of α and power, and to other asymptotically normal test statistics. For $0 < a < 1$, let z_a denote the $(1 - a)$th quantile of a standard normal distribution. The most important sample size/power principle is the following 'EZ' principle, so named because it involves the expected value of the z-statistic (EZ).

Principle 8.1. The EZ Principle (it's easy!) *Power $1 - \beta$ for a one-tailed test at level $\alpha/2$ or a two-tailed test at level α requires the expected z-statistic to satisfy:*

$$\boxed{\mathrm{E}(Z) = z_{\alpha/2} + z_\beta,} \tag{8.2}$$

We often use a two-tailed test at level 0.05, so $z_{\alpha/2}$ is 1.96. The most common values of power are between 0.80 and 0.90 (i.e., type II error rates β between 0.10 and 0.20). For these power values, z_β is given in Table 8.1.

Table 8.1: Values of z_β for power 0.80, 0.85, or 0.90.

Power	0.80	0.85	0.90
z_β	0.84	1.04	1.28

From the EZ principle flows everything of interest about power and sample size. Equation (8.2) emphasizes that the only thing that matters is the expected z-score. Table 8.1 shows that if the expected z-score is $1.96 + 0.84 = 2.80$, $1.96 + 1.04 = 3$, or $1.96 + 1.28 = 3.24$, then power for a two-tailed t-test at $\alpha = 0.05$ or a one-tailed t-test at $\alpha = 0.025$ will be approximately 80%, 85%, or 90%. If the expected z-score is substantially smaller, there is an error in the sample size calculation. We will see that the EZ principle applies to many other asymptotically normal test statistics used in clinical trials.

We now illustrate the use of the EZ principle to compute sample size, power, and the detectable effect in a clinical trial that uses a 2-sample t-test. The per-arm sample size to achieve power $1 - \beta$ for a two-tailed t-test at level α or a one-tailed t-test at level $\alpha/2$ can be obtained by replacing $\mathrm{E}(Z)$ by $\delta/(2\sigma^2/n)^{1/2}$ and solving Equation (8.2) for n. Solving

$$\frac{\delta}{\sqrt{2\sigma^2/n}} = (z_{\alpha/2} + z_\beta) \tag{8.3}$$

for n yields a per-arm sample size of

$$n = \frac{2\sigma^2(z_{\alpha/2} + z_\beta)^2}{\delta^2}. \tag{8.4}$$

Example 8.2. Consider a clinical trial comparing two diets with respect to change in diastolic blood pressure from baseline to 6 weeks. From a prior clinical trial, we estimate the standard deviation of change in diastolic blood pressure to be 5 mmHg. We want 90% power to detect a between-diet difference of $\delta = 3$ mmHg.

Use Equation (8.4) with $z_{\alpha/2} = 1.96$, $z_\beta = 1.28$, $\delta = 3$ and $\sigma = 5$:

$$n = \frac{2(5^2)(1.96 + 1.28)^2}{3^2} = 58.32.$$

Since n must be an integer, we round up to 59 to be conservative. This tells us we need 59 people in each of the two arms, or 118 total. $\quad\square$

We can also solve Equation 8.3 for other quantities of interest. For instance, suppose that in Example 8.2, we can afford only 80 people total, $n = 40$ per arm. A relevant question might then be: what size treatment effect can we detect with 40 per arm and 90% power? We solve Equation 8.3 for δ:

$$\delta = (z_{\alpha/2} + z_\beta) \sqrt{2\sigma^2/n}. \tag{8.5}$$

Substituting $z_{\alpha/2} = 1.96$, $z_\beta = 1.28$, $n = 40$, and $\sigma = 5$ into Equation (8.5) yields $\delta = 3.62$. In other words, with a sample size of 40 per arm, we have 90% power if the true difference between arms is 3.62 mmHg.

We can also use Equation (8.3) to compute power for the originally hypothesized difference of 3 mmHg with 40 people per arm. Rewrite Equation 8.3 so that the term involving β is on one side and everything else is on the other side:

$$\frac{\delta}{\sqrt{2\sigma^2/n}} - z_{\alpha/2} = z_\beta.$$

Now take Φ of both sides of the equation and remember that z_β is defined to be the $(1-\beta)$th quantile of a standard normal distribution:

$$\Phi\left\{ \frac{\delta}{\sqrt{2\sigma^2/n}} - z_{\alpha/2} \right\} = \Phi(z_\beta) = 1 - \beta.$$

In other words,

$$\text{Power} = \Phi\left\{ \frac{\delta}{\sqrt{2\sigma^2/n}} - z_{\alpha/2} \right\}. \tag{8.6}$$

Substituting $n = 40$, $\delta = 3$, $\sigma = 5$, and $z_{\alpha/2} = 1.96$, we obtain power

$$\Phi\left\{ \frac{3}{\sqrt{2(5)^2/40}} - 1.96 \right\} = \Phi(0.723) = 0.765.$$

Sample size and power can also be computed in a trial with unequal sample sizes, as illustrated in the following example.

Example 8.3. Suppose that the trial in Example 8.2 used 2:1 randomization to treatment or control. If n denotes the control sample size, then $2n$ is the sample size in the treatment arm. The expected z-score is

$$\text{E}(Z) = \frac{\delta}{\sqrt{\sigma^2\{1/n + 1/(2n)\}}} = \frac{\sqrt{n}\delta}{\sqrt{\sigma^2\{1 + 1/2\}}}.$$

For 90% power, equate the expected z-score to $1.96 + 1.28 = 3.24$ and solve for n:

$$\frac{\sqrt{n}\delta}{\sqrt{\sigma^2\{1 + 1/2\}}} = 3.24; \quad n = \frac{(3.24)^2(3/2)\sigma^2}{\delta^2}.$$

Substituting $\delta = 3$ and $\sigma = 5$ yields $n = 43.74$. Therefore, the sample sizes in the control and treatment arms should be 44 and 88, respectively. The total sample size of $44 + 88 = 132$ is larger than the figure 118 obtained in Example 8.2. This makes sense because 2:1 randomization is less efficient than 1:1 randomization. □

8.2.1 Important Takeaways from the EZ Principle

Formulas (8.4), (8.5), and (8.6) for sample size, detectable effect, and power all arose from the EZ principle and Equation (8.2). Two important points about Equation (8.2) and its sequelae are as follows:

1. Because Equation (8.2) is based on a large sample approximation, **the resulting sample size (8.4) cannot be trusted if it is small.**

2. | If δ equals its hypothesized value, the expected z-score is very large. |

Regarding point 1, a small sample size arises when the assumed treatment effect is extremely large. For instance, in Example 8.2, suppose that the assumed treatment effect were 15 instead of 3. The sample size from Equation (8.4) is

$$n = \frac{2(5^2)(1.96 + 1.28)^2}{15^2} = 2.33.$$

That would suggest that only 3 participants per arm are needed. But Equation (8.4) is based on a large sample approximation, which cannot be applied if n is 3. In settings like this with a very large treatment effect, sample size can be computed using the exact method in Section 8.6.

Point 2 is under-appreciated. If the sample size assumptions are correct and power is 90%, we expect to see a z-score of $1.96 + 1.28 = 3.24$, with a corresponding two-tailed p-value of 0.001. If we instead see a barely statistically significant z-score of 1.96, then the observed treatment effect was much smaller than originally anticipated. This fact is sometimes used to malign hypothesis testing as not being reproducible, as in the following argument. Suppose that a z-score of 1.96 is observed, and assume that the true treatment effect, $\mu_C - \mu_T$, is the observed effect, $\bar{Y}_C - \bar{Y}_T$. Then the expected z-score was $(\mu_C - \mu_T)/(2\sigma^2/n)^{1/2} = (\bar{Y}_C - \bar{Y}_T)/(2\sigma^2/n)^{1/2} = 1.96$. From Equation (8.6), power was approximately $\Phi(1.96 - 1.96) = \Phi(0) = 1/2$. If we attempt to replicate the trial using the same sample size, **and the observed treatment effect in the first trial is the true effect**, there is a 50% probability that the second trial will not be statistically significant. In other words, there is a 50% chance of failing to replicate the result of the first trial. But if the observed effect from the first trial was the true effect, then the true effect was much smaller than anticipated. In that case, we should increase the sample size in the second trial to replicate the result of the first. It is not surprising that repeating a trial that had only 50% power could result in the opposite conclusion!

8.3 EZ Principle Applied More Generally

Many test statistics used in clinical trials are of the form

$$Z = \frac{\hat{\delta}}{\widehat{se}(\hat{\delta})}, \tag{8.7}$$

where $\hat{\delta}$ is an estimator of the treatment effect and $\widehat{se}(\hat{\delta})$ is an estimator of the standard error of $\hat{\delta}$. The reasoning underlying the EZ principle and Equation (8.2) applies to any z-score of the form (8.7) as long as the following conditions hold:

Key conditions when the sample size is large:

1. $\hat{\delta}/se(\hat{\delta})$ is approximately normal with mean θ and variance 1. Here, the denominator is the true, not estimated, standard error of $\hat{\delta}$.

2. The ratio of estimated to true standard errors is close to 1. More specifically, $\widehat{\mathrm{se}}(\hat{\delta})/\mathrm{se}(\hat{\delta})$ converges to 1 (in probability).

3. $\theta = 0$ under the null hypothesis and $\theta > 0$ if treatment is effective.

Whenever the key conditions are satisfied, approximate power can be computed from the EZ principle using the same steps we used to arrive at Equation (8.6). Isolating the term involving β on one side of the equation, moving all other terms to the opposite side, and taking Φ of both sides yields

$$\Phi\left\{\mathrm{E}(Z) - z_{\alpha/2}\right\} = \Phi(z_\beta) = 1 - \beta.$$

The right side is power, so

$$\mathrm{Power} = \Phi\left\{\mathrm{E}(Z) - z_{\alpha/2}\right\}. \tag{8.8}$$

Likewise, we can find the detectable effect for a given level of power by substituting $\delta/\mathrm{se}(\hat{\delta})$ for $\mathrm{E}(Z)$ in (8.2) and solving for δ. From

$$\frac{\delta}{\mathrm{se}(\hat{\delta})} = z_{\alpha/2} + z_\beta,$$

we see that

$$\delta = (z_{\alpha/2} + z_\beta)\mathrm{se}(\hat{\delta}). \tag{8.9}$$

The next several sections illustrate the calculations applied to many common clinical trial settings.

8.3.1   1-Sample t-test

The EZ principle can be used in a paired setting such as that of the COMMIT trial of Example 6.1. Recall that communities were pair-matched and one member of each pair was assigned to the smoking Intervention, the other to the Control. Let $D_1, \ldots, D_n$ be the difference between Intervention and Control communities in the ith pair. The estimator and its standard error are

$$\hat{\delta} = \bar{D}, \quad \text{and} \quad \mathrm{se} = \sqrt{\sigma^2/n},$$

where σ is the standard deviation of a pairwise difference D_i. The z-score $Z = \hat{\delta}/\mathrm{se}$ has variance 1 and mean

$$\theta = \frac{\delta}{\sqrt{\sigma^2/n}} = \frac{\sqrt{n}\,\delta}{\sigma}.$$

For power $1 - \beta$ with a two-tailed test at level α or a one-tailed test at level $\alpha/2$, we solve

$$\frac{\sqrt{n}\,\delta}{\sigma} = z_{\alpha/2} + z_\beta.$$

The required number of pairs is

$$n = \frac{\sigma^2(z_{\alpha/2} + z_\beta)^2}{\delta^2}. \tag{8.10}$$

For example, suppose we want to test a new community intervention to improve smoking quite rates using the same paired design as COMMIT. We can use the standard deviation of paired differences from COMMIT, 0.045 to estimate σ. If we want 90% power to detect a 3 percentage point improvement in the smoking quit rate in Intervention versus Control communities, then $\delta = 0.03$, $z_{\alpha/2} = 1.96$, and $z_\beta = 1.28$. We need

$$n = \frac{(0.045)^2(1.96 + 1.28)^2}{(0.03)^2} = 23.62.$$

Rounding up, we see that 24 pairs are required.

If only 20 pairs are available, approximate power can be obtained from (8.8) as

$$\text{Power} = \Phi\{E(Z) - 1.96\} = \Phi\left\{\frac{\delta}{\sqrt{\sigma^2/n}} - 1.96\right\}$$

$$= \Phi\left\{\frac{0.03}{\sqrt{(0.045)^2/20}} - 1.96\right\} = \Phi(1.021)$$

$$= 0.85. \tag{8.11}$$

Although we do not have 90% power with only 20 communities, we still achieve a respectable level of power, 85%.

Alternatively, we can find the difference in smoking quit probabilities detectable with 20 communities and 90% power by using (8.9):

$$\delta = (1.96 + 1.28)\sqrt{(0.045)^2/n} = 0.033.$$

In other words, although we do not have 90% power to detect a 3 percentage point difference with only 20 communities, we do have 90% power for a 3.3 percentage point difference.

8.3.2 Test of Proportions

The EZ principle can be used to compute sample size and power for a test of proportions. Substitute the expected proportions for $\hat{p}_C$ and $\hat{p}_T$ in the usual z-statistic formula, equate to $z_{\alpha/2} + z_\beta$, and solve for the per-arm sample size n:

$$\frac{p_C - p_T}{\sqrt{2\bar{p}(1 - \bar{p})/n}} = z_{\alpha/2} + z_\beta$$

$$\sqrt{n}(p_C - p_T) = (z_{\alpha/2} + z_\beta)\sqrt{2\bar{p}(1 - \bar{p})}$$

$$n = \frac{2(z_{\alpha/2} + z_\beta)^2 \bar{p}(1 - \bar{p})}{(p_C - p_T)^2}, \tag{8.12}$$

where $\bar{p} = (\hat{p}_C + \hat{p}_T)/2$.

Example 8.4. In the Pamoja Tulinde Maishe (PALM) trial in Ebola virus disease in the Democratic Republic of the Congo, the primary outcome was 28-day mortality. The expected event probability in the control arm was 0.30. The trial was powered for a large relative treatment benefit of 50%. That is, the 28-day mortality probability in a given treatment arm was assumed to be $(1 - 0.50)(0.30) = 0.15$. Therefore, $\bar{p} = (0.30 + 0.15)/2 = 0.225$. Although the primary analysis used Boschloo's test instead of the usual z-test of proportions, the two tests are asymptotically equivalent. Therefore, we proceed as if the usual z-test of proportions were being used.

Suppose we want 85% power, so $\beta = 0.15$ and $z_\beta = 1.04$. Formula (8.12) yields a sample size of

$$\frac{2(1.96 + 1.04)^2(0.225)(1 - 0.225)}{(0.30 - 0.15)^2} = 139.5.$$

We round up to 140 per arm, 280 total to achieve 85% power. □

Power for a given number of people can be obtained from (8.8) as

$$\text{Power} = \Phi \left\{ \frac{p_C - p_T}{\sqrt{\frac{2\bar{p}(1-\bar{p})}{n}}} - z_{\alpha/2} \right\}. \tag{8.13}$$

For example, suppose that in Example 8.4, the Ebola virus ends with only 100 participants per arm. Then power is approximately

$$\Phi \left\{ \frac{0.30 - 0.15}{\sqrt{\frac{2(0.225)(0.775)}{100}}} - 1.96 \right\} = \Phi(2.540 - 1.960) = 0.72.$$

That is, power is approximately 72% if there are 100 participants per arm.

The test of proportions setting is slightly different from other settings in that the variance of $\hat{\delta} = \hat{p}_C - \hat{p}_T$ differs depending on whether the null or alternative hypothesis is true. This has given rise to two alternative sample size formulas discussed in the Appendix at the end of the chapter. All three formulas give very similar sample sizes. We prefer formula (8.12) because it is slightly more conservative than the other two.

8.3.3   Logrank Test

Sample size for the logrank test differs slightly from the other settings considered in that it is in terms of number of events rather than number of people. Recall from (7.9) that the logrank z-score is

$$Z = \frac{\sum_{i=1}^{d}(O_i - E_i)}{\sqrt{\sum_{i=1}^{d} V_i}}.$$

Also, from the O minus E except after V principle (Principle 7.1), $\sum_{i=1}^{d}(O_i - E_i)/\sum_{i=1}^{d} V_i$ estimates the control to treatment log hazard ratio. Therefore, the logrank z-score is

$$Z = \frac{\sum_{i=1}^{d}(O_i - E_i)}{\sqrt{\sum_{i=1}^{d} V_i}} = \left\{ \frac{\sum_{i=1}^{d}(O_i - E_i)}{\sum_{i=1}^{d} V_i} \right\} \sqrt{\sum_{i=1}^{d} V_i} \approx \ln(\widehat{HR}) \sqrt{\sum_{i=1}^{d} V_i}.$$

Now consider $\sum_{i=1}^{d} V_i$. At the ith death, V_i is $n_{Ci} n_{Ti}/(n_{Ci} + n_{Ti})^2$, where n_{Ci} and n_{Ti} are the numbers of patients at risk in the control and treatment arms, respectively, just prior to the ith death. At the first death, the numbers at risk in the two arms should be nearly identical (assuming 1-1 randomization), so $V_1 = (1/2)(1-1/2) = 1/4$. At subsequent deaths, the numbers at risk in the two arms may separate somewhat if treatment is effective. Still, for treatment effects observed in clinical trials, n_{C_i} and n_{T_i} should be approximately the same and V_i should be approximately $(1/2)(1 - 1/2) = 1/4$. Therefore, $\sum_{i=1}^{d} V_i \approx d/4$ and

$$Z \approx \ln(\widehat{HR}) \sqrt{d/4}$$

$$E(Z) \approx \ln(HR) \sqrt{d/4}. \tag{8.14}$$

Equating the expected z-score to $z_{\alpha/2} + z_\beta$ and solving for d yields

$$d = \frac{4(z_{\alpha/2} + z_\beta)^2}{\{\ln(HR)\}^2}. \tag{8.15}$$

Equation (8.15) is the number of events needed to have power $1 - \beta$ for a two-tailed logrank test at level α or a one-tailed logrank test at level $\alpha/2$.

For example, suppose we want 90% power if treatment reduces the hazard for the primary outcome by 25%. That means that the treatment to control hazard ratio is $1 - 0.25 = 0.75$, and the control to treatment hazard ratio is $1/0.75 = 4/3$. The number of primary endpoints needed is approximately

$$d = \frac{4(1.96 + 1.28)^2}{\{\ln(4/3)\}^2} = 507.37.$$

In other words, approximately 508 events are required.

The number of people required for 508 events can be determined based on the assumed event rate and treatment effect. The simplest and most common method assumes an exponential distribution for time to event in each arm. Let λ_C be the exponential parameter in the control arm, so the density and distribution function for time to event are

$$f(t) = \lambda_C \exp(-\lambda_C t) \quad \text{and} \quad F(t) = 1 - \exp(-\lambda_C t).$$

For example, if we anticipate a 10% event rate per year, then we solve $1 - \exp(-\lambda_C \cdot 1) = 0.10$ for λ_C. This yields $\lambda_C = -\ln(1 - 0.90) = 0.1054$. A 25% reduction in hazard from treatment means that the hazard rate in the treatment arm is $(1 - 0.25)(0.1054) = 0.0791$. Suppose that there will be 2 years of recruitment followed by a minimum of 4 years of follow-up. That is, a patient recruited right after the study opened would be followed for $2 + 4 = 6$ years, whereas someone recruited after 2 years would be followed for $0 + 4 = 4$ years. "On average", a patient arrives at the halfway point of recruitment, 1 year, and is followed for $1 + 4 = 5$ years. Therefore, with n patients per arm followed for an average of 5 years, the expected numbers, E_C and E_T, of deaths in the two arms are

$$E_C = \{1 - \exp(-0.1054)\}n; \quad E_T = \{1 - \exp(-0.0791)\}n.$$

The total expected number of events is $E_C + E_T = \{2 - \exp(-0.1054) - \exp(-0.0791)\}n$. Equate $E_C + E_T$ to 508 and solve for n:

$$n = \frac{508}{\{2 - \exp(-0.1054) - \exp(-0.0791)\}} = 2884.92.$$

Therefore, the trial requires 2885 people per arm, 5770 total.

Power for a given number of events can be computed using Formula (8.8):

$$\text{Power} = \Phi\left\{E(Z) - z_{\alpha/2}\right\} \approx \Phi\left\{\ln(\text{HR})\sqrt{d/4} - z_{\alpha/2}\right\}. \qquad (8.16)$$

For instance, in the example above, if there are 450 events instead of 508, power is approximately

$$\Phi\left\{\ln(4/3)\sqrt{450/4} - 1.96\right\} = \Phi(1.091) = 0.86.$$

8.3.4 Cluster-Randomized Trials

The EZ principle also applies to clinical trials in which the unit of randomization is a cluster instead of an individual. The only difference from a sample size/power standpoint between individual- and cluster-randomized trials is that the correlation between repeated measurements in a cluster-randomized trial must be accounted for.

Let X be the endpoint, continuous or binary, measured on each of m individuals within a cluster. The endpoint for the cluster is the average, $Y = \bar{X} = (1/m)\sum_{i=1}^{m} X_i$. Under the assumption that all pairs of observations within a cluster have the same correlation ρ, the variance of Y is:

$$\sigma_Y^2 = \mathrm{var}\left(\frac{1}{m}\sum_{i=1}^{m}X_i\right) = \left(\frac{1}{m^2}\right)\mathrm{var}\left(\sum_{i=1}^{n}X_i\right)$$

$$= \left(\frac{1}{m^2}\right)\mathrm{cov}\left(\sum_{i=1}^{n}X_i,\sum_{j=1}^{n}X_j\right) = \left(\frac{1}{m^2}\right)\sum_{i=1}^{n}\sum_{j=1}^{n}\mathrm{cov}(X_i,X_j)$$

$$= \left(\frac{1}{m^2}\right)\left\{\sum_{i=1}^{m}\mathrm{var}(X_i) + \sum\sum_{i\neq j}\mathrm{cov}(X_i,X_j)\right\}$$

$$= \left(\frac{1}{m^2}\right)\left\{m\sigma_X^2 + m(m-1)\mathrm{cov}(X_1,X_2)\right\}$$

$$= \left(\frac{1}{m^2}\right)\left\{m\sigma_X^2 + m(m-1)\rho\sigma_X^2\right\}$$

$$= \left(\frac{\sigma_X^2}{m}\right)\left\{1 + (m-1)\rho\right\}. \tag{8.17}$$

In the binary outcome setting with $P(X=1)=p$, $\sigma_X^2 = p(1-p)$.

Note that the variance of $Y = \bar{X}$ in this correlated outcome setting is the variance of $Y = \bar{X}$ in the independent outcome setting times the *variance inflation factor*

$$\mathrm{VIF} = 1 + (m-1)\rho.$$

Even if the correlation ρ is small, it cannot be ignored. For example, if $\rho = 0.1$ and there are 100 observations per cluster, the variance inflation factor is $1 + 99(0.1) = 10.9$, meaning that the true variance of Y is more than 10 times larger than if we naively ignore the correlation. Another way to see the impact of the correlation is to note that $\mathrm{var}(Y)$ tends to 0 as $m \to \infty$ if $\rho = 0$, but tends to $\rho\sigma_X^2$ as $m \to \infty$ if $\rho \neq 0$.

Sample size, power, and detectable effect for a cluster-randomized trial with n clusters are exactly the same as for an individual-randomized trial of n people using a t-test, with σ^2 in the individual-randomized trial replaced by Expression (8.17).

Example 8.5. In some trials of infectious disease, a "case" (someone with the disease) is identified, and the "ring" of close contacts of that person are identified as being at high risk of contracting the disease. One option for testing whether a vaccine works is to randomize each cluster to the same condition, either all receive immediate vaccination or all receive delayed vaccination. This was the approach taken in the Ring Vaccination trial testing the rVSV-ZEBOV Ebola virus vaccine in Guinea in Western Africa (Henao-Restrepo, Camacho, Longini et al., 2017).

Suppose we want to determine sample size for a ring type trial in an infectious disease. Assume that the primary outcome for each ring is the proportion of members in the ring who contract the disease within 2 months. Let X_i be the indicator that individual i contracts the disease within 2 months. Assume that, in the absence of an effective vaccine, $P(X_i = 1) = 0.15$, and the average ring size is expected to be $m = 20$ people. The correlation between X_i and X_j is expected to be 0.10 for any pair of members of a ring. From (8.17), the variance of a typical ring proportion $Y = (1/20)\sum_{i=1}^{20}X_i$ is

$$\frac{(0.15)(0.85)}{20}\{1 + 19(0.1)\} = 0.0185.$$

Suppose we want 85% power if the vaccine reduces the probability of the disease by 60%. In that case, the expected value of the proportion with disease in the vaccine arm is $(1 - 0.60)(0.15)$, and the expected difference between delayed and immediate vaccination arms is $\delta = (0.15) - (0.15)(1 - 0.60) = 0.09$. Use Formula (8.4) with $z_{\alpha/2} = 1.96$, $z_\beta = 1.04$, $\delta = 0.09$, and $\sigma^2 = 0.0185$:

$$n = \frac{2(0.0185)(1.96 + 1.04)^2}{(0.09)^2} = 41.11.$$

This shows that approximately 42 rings in each arm are required. $\qquad\square$

8.3.5 In a Nutshell

Table 8.2 summarizes the expected z-score approach to sample size calculation in trials with different types of endpoints. The EZ principle can be used in conjunction with the expected z-score to quickly check a power calculation. Substitute parameter values expected in the trial; if the expected z-score is not approximately 2.80, 3.00, or 3.24, then power is not approximately 80, 85, or 90%.

Table 8.2: Examples of test statistics of the form (8.7) satisfying the key conditions.

	Estimator $\hat\delta$	$\widehat{se}(\hat\delta)$	$\theta = \mathrm{E}(Z)$
1-sample t-test	$\bar{D}$	$\frac{s_D}{\sqrt{n}}$	$\frac{\sqrt{n}\,\delta}{\sigma_D}$
2-sample t-test	$\bar{Y}_C - \bar{Y}_T$	$\sqrt{\frac{2}{n}}s_Y$	$\frac{\sqrt{\frac{n}{2}}\,\delta}{\sigma_Y}$
cluster randomized t-test, correlation ρ n clusters of size m	$\bar{Y}_C - \bar{Y}_T$ $Y = \frac{1}{m}\sum_{i=1}^m X_i$	$\sqrt{\frac{2}{n}}s_Y$	$\frac{\sqrt{\frac{n}{2}}\,\delta}{\sigma_Y}$ $\sigma_Y^2 = \left(\frac{\sigma_X^2}{m}\right)$ $\{1 + (m-1)\rho\}$
Linear/logistic reg	$\hat\beta$	$\widehat{se}(\hat\beta)$	$\frac{\beta}{se(\hat\beta)}$
proportions	$\hat{p}_C - \hat{p}_T$	$\sqrt{\frac{2\hat{p}(1-\hat{p})}{n}}$	$\frac{p_C - p_T}{\sqrt{\frac{2p(1-p)}{n}}}$
logrank, d events	$\frac{\sum_{i=1}^d (O_i - E_i)}{\sum_{i=1}^d V_i}$ estimates $\ln(HR)$	$\frac{1}{\sqrt{\sum_{i=1}^d V_i}} \approx \sqrt{4/d}$	$\ln(HR)\sqrt{\frac{d}{4}}$

8.4   Nonzero Nulls

In some cases, we are interested in testing a nonzero null hypothesis. For example, in a vaccine trial, participants who do not yet have a disease are given a vaccine that could have side effects or other adverse effects. Consequently, we may want to prove not only that vaccine reduces the incidence of a disease, but that it reduces the incidence by at least 30%, for example. Another example with a nonzero null hypothesis is a noninferiority trial. The goal is not to demonstrate superiority of a new drug to the standard drug, but to demonstrate that the new drug is not more than 0.10 worse than the standard drug, for example. If p_N and p_S denote the probabilities of event on the new and standard drugs, and $\delta = p_S - p_N$, we would formulate the null and alternative hypotheses as $H_0 : \delta \leq -0.10$ versus $H_1 : \delta > -0.10$.

We can easily convert a nonzero null hypothesis $H_0 : \delta = \delta_0$ to the zero null hypothesis $H_0 : \delta - \delta_0 = 0$. Therefore, sample size and power can be computed using the expected z-score method, but now the z-score is

$$Z = \frac{\hat{\delta} - \delta_0}{\widehat{se}(\hat{\delta})}.$$

Example 8.6. Sample size for a noninferiority trial   Consider a tuberculosis trial in which the cure rate after 6 months of treatment in a difficult to treat population is expected to be 90%. We wish to test whether a 4-month regimen can produce results "almost as good," meaning that the cure rate with 4 months of treatment is not more than 5 percentage points worse than with 6 months of treatment. Denote the probability of relapsing on 4 and 6 months of treatment by p_4 and p_6, and let $\delta = p_6 - p_4$. Then the null and alternative hypotheses are $H_0 : \delta \leq -0.05$ versus $H_0 : \delta > -0.05$. The z-score is

$$Z = \frac{\hat{p}_6 - \hat{p}_4 - (-0.05)}{\sqrt{\frac{\hat{p}_6(1-\hat{p}_6)+\hat{p}_4(1-\hat{p}_4)}{n}}} = \frac{\hat{p}_6 - \hat{p}_4 + 0.05}{\sqrt{\frac{\hat{p}_6(1-\hat{p}_6)+\hat{p}_4(1-\hat{p}_4)}{n}}}.$$

We want to compute power with 400 per arm if the true relapse probability is 0.10 in each arm. Substitute 400 for n and 0.10 for $\hat{p}_4$ and $\hat{p}_6$ to approximate the expected z-score.

$$E(Z) = \frac{(0.10) - (0.10) + 0.05}{\sqrt{\frac{2(0.10)(0.90)}{400}}} = 2.357.$$

For a 1-tailed test at level 0.05, $z_\alpha = 1.645$, so power is approximately

$$\Phi(2.357 - 1.645) = \Phi(0.712) = 0.76.$$

Therefore, power is lower than the conventionally accepted level of 0.80 or greater.

□

8.5   Practical Aspects of Sample Size Calculations

Thus far we have focused on the calculation of sample size and power, but have said nothing about how to estimate the parameters needed for the calculation. This section is devoted to the practical aspects of sample size calculations. Regardless of the setting (comparison of means, proportions, or survival), we must specify the treatment effect δ and *nuisance parameters*, quantities that are not of primary interest, but must nevertheless be estimated.

For example, if the primary outcome is continuous and a t-test is used, sample size depends on the between-arm difference in means, $\delta = \mu_T - \mu_C$, and the common standard deviation σ, the nuisance parameter. If the primary endpoint is binary and a large sample z or chi-squared test is used, sample size depends on the between-arm difference in probabilities of events, $\delta = p_T - p_C$, and the control probability of event, p_C. Here, p_C is the nuisance parameter. Keep in mind, as you read this section, that nuisance parameters are handled very differently than the treatment effect. Nuisance parameters must be accurately **estimated**, whereas the treatment effect used to power a trial might be estimated or might be determined as the smallest effect that is deemed worthy of detection.

8.5.1 Test of Means

Estimation of Nuisance Parameter

For the t-test, we usually assume a common standard deviation σ between the two arms. The rule to follow is this:

Err on the side of overestimating σ.

The reason is that the sample size function (8.4) is an increasing function of σ. Overestimating σ means using a sample size that is larger than necessary, ensuring higher than the desired power level. On the other hand, underestimating σ results in a sample size too small and power too low. The best way to get a reasonable estimate of σ is from a similar clinical trial, if there is one. It is not generally a good idea to use, without alteration, an estimate of standard deviation from an observational study. An interventional clinical trial changes the normal routine of participants by assigning them to a new treatment or control treatment. Changing someone's routine could very well increase variability. It is far better to estimate σ from a randomized clinical trial.

It may be difficult to find a comparable clinical trial. For example, suppose the outcome in the current trial is change in systolic blood pressure from baseline to 8 weeks. The relevant standard deviation is the standard deviation of a change over 8 weeks. We might have data from a clinical trial whose primary outcome was change in systolic blood pressure from baseline to 4 weeks. Using the estimate from the 4-week trial without modification is not advisable because the standard deviation of a change over some duration of time often increases with the duration. Therefore, using the standard deviation of 4-week change will probably underestimate σ. If the situation were reversed, i.e., the planned trial will use a 4-week change and the prior trial used an 8-week change, we might use that estimate on the grounds that it should be conservative (that is, it would, if anything, overestimate σ).

Articles reporting results of trials that use a change from baseline often make the same mistake; they report the mean and standard deviation at baseline and at the end of study, without reporting the standard deviation of the **change** from baseline to end of study. Investigators planning a new trial cannot readily use the information to estimate the standard deviation of change. However, most articles report a confidence interval, from which we can back calculate the standard deviation. If the reported estimate and $100(1-\alpha)\%$ confidence interval are $\hat{\delta}$ and (L, U). Then $U - \hat{\delta}$ and $\hat{\delta} - L$ both estimate $t_{n-1,\alpha/2}s/\sqrt{n}$ in a paired data setting and $t_{n_T+n_C-2,\alpha/2}s\sqrt{1/n_T + 1/n_C}$ in a two-sample trial, where $t_{\nu,\alpha/2}$ is the $(1-\alpha/2)$th quantile of a t-distribution with ν degrees of freedom. Back calculating s in a paired setting yields

$$s = \frac{\sqrt{n}\left(U - \hat{\delta}\right)}{t_{n-1,\alpha/2}} \text{ or } s = \frac{\sqrt{n}\left(\hat{\delta} - L\right)}{t_{n-1,\alpha/2}}.$$

In the two-sample setting, the two estimates of the common standard deviation are

$$s = \frac{U - \hat{\delta}}{t_{n_T+n_C-2,\alpha/2}\sqrt{1/n_T + 1/n_C}} \text{ or } s = \frac{\hat{\delta} - L}{t_{n_T+n_C-2,\alpha/2}\sqrt{1/n_T + 1/n_C}}.$$

For example, suppose that the estimate and 95% confidence interval for a trial with 10 and 12 people in the treatment and control arms are 6.5 and $(4.6, 8.5)$, respectively. Then $\alpha = 0.05$ and there are $10 + 12 - 2 = 20$ degrees of freedom. The critical value $t_{0.05/2,20} = t_{0.025,20}$ is 2.086, so the estimates of s are

$$\frac{8.5 - 6.5}{2.086\sqrt{1/10 + 1/12}} = 2.239 \text{ or } \frac{6.5 - 4.6}{2.086\sqrt{1/10 + 1/12}} = 2.127.$$

The estimates differ somewhat because of roundoff error for the numbers reported in the article. To be conservative, we would use the larger standard deviation estimate of 2.239.

Another method of estimating the standard deviation of change from standard deviations reported at the separate time points can be used if the correlation ρ between baseline and end of study measurements is known. The standard deviation of change can be estimated as $\{2\sigma^2(1 - \rho)\}^{1/2}$ (Equation 4.8). For example, suppose that a trial reports standard deviations of 9.747 and 10.247 at baseline and end of trial, respectively. The average of the two variances is $\{(9.747)^2 + (10.247)^2\}/2 \approx 100$, so the standard deviation at a given time point is estimated as $\sqrt{100} = 10$. If the correlation between baseline and end of study measurements is known to be approximately 0.75, then the standard deviation of change is estimated to be $\{2(10)^2(1 - 0.75)\}^{1/2} = 7.07$.

Specification of Treatment Effect

There is a choice in how to select the treatment effect for sample size/power calculations. One option is to specify the treatment effect that was observed in a similar clinical trial. That would be logical if the intent is to replicate the trial in a somewhat different population, for example. But another option is to specify the minimum effect that would be worthy of detection. In a drug trial, there are almost always side effects and other adverse effects. Consequently, to justify the use of such a drug, we should be able to demonstrate a relatively large benefit on the target of therapy, say blood pressure. On the other hand, in a trial comparing two diets, we expect fewer adverse effects. Even if one diet lowers blood pressure by a very modest amount relative to another diet, that might be worthwhile from a public health standpoint. Therefore, whereas a drug trial might anticipate a relatively large effect on blood pressure (e.g., 5 mmHg), a diet trial might be powered for a smaller effect like 2 mmHg.

8.5.2   Test of Proportions

For the test of proportions, we must specify the probability of the primary endpoint in the control and treatment arms. We often regard the control probability p_C as the nuisance parameter. For the purpose of sample size calculations, we specify the treatment effect as either $p_T - p_C$ or $p_C - p_T$, whichever would be expected to be positive if treatment is effective. That is, we use $p_T - p_C$ if the outcome is a good thing like response to treatment, and $p_C - p_T$ if the outcome is a bad thing like death within 28 days. Rather than specifying a given difference like 0.10 between control and treatment probabilities of events, we often think in terms of a given relative reduction in event probability. For example, we might specify that the control probability is expected to be 0.20, and we wish to detect a 25% relative reduction in the treatment arm. That is, we expect the probability of event in the treatment arm to be $(1 - 0.25)(0.20) = 0.15$.

Estimation of Nuisance Parameter

When the treatment effect is expressed as a given relative reduction in event probability, such as 25%, the sample size formula (8.12) increases as p_C decreases. Therefore, to be conservative, we should follow this rule:

Err on the side of underestimating p_C.

That way, we may end up with more patients than necessary, but that will give even more power. Underestimating p_C is easier said than done. Event rate estimates taken from observational studies will almost always overestimate the rate in a clinical trial. Participants who volunteer for clinical trials tend to be more health-conscious than the general population. Participants in a clinical trial often receive more care than they would have outside the trial. Therefore, event rate estimates from observational studies need to be reduced to reflect a healthy volunteer effect and a better background care effect. If the observational data was from years ago, one must also account for improvement of care over time. Such adjustments to event rates are somewhat arbitrary, so it would be far better to use an event rate from a similar clinical trial conducted at roughly the same time.

8.5.3 Specification of Treatment Effect

As mentioned earlier, the difference in proportions δ used in sample size/power calculations is often arrived at indirectly by specifying a control event rate and a given relative reduction from treatment. Relative reductions of 25% or more are generally considered large effects, whereas relative reductions of 15% or less are considered small. The treatment effect on a primary endpoint that is closely related to the mechanism of action of the intervention should be larger than the effect on a more distant outcome. For example, in a cardiovascular trial, a cholesterol lowering medication would be expected to have a larger effect on heart attacks than on overall mortality. After all, many things could cause death, only some of which may be affected by treatment.

The same reasoning that was used in trials with a continuous outcome apply to binary outcome trials as well. A treatment that is expected to have adverse effects would need to have a relatively large effect to be deemed worthwhile, whereas a more benign treatment could be worthwhile even if it had a smaller effect.

8.6 Exact Power

Thus far we have demonstrated approximate sample size and power calculations using asymptotic formulas, but power can be computed exactly for some tests.

8.6.1 t-Tests

Power for the t-test can be computed using the noncentral t-distribution. The following R program can be used to compute power for either a one-sample or two-sample t-test.

```
# One sample t
n<-15                          # sample size
delta<-8                       # mean
sig<-10                        # standard deviation
df<-n-1                        # degrees of freedom for a one-sample test
alpha<-0.05                    # two-tailed test at level alpha
crit<-qf(1-alpha,1,df)         # critical value for F (square of t)
noncent<-sqrt(n)*delta/sig     # noncentrality parameter for t
```

```
noncenf<-noncent^2                    # noncentrality parameter for F
pow<-round(1-pf(crit,1,df,noncenf),
digits=3)                             # power
pow


# Two sample t
n1<-20                                # sample size, arm 1
n2<-20                                # sample size, arm 2
delta<-10                             # difference of means
sig<-11                               # common standard deviation
df<-n1+n2-2                           # degrees of freedom for a two-sample test
alpha<-0.05                           # two-tailed test at level alpha
crit<-qf(.95,1,df)                    # critical value for F (square of t)
noncent<-delta/sqrt(sig^2*(1/n1+1/n2))  # noncentrality parameter for t
noncenf<-noncent^2                    # noncentrality parameter for F
pow<-round(1-pf(crit,1,df,noncenf),
digits=3)                             # power
pow
```

For example, the one-sample program above shows power when the sample size, mean, and standard deviation are $n = 15$, $\mu = 8$, and $\sigma = 10$. Running this R program yields power 0.821. Simply change the numbers to fit the circumstances of the given trial.

The two-sample test shows power when the sample sizes, difference in means, and common standard deviation are $n = 20$ per arm, $\delta = \mu_1 - \mu_2 = 10$, and $\sigma = 11$. Running this program yields power 0.80. Again, change the numbers to fit the circumstances of the given trial.

8.6.2   Exact Power for Fisher's Exact Test

For Fisher's exact test, we can compute exact power by using the event probabilities in each arm to calculate the probability of each possible outcome, and then summing the probabilities of outcomes that yield a p-value of α or less. The following R program does this.

```
fishy<-function(n0,n1,p0,p1,alpha){
# This program computes exact power for Fisher's exact test

# alpha is the alpha level for the test
# n0 and n1 are the sample sizes in groups 0 and 1
# p0 and p1 are probabilities in groups 0 and 1

power<-0
for(i0 in 0:n0){
    for(i1 in 0:n1){
       datmat<-matrix(c(i0,n0-i0,i1,n1-i1),nrow=2,byrow=T)
       pval<-fisher.test(datmat,alternative="two.sided")$p.value
       if(pval<=alpha) power<-power+dbinom(i0,n0,p0)*dbinom(i1,n1,p1)
    }
}
power<-round(power,digits=3)
return(paste("power for test of |p1-p0|>0 is", power))
```

```
}

# SUPPLY THE KEY PARAMETERS IN THE NEXT LINE
n0<-30; n1<-30; p0<-.50; p1<-.15; alpha<-0.05

fishy(n0,n1,p0,p1,alpha)
```

The program above gives power for a two-tailed Fisher's exact test at $\alpha = 0.05$ with 30 patients per arm when the control and treatment probabilities of events are 0.50 and 0.15, respectively. Running this program yields power 0.777. Change the above numbers to fit the circumstances of the specific trial.

8.7 Adjusting for Noncompliance and Other Factors

Several papers (e.g., Lakatos, 1986; Lakatos, 1988) attempt to adjust sample size calculations for noncompliance, dropout, and other factors. This requires specification of (1) the treatment effect under ideal conditions, i.e., with perfect compliance and no missing data, and (2) the rates of noncompliance, dropout, and so on. The approach divides time into tiny intervals; within each interval, a patient can be in any of several states. For example, consider a relatively simple setting in which patients assigned to either arm might drop out of the study, and patients assigned to the treatment arm might stop taking treatment. During any tiny interval of time, a patient in the control arm could be in one of three states: (1) event, (2) no event, but still in follow-up, or (3) no event, no longer in follow-up. A patient in the treatment arm could be one of four states: (1) event, (2) no event, in follow-up, and on treatment, (3) no event, in follow-up, and off treatment, (4) no event, no longer in follow-up. For a patient who is still in follow-up, the probability of having an event in a tiny time interval is calculated based on whether the patient is on or off treatment during that interval. The clinical trial is then simulated a large number of times, and the proportion of trials resulting in a statistically significant difference is used to estimate power.

We do not favor the approach in the preceding paragraph. Rates of noncompliance, loss to follow-up, etc., are difficult to predict. The process of estimating the treatment effect by trying to estimate multiple unknown rates is analogous to trying to estimate someone's weight by adding the estimated weights of their fingers, toes, and so on. The error in estimating weights of separate body parts is likely to be much greater than the error in just giving a 'ballpark' estimate of overall weight. Likewise, the error in estimating things like noncompliance, loss to follow-up is likely to be greater than the error in estimating the total attenuation of treatment effect caused by all factors combined. Furthermore, the models assume that patients who stop complying with treatment have the same event rate as a randomly selected control patient. In reality, patients who discontinue treatment may be very different from randomly selected control patients. We prefer the much simpler method of computing sample size for a given *net* reduction in event rate. Thus, if we expect a reduction of 25% under ideal conditions, we might power the trial for a 20% net reduction.

Exercises

1. Why is it important to have high power in a clinical trial?

2. Which one of the following is a correct statement summarizing the meaning of 90% power for a treatment difference of size 5 in a test of $H_0 : \delta = 0$ versus the alternative hypothesis $H_1 : \delta \neq 0$?

(a) If the observed treatment effect is 5, there is a 90% chance of a statistically significant result.

(b) If the true treatment effect is 5, there is a 90% chance of a statistically significant result.

(c) If the true treatment effect is 5, there is a 90% chance that the observed effect will be at least 5.

(d) If the observed treatment effect is at least 5, there is a 90% chance that the true treatment effect is at least 5.

(e) If the null hypothesis is true, there is a 90% chance that the result will not be statistically significant.

3. The sample size section for a clinical trial that used a two-sample t-test claimed that 50 people per arm would give 90% power. The expected treatment effect and standard deviation were 2 and 10, respectively. Is this calculation approximately correct? Justify your answer.

4. The sample size section for a clinical trial that used a z-test of proportions claimed that 200 people per arm would give 80% power. The event probabilities in the control and treatment arms are expected to be 0.20 and 0.10, respectively. Is the sample size calculation approximately correct?

5. In a clinical trial using a two-sample test to compare arms, suppose that a sample size of 10 per arm is used and the standard deviation is 5.

(a) Use the key equation (8.2) to approximate power to detect a treatment difference of 6.

(b) Use the program in Section 8.6 to compute exact power to detect a treatment difference of 6.

(c) Now repeat (a) for a sample size of 20 per arm.

(d) Repeat (b) for a sample size of 20 per arm.

(e) Why are (c) and (d) closer to each other than (a) and (b)?

6. Consider a clinical trial using Fisher's exact test to compare probabilities p_T and p_C of events in the treatment and control arms. Suppose that $p_C = 0.40$ and $p_T = 0.20$ and the sample size is 75 per arm.

(a) Use the key equation (8.2) to approximate power.

(b) Use the program in Section 8.6 to compute exact power.

7. In a survival trial, approximately how many events are required for 85% power to detect a treatment to control hazard ratio of 0.50?

8. In a cluster-randomized trial, suppose that the number of people in each cluster is 50.

(a) Is the number of clusters required for a given power level an increasing or decreasing function of the correlation ρ between two observations within a cluster?

(b) If you calculate the number of clusters by assuming $\rho = 0$, but the truth is that $\rho > 0$, will your answer be an underestimate or overestimate of the number of clusters actually needed?

9. Suppose that power to detect a given treatment effect is 90%. What is the power to detect an effect that is 30% smaller?

10. Suppose that power to detect a given effect in a t-test is 80%. What is power if the standard deviation is only half as large as anticipated?

8.8 Appendix: Other Sample Size Formulas for Two Proportions

Sample size formula (8.12) was based on the *score statistic*, with variance of $\hat{p}_C - \hat{p}_T$ estimated under the null hypothesis. The *Wald statistic*,

$$Z_W = \frac{\hat{p}_C - \hat{p}_T}{\sqrt{\hat{p}_C(1 - \hat{p}_C)/n_C + \hat{p}_T(1 - \hat{p}_T)/n_T}},$$

uses a variance that does not assume the null hypothesis. Substituting the expected values of $\hat{p}_T$ and $\hat{p}_C$ under the alternative hypothesis yields the sample size formula

$$n = \frac{(z_{\alpha/2} + z_\beta)^2 \{p_C(1 - p_C) + p_T(1 - p_T)\}}{(p_C - p_T)^2}. \tag{8.18}$$

The most common per-arm sample size formula for the test of proportions merges features of the score and Wald statistic:

$$n = \frac{\left\{ z_{\alpha/2}\sqrt{2p(1 - p)} + z_\beta\sqrt{p_C(1 - p_C) + p_T(1 - p_T)} \right\}^2}{(p_C - p_T)^2}. \tag{8.19}$$

The three formulas are asymptotically equivalent, even though they are always ordered in the following way:

$$(8.18) \leq (8.19) \leq (8.12). \tag{8.20}$$

To see this, note that the function $f(p) = p(1-p)$ is concave, which implies that $(1/2)f(p_C) + (1/2)f(p_T) \leq f(\bar{p}) = f\{(p_C + p_T)/2\}$. Consequently, $p_T(1 - p_T) + p_C(1 - p_C) \leq 2\bar{p}(1 - \bar{p})$. This implies that the sample sizes in the three formulas are ordered as in (8.20)

The most conservative of the three sample size formulas is (8.12) because it gives the largest sample size.

8.9 Summary

1. If power is high, a null result makes us confident that the treatment effect is not as large as originally hypothesized.

2. Formulas for sample size, power, and detectable effect for a two-tailed test at level α or a one-tailed test at level $\alpha/2$ all flow from the EZ principle: for power $1 - \beta$ for a one-tailed test at level $\alpha/2$ or a two-tailed test at level α,

$$\mathrm{E}(Z) = z_{\alpha/2} + z_\beta. \tag{8.21}$$

3. Equation (8.21) makes it easy to check sample size calculations: substitute values expected for nuisance parameters and the treatment effect into the z-score equation. This 'expected' z-score should be approximately $z_{\alpha/2} + z_\beta$.

4. If the assumptions underlying the sample size calculation are correct, we expect to see a very large z-score and very small p-value. If the actual z-score is barely significant, the observed treatment effect was much smaller than hypothesized.

5. Sample size calculations require accurate **estimation** of nuisance parameters and **specification** of the treatment effect. The treatment effect could be based either on estimates from other trials or based on the smallest effect that is clinically meaningful.

6. The treatment effect for which a trial is powered should reflect the treatment's expected adverse event profile; the more side effects or adverse events expected, the larger the treatment effect should be to justify use of that treatment.

7. For a continuous outcome analyzed using a t-test, it is better to overestimate than underestimate the variance.

8. For a binary outcome powered for a fixed relative effect (e.g., a 25% reduction), it is better to underestimate than overestimate the control event probability.

Chapter 9

Monitoring

9.1 Introduction

Clinical trials are monitored throughout by a *Data and Safety Monitoring Board (DSMB)*, a group of outside experts who make recommendations to the trial sponsor about whether to continue as is, make a change such as dropping an arm, or stop the study. The sponsor makes the final decision, but they almost always accept the recommendations of the DSMB. The board typically consists of between 4 and 10 members: doctors, one or two statisticians, and an ethicist. Their most important responsibility is to ensure the safety of participants in the trial. A more mundane responsibility is to monitor general conduct to ensure that outcomes are being measured properly, forms are being submitted in a timely fashion, data are being transcribed correctly, and so on. Statistical aspects of monitoring relate to efficacy, safety, and futility: has the treatment demonstrated clear superiority over control, are there compelling safety concerns that preclude use of the drug, or are results so unpromising that there is no point in continuing? Because trials are monitored at *interim analyses* (also called *interim looks*) after groups of data accrue, the term *group-sequential monitoring* is used.

Decisions of a DSMB can be very difficult. The board must weigh two sometimes competing ethical principles: (1) *individual ethics*: preserve the safety and wellbeing of individuals in the trial and (2) *collective ethics*: consider the impact of decisions on the collective good of people outside the trial. For instance, when a DSMB recommends stopping a trial because the treatment appears to be superior to control, they think primarily about patients inside the trial. Stopping and unblinding the trial may allow patients in the control arm to start taking the beneficial medication. But stopping before the evidence is sufficient to convince the medical community may not change medical practice. That could negatively affect the care of people outside the trial. Members of a DSMB may disagree on what recommendation to make. That is when good communication between members becomes paramount. There is a reason that a DSMB is composed of experts in different fields. You, as a statistician, must find a way to explain statistical concepts in simple terms to other members, just as they must explain biology, immunology, and medical concepts to allow you to make the most informed decision. A DSMB should always try to reach a unanimous decision. A split decision is difficult for a sponsor to interpret. Service on a DSMB, while difficult at times, is also very rewarding. Embrace the challenge!

DOI: 10.1201/9781315164090-9

9.2   Efficacy Monitoring

9.2.1   Brief History of Efficacy Boundaries

In the 1960s and early 1970s, clinical trials often used the same criterion for stopping at interim analyses as at the final analysis. They stopped if the p-value ever dropped below 0.05. The problem with this procedure is that the *familywise error rate*, the probability of at least one false rejection of the null hypothesis, exceeds α. Just as an unskilled dart thrower will hit the bull's eye given enough throws, an ineffective treatment will appear beneficial with enough interim analyses using the same level of evidence at each. In the words of British economist Ronald Coase, "if you torture the data long enough, it will confess to anything."

Table 9.1 shows the probability of falsely declaring a treatment difference at least once among k analyses using a two-tailed z-test at level 0.01 or 0.05. As we will see in Section 9.2.2, Table 9.1 and the other tables in this section apply asymptotically for a wide range of different z-statistics. Even with only two analyses, the actual type I error rate for a trial intended to have $\alpha = 0.05$ is 0.083 when there is an equal amount of information between successive looks (we define "information" precisely later; for now, think of sample size). Things can be even worse with unequal amounts of information between successive looks. For example, with 10 looks, the actual type I error rate for an $\alpha = 0.05$ test is 0.193 for equally-spaced looks and 0.401 for the worst case timing of looks.

Table 9.1: type I error rate if the null hypothesis is rejected whenever the two-tailed p-value drops below the intended level, 0.01 or 0.05. The analysis times are either equally spaced or at their worst case configuration in terms of alpha inflation.

# Looks (k)	Reject H_0 if $p \leq 0.01$		Reject H_0 if $p \leq 0.05$	
	Equally Spaced	Worst Case	Equally Spaced	Worst Case
2	0.018	0.020	0.083	0.098
3	0.024	0.030	0.107	0.143
4	0.029	0.039	0.126	0.185
5	0.033	0.049	0.142	0.226
6	0.036	0.059	0.155	0.265
7	0.040	0.068	0.166	0.302
8	0.042	0.077	0.176	0.337
9	0.045	0.086	0.185	0.370
10	0.047	0.096	0.193	0.401
20	0.064	0.182	0.248	0.642

The solution to the alpha inflation problem is to require stronger evidence to stop at an interim analysis than would be required with a single analysis of data. An early suggestion by Pocock (1977) assumes equal spacing of looks in terms of information. The Pocock boundary uses the same z-score cutoff at each analysis, where that cutoff is selected to make the familywise error rate α. Table 9.2 shows the z-score and p-value cutoffs for two-tailed tests at an overall alpha of 0.01, 0.05, or 0.10. For example, for a 4-look trial at $\alpha = 0.01$, the trial is stopped at any look if the absolute value of the z-score is 2.939 or greater. Equivalently, the trial is stopped if the two-tailed p-value is 0.0033 or less. A serious drawback to the Pocock procedure is that the level of evidence required at the end of the trial is much greater than if there were no monitoring. In this example, the p-value cutoff at the end of the trial, 0.0033, is about three times smaller than if there were no monitoring. For this reason, Pocock now recommends against his procedure.

Table 9.2: Two-tailed boundaries for the absolute value of the z-score or the two-tailed p-value for the Pocock procedure.

# Looks (k)	$\alpha = 0.01$	$\alpha = 0.05$	$\alpha = 0.10$
1	2.576	1.960	1.645
	0.0100	0.0500	0.1000
2	2.772	2.178	1.875
	0.0056	0.0294	0.0608
3	2.873	2.289	1.992
	0.0041	0.0221	0.0464
4	2.939	2.361	2.067
	0.0033	0.0182	0.0387
5	2.986	2.413	2.122
	0.0028	0.0158	0.0338
6	3.023	2.453	2.164
	0.0025	0.0142	0.0305
7	3.053	2.485	2.197
	0.0023	0.0130	0.0280
8	3.078	2.512	2.225
	0.0021	0.0120	0.0261
9	3.099	2.535	2.249
	0.0019	0.0112	0.0245
10	3.117	2.555	2.270
	0.0018	0.0106	0.0232

A better option is to require extremely strong evidence to stop very early. Strange results can happen early in a trial when staff may be less familiar with a complex protocol, for example. We would not want to stop early, only to find out that an apparent treatment effect was really the result of misinterpretation of protocol procedures. For this reason, early boundaries should be quite high. Another advantage of high early boundaries is that they allow the boundary at the end of the trial to be close to what it would be with no monitoring. The *Haybittle-Peto boundary*, slightly modified from its first description in Haybittle (1971), is based on the Bonferroni inequality. At each of $k - 1$ interim analyses, stopping for efficacy requires a p-value of 0.001 or less. At the final analysis, the p-value is required to be $\leq \alpha - (k - 1)(0.001)$. For example, if $\alpha = 0.05$ and there are three interim and one final analysis, we stop at any interim analysis if $p \leq 0.001$, and at the final analysis if $p \leq 0.05 - 3(0.001) = 0.047$. By the Bonferroni inequality, the probability of at least one false declaration that treatment has an effect is

$$P[\cup_{i=1}^{4}\{\text{Reject } H_0 \text{ at analysis } i\}] \leq \sum_{i=1}^{4} P\{\text{Reject } H_0 \text{ at analysis } i\}$$

$$= 3(0.001) + 0.05 - 3(0.001) = 0.05.$$

Three advantages of the Haybittle-Peto method are: (1) simplicity–no computer programs are needed, (2) the boundaries are guaranteed to control the familywise error rate regardless

of the joint distribution of the test statistic over time, and (3) the looks do not need to be
equally-spaced in terms of information.

A disadvantage of the Haybittle-Peto method is that the change in required p-values from
0.001 at an interim analysis to close to 0.05 at the final analysis is abrupt. For example,
consider a trial using a test of proportions, and suppose there are four equally-spaced
analyses. Suppose that the p-value at the third analysis is 0.005, not quite small enough
to declare a difference. Suppose that more of the remaining events occur in the treatment
group than in the control group, but because the p-value was so small at the third analysis,
the final p-value crosses its boundary of 0.047 (Figure 9.1). It seems illogical that we were
not convinced of the treatment's benefit at the third analysis, but now that we have seen
a partial reversal of results from the third to the final analysis, we are convinced! We call
this the *reversal of fortune problem.*

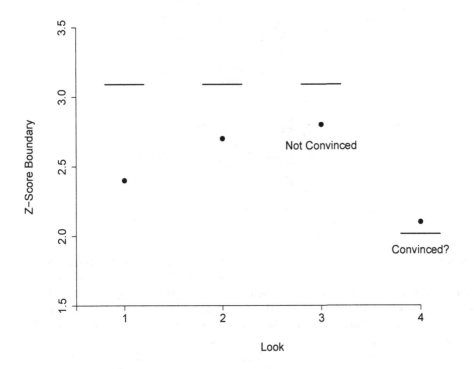

Figure 9.1: Haybittle-Peto boundary and observed z-scores for a trial with three interim and one final
analysis. The boundary is first crossed at the end, after a partial reversal of results.

We now have a conundrum. On one hand, we want boundaries to be high early and then
decrease as the trial progresses. On the other hand, we want to avoid the reversal of fortune
problem described in the preceding paragraph. It can be shown that for equally-spaced looks,
the   steepest   descending
z-score boundaries c_i that avoid the reversal of fortune problem are obtained by making c_i proportional to $1/i^{1/2}$. This condition, coupled with the requirement that the overall
type I error rate is α, leads to a unique boundary, the *O'Brien-Fleming boundary.* (O'Brien
and Fleming, 1979). The z-score and p-value required to stop at each of the k equally-
spaced looks are shown in Table 9.3 for $k = 1, 2, \ldots, 10$ equally spaced looks. For instance,
with a 6-look trial, the absolute value of the z-score must be ≥ 5.029 (two-tailed p-value

Table 9.3: Two-tailed boundaries for the absolute value of the z-score or the two-tailed p-value for the O'Brien-Fleming procedure at $\alpha = 0.05$. Row k contains the boundaries for k equally-spaced analyses, $k = 1, 2, \ldots, 10$.

k	1	2	3	4	5	6	7	8	9	10
1	1.960									
	0.0500									
2	2.796	1.977								
	0.0052	0.0480								
3	3.471	2.454	2.004							
	0.0005	0.0141	0.0451							
4	4.048	2.862	2.337	2.024						
	5×10^{-5}	0.0042	0.0194	0.0430						
5	4.562	3.226	2.634	2.281	2.040					
	5×10^{-6}	0.0013	0.0084	0.0225	0.0414					
6	5.029	3.556	2.903	2.514	2.249	2.053				
	5×10^{-7}	0.0004	0.0037	0.0119	0.0245	0.0401				
7	5.458	3.860	3.151	2.729	2.441	2.228	2.063			
	5×10^{-8}	0.0001	0.0016	0.0064	0.0146	0.0259	0.0391			
8	5.861	4.144	3.384	2.930	2.621	2.393	2.215	2.072		
	5×10^{-9}	3×10^{-5}	0.0007	0.0034	0.0088	0.0167	0.0268	0.0383		
9	6.240	4.412	3.603	3.120	2.791	2.547	2.358	2.206	2.080	
	4×10^{-10}	1×10^{-5}	0.0003	0.0018	0.0053	0.0109	0.0184	0.0274	0.0375	
10	6.600	4.667	3.810	3.300	2.951	2.694	2.494	2.333	2.200	2.087
	4×10^{-11}	3×10^{-6}	0.0001	0.0010	0.0032	0.0071	0.0126	0.0196	0.0278	0.0369

$\leq 5 \times 10^{-7}$) at the first look, 3.556 (two-tailed p-value ≤ 0.0004) at the second look,..., 2.053 (two-tailed p-value ≤ 0.0401) at the sixth look. Note that the O'Brien-Flemingry, like the Pocock boundary, requires looks to be equally-spaced in terms of information.

Figure 9.2 compares the Pocock, O'Brien-Fleming, and Haybittle-Peto boundaries for four equally spaced looks. The two procedures with high early boundaries, O'Brien-Fleming and Haybittle-Peto, have a final boundary close to 1.96.

The Pocock and O'Brien-Fleming boundaries are two members of the *Wang-Tsiatis family* of group-sequential boundaries $c_i = c(i/k)^{\Delta - 0.5}$, $0 \leq \Delta \leq 0.5$. $\Delta = 0$ produces the O'Brien-Fleming boundary, while $\Delta = 0.5$ produces the Pocock boundary. Values of Δ in the open interval $(0, 0.5)$ produce boundaries intermediate between those of O'Brien-Fleming and Pocock.

As we have seen, some early procedures like Pocock or O'Brien-Fleming require equal spacing of looks in terms of information. The problem is that DSMBs meet according to the busy schedules of their members. The amount of information between successive DSMB meetings may or may not be equal. Lan and DeMets (1983) solved this problem by specifying an increasing *alpha spending function* $\alpha^*(t)$ dictating the cumulative amount of alpha to spend when the proportion of information is t. At the beginning and end of the trial, $t = 0$ and $t = 1$, so $\alpha^*(0) = 0$ and $\alpha^*(1) = \alpha$. The latter constraint ensures that all of the alpha is eventually spent. The spending function is used to find boundaries such that the cumulative crossing probability by time t is $\alpha^*(t)$. Construction of a one-tailed upper boundary is as follows. At the first analysis, determine c_1 such that $P(Z(t_1) > c_1) = \alpha^*(t_1)$. At the second analysis, determine c_2 such that $P\{Z(t_1) > c_1 \text{ or } Z(t_2) > c_2\} = \alpha^*(t_2)$. At the third analysis, determine c_3 such that $P\{Z(t_1) > c_1 \text{ or } Z(t_2) > c_2 \text{ or } Z(t_3) > c_3\} = \alpha^*(t_3)$, and so on. More details of boundary construction are given in Section 9.2.4. The important point is that

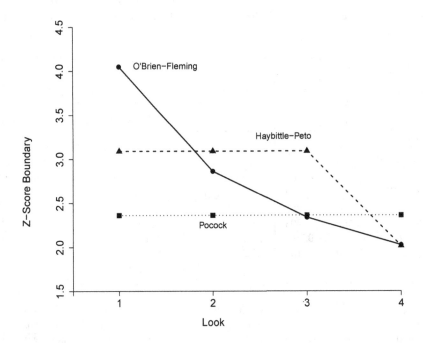

Figure 9.2: A graphical comparison of the Pocock, O'Brien-Fleming, and Haybittle-Peto boundaries for a trial with four equally-spaced looks.

critical values are determined iteratively based only on the current and previous analysis times and the spending function. Analysis times need not be equally-spaced or even pre-specified. In fact, even the number of interim analyses need not be pre-specified, although it is good practice to do so. Slud and Wei (1982) had suggested a similar idea of spending different cumulative amounts of alpha at different interim looks, but the increments of alpha were fixed in advance instead of being tied to fractions of information as they are in the Lan-DeMets formulation.

9.2.2   Z-scores, B-Values, and Information

We alluded to the fact that all of the tables in Section 9.2.1 apply not only to t-tests, but to z-tests of proportions, the logrank statistic and Cox models, z-statistics formed from maximum likelihood estimators, and many other asymptotically normal test statistics. Lan and Zucker (1993) unify all of these settings using so-called *B-values*. See also Proschan, Lan, and Wittes (2006) or Jennison and Turnbull (2000).

Introduction to B-Values through the Paired t-Test

We begin with the setting of monitoring a trial with paired differences. Let D_i be the treatment minus control difference for the ith pair. Assume, for simplicity, that D_i is normally distributed with mean δ and known variance σ^2. Without loss of generality, let $\sigma^2 = 1$. The trial will continue until N pairs have been evaluated, at which time the z-score will be $Z_N = S_N/\{\text{var}(S_N)\}^{1/2} = S_N/N^{1/2}$, where $S_N = \sum_{i=1}^{N} D_i$.

We decompose the final z-score Z_N in terms of interim results after $n < N$ pairs as follows:

$$Z_N = \frac{S_N}{\sqrt{N}} = \frac{S_n + S_N - S_n}{\sqrt{N}} = \frac{S_n}{\sqrt{N}} + \frac{S_N - S_n}{\sqrt{N}}. \tag{9.1}$$

We call

$$t = n/N$$

the *information time* or *information fraction*, the fraction of the trial that has been completed after n of N pairs have been evaluated. The beginning and end of the trial correspond to $t = 0/N = 0$ and $t = N/N = 1$, respectively. Define the *B-value* at information fraction t by

$$B(t) = \frac{S_n}{\sqrt{N}}. \tag{9.2}$$

The reason for calling $B(t)$ a B-value will become clear shortly. Note that if the denominator were $n^{1/2}$ instead of $N^{1/2}$, we would have the interim z-score.

Next, we write decomposition (9.1) as a decomposition of B-values as follows. The left side of (9.1) is $Z_N = B(N/N) = B(1)$, while the right side is

$$B(t) + \frac{S_N}{\sqrt{N}} - \frac{S_n}{\sqrt{N}} = B(t) + B(1) - B(t).$$

Thus, (9.1) is equivalent to

$$B(1) = B(t) + B(1) - B(t),$$

where $B(t)$ is the B-value at the interim analysis. Also, S_n is a function of $D_1, \ldots, D_n$, while $S_N - S_n = \sum_{i=n+1}^{N} D_i$ is a function of $D_{n+1}, \ldots, D_N$. Because the D_i are iid, S_n and $S_N - S_n$ are independent, which makes $B(t)$ and $B(1) - B(t)$ independent.

We can generalize to multiple interim analyses as follows. Let $n_1 < n_2 < \ldots < n_k = N$ correspond to the $k - 1$ interim analyses and one final analysis. With $B(t_i)$ defined by $S_{n_i}/N^{1/2}$, write

$$B(1) = B(t_1) + \{B(t_2) - B(t_1)\} + \{B(t_3) - B(t_2)\} + \ldots + \{B(1) - B(t_{k-1})\}. \tag{9.3}$$

The increments $B(t_1), \{B(t_2) - B(t_1)\}, \ldots, \{B(t_k) - B(t_{k-1})\}$ are independent.

We next compute the mean and variance of $B(t)$. Because the D_i have mean δ,

$$E\left(\frac{S_n}{\sqrt{N}}\right) = \frac{n\delta}{\sqrt{N}} = \left(\sqrt{N}\,\delta\right)(n/N) = \theta t,$$

where $\theta = N^{1/2}\delta$ is the expected value of the z-score at the end of the trial and $t = n/N$ is the information fraction. The variance of $B(t)$ is

$$\mathrm{var}\left(\frac{S_n}{\sqrt{N}}\right) = \frac{\mathrm{var}(S_n)}{N} = \frac{n}{N} = t.$$

We have shown that the stochastic process $B(t)$ has the following properties:

B1: Whenever $t_1 \leq t_2 \leq \ldots \leq t_k$, the increments $B(t_1), \{B(t_2) - B(t_1)\}, \ldots, \{B(t_k) - B(t_{k-1})\}$ are independent (*independent increments property*) and normally distributed.

B2: $E\{B(t)\} = \theta t$, where θ is the expected value of the z-statistic at the end of the trial.

B3: $\mathrm{var}\{B(t)\} = t$.

These three properties also imply:

B4: If $s \le t$, then $\text{cov}\{B(s), B(t)\} = s$.

B5: If $s \le t$, $\text{E}\{B(t) - B(s)\} = \theta(t - s)$ and $\text{var}\{B(t) - B(s)\} = t - s$.

We simulated $k = 10$ equally-spaced B-values $B(0.10), B(0.20), \ldots, B(0.90)$, $B(1)$ under the null hypothesis $\theta = 0$ by first generating the 10 increments $B(t_i) - B(t_{i-1})$ as iid $N(0, 0.10)$ and forming cumulative sums: $B(t_j) = \sum_{i=1}^{j}\{B(t_i) - B(t_{i-1})\}$, $i = 1, \ldots, 10$ (remember that $B(0)$ is defined to be 0). The left side of Figure 9.3 is a line plot joining the observed B-values. We repeated this exercise with $k = 500$, resulting in the extremely jagged plot on the right side of Figure 9.3. As $k \to \infty$, the time points $1/k, 2/k, \ldots$ saturate the unit interval $(0, 1)$, and the limiting stochastic process $B(t)$ is a random function satisfying properties B1–B3. This random function is called *Brownian motion with drift θ*. The "B" of B-value stands for Brownian motion. A given Brownian motion path is continuous but infinitely jagged in the sense that $B(t)$ is not differentiable for any value of t! When we monitor a clinical trial using (9.2), we are observing a Brownian motion at discrete time points.

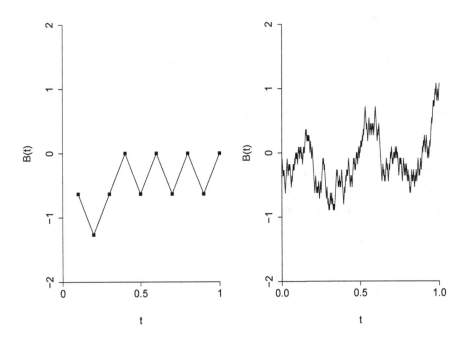

Figure 9.3: Left: Observed B-values from a Brownian motion with drift 0 at $k = 10$ equally spaced points joined by lines. Right: Observed B-values at $k = 500$ equally spaced points joined by lines.

Brownian motion has been studied by mathematicians and physicists alike. In fact, the great Albert Einstein made significant contributions to its theory and applications (Einstein, 1956). One advantage of using the B-value formulation to monitor clinical trials is that we can borrow from the many results about Brownian motion derived by these scientific masters.

Here is a brief review of what we have just developed for monitoring a clinical trial in a paired data setting with variance 1. At an interim analysis, the amount of information contained in the estimator $\bar{D}$ is measured by the number of pairs, n, that have been evaluated. The fraction of information is $t = n/N$, where N is the sample size at the end of the trial. Monitoring the trial corresponds to monitoring a z-score $Z(t)$ or, equivalently, the B-value $B(t)$, at discrete information fractions $t_1, \ldots, t_k$. Although we defined the B-value by (9.2), that definition is equivalent to

$$B(t) = \sqrt{t}Z(t).$$

Therefore, the B-value is a straightforward transformation of the z-score.

We made the simplifying assumption that $\sigma^2 = 1$, which is usually not true. Therefore, we must generalize the concept of the information contained in $\bar{D}$ to other values of σ^2. When $\sigma^2 = 1$, the variance of $\bar{D}_n$ is $1/n$, so n is actually the inverse of the variance of $\bar{D}_n$. We can use this inverse variance definition for arbitrary σ^2. Define the information I contained in $\bar{D}$ as

$$I = \frac{1}{\text{var}(\bar{D})}. \tag{9.4}$$

Note that, for a fixed number of pairs n, the amount of information increases as σ^2 decreases. The *information fraction* at an interim analysis is defined as $n/N = I/I_{\text{end}}$, where I is the information at the interim analysis and I_{end} is the information at the end of the trial. Notice that σ^2 cancels out when we compute the ratio I/I_{end}, so the information fraction is again n/N, the ratio of the current sample size to the sample size at the end of the trial.

Example 9.1. Crossover example In crossover trials of the effects of different salt levels on blood pressure, each participant is randomized to either a low salt followed by a high salt diet or vice versa. Blood pressure is measured at the end of each diet period. Let D_i be the difference in blood pressure on the low versus high salt diet for participant i. The trial will continue until 100 people are evaluated for the primary endpoint. At an interim analysis, suppose that 50 people have been randomized, but only 37 have completed both salt levels. Even though people who have completed only one salt level give some information about $\text{var}(\bar{D})$, the simplest approach uses the data from those completing both levels to compute $\text{var}(\bar{D})$. The current information is $I = 1/\text{var}(\bar{D}_{37}) = 1/(\sigma^2/37) = 37/\sigma^2$. To estimate the information, we would need to estimate σ^2. However, we do not need to estimate σ^2 to calculate the information fraction, $t = (37/\sigma^2)/(100/\sigma^2) = 37/100$. The information fraction is simply the proportion of patients who have completed the trial. Even though the trial is 50% complete in terms of enrollment, it is 37% complete in terms of information. □

More General Settings

Although we have considered the case of paired differences, the same Brownian motion framework arises with many different statistics, including paired and unpaired t-statistics, the z-test comparing proportions, tests based on a maximum likelihood estimator, and the logrank test and Cox proportional regression models. We will take the same approach in all of these settings: estimate the fraction of information at interim analyses and monitor the z-score or B-value the same way we did in the paired difference setting. The z-score is

$$Z = \frac{\hat{\delta}}{\widehat{\text{se}}(\hat{\delta})} \approx \frac{\hat{\delta}}{\text{se}(\hat{\delta})},$$

where $\hat{\delta}$ is the treatment effect estimator and $\text{se}(\hat{\delta})$ and $\widehat{\text{se}}(\hat{\delta})$ are its standard error and estimated standard error, respectively. We define the *information I* contained in the estimator $\hat{\delta}$ as

$$I = \frac{1}{\widehat{\text{var}}(\hat{\delta})} \approx \frac{1}{\text{var}(\hat{\delta})}. \tag{9.5}$$

Remark 9.2. *For an arbitrary estimator $\hat{\delta}$, think of $\hat{\delta}$ and $I\hat{\delta}$ as being analogous to the sample mean and sum, respectively, of I iid normal observations with mean δ and variance 1.*

Remark 9.2 may seem strange because I defined by (9.5) need not be an integer, but the analogy is still useful. For example, the variances of $\hat{\delta}$ and $I\hat{\delta}$ are $1/I$ and $I^2\text{var}(\hat{\delta}) = I^2/I = I$, which are identical to the variance of a sample mean and sum of I iid $N(\delta, 1)$ observations. The analogy also carries over to joint distributions. Think about monitoring an estimator $\hat{\delta}$ at k different analyses corresponding to information levels $I_1, \ldots, I_k$. It can be shown that the joint distribution of $\hat{\delta}_1, \ldots, \hat{\delta}_k$, and of $I_1\hat{\delta}_1, \ldots, I_k\hat{\delta}_k$, are approximately those of cumulative sample means and sums of $I_1, \ldots, I_k$ iid $N(\mu, 1)$ observations. For example, $I\hat{\delta}$ has approximately independent increments when sample sizes are large.

More important than information is the *information fraction*, t defined as

$$t = \frac{I}{I_{\text{end}}}, \tag{9.6}$$

where I and I_{end} are the information levels currently and at the end of the trial, respectively. As in the paired t-test setting, the B-value is defined as

$$B(t) = \sqrt{t}Z(t), \text{ where } Z(t) = \frac{\hat{\delta}(t)}{\text{se}\{\hat{\delta}(t)\}}. \tag{9.7}$$

Theorem 9.3. *In clinical trial settings using either paired or unpaired t-statistics, z-tests of proportions, tests based on maximum likelihood estimators or minimum variance unbiased estimators, or survival tests such as the logrank or Cox model, the B-value defined by (9.7) has the same asymptotic joint distribution over information time t as Brownian motion with drift θ, where θ is the expected z-score at the end of the trial. Accordingly, the same z-score boundaries asymptotically control the type I error rate in all of these settings.*

We omit the proof of Theorem 9.3. Details are found in Lan and Zucker (1993), Jennison and Turnbull (2000), and Proschan, Lan, and Wittes (2006). The result is not surprising in light of Remark 9.2, which suggests that we can transform an arbitrary estimator back to the sample mean case, for which we have already established that Brownian motion is a good approximation.

We can monitor clinical trials using either the z-score or B-value. Each is a monotone transformation of the other. We give examples to illustrate computation of the information fraction in different settings, culminating in summary Table 9.4.

Example 9.4. Model-based estimators.   This example shows how to monitor when a model is used to estimate the treatment effect adjusted for between-arm differences in baseline covariates. The example deals with linear models, but the same approach can be used for logistic regression and other settings in which the estimator is asymptotically normally distributed. Consider a parallel arm trial using a linear model to compare blood pressure in a treatment and control diet, adjusting for covariates. The model is $Y = \beta_0 + \beta_1 x_1 + \ldots + \beta_p x_p + \epsilon$, where Y is end of study blood pressure, x_1 is the treatment indicator taking value 0 for control and 1 for treatment, and $x_2, \ldots, x_p$ are baseline covariates such as baseline blood pressure, age, gender, etc. The term ϵ_i is a mean 0 random error. The treatment effect estimator is $\hat{\beta}_1$. Suppose that at an interim analysis, the adjusted treatment effect estimate $\hat{\beta}_1$ and its estimated standard error are

$$\hat{\beta}_1 = 2.0; \;\; \text{se}(\hat{\beta}_1) = 1.5.$$

The current information is $I = 1/\text{var}(\hat{\beta}_1) = 1/1.5^2 = 0.444$. We do not know precisely how much information there will be at the end of the trial, so how can we estimate the information fraction t? Use the fact that the information at any given analysis should be proportional to sample size. Therefore, the information fraction is approximately the ratio

$$t = n_{\text{tot}}/N_{\text{tot}}$$

of total sample sizes currently and at the end of the trial. This applies under equal or unequal randomization. If the current sample size is 52 and the trial will ultimately enroll 200, the information fraction is $t = 52/200 = 0.26$.

The current z-score and B-value are

$$Z(0.26) = 2.0/1.5 = 1.333 \quad \text{and} \quad B(0.26) = \sqrt{.26}\,(1.333) = 0.680.$$

The B-value formulation is particularly useful for seeing if the current treatment effect is better or worse than the originally hypothesized effect. Suppose that the trial was originally powered at 85%. From Chapter 8, the expected z-score at the end of the trial for 85% power is $1.96 + 1.04 = 3$. Therefore, if the assumptions underlying the sample size calculations are correct, the expected B-value is $3t = 3(0.26) = 0.78$. The current B-value of 0.68 is close to, but slightly less than, what we expect it to be (Figure 9.4).

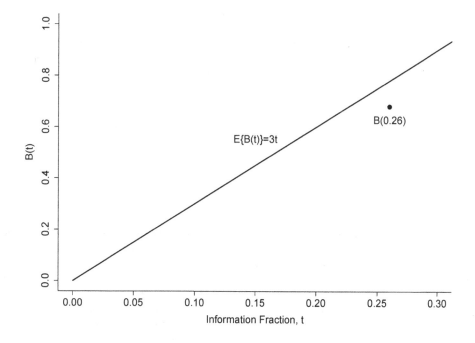

Figure 9.4: The observed B-value $B(0.26)$ and the expected value of $B(t)$, $3t$ (line), under the originally hypothesized treatment effect.

The joint distribution of B-values and z-scores over information time are the same for this linear model setting as for t-tests. Therefore, the same z-score boundaries can be used in the two settings. For example, if this is the first of four roughly equally-spaced looks and we are using the O'Brien-Fleming method, we compare the observed z-score, 1.333, to its boundary value of 4.048 from Table 9.3. The observed z-score is well below its boundary, so the trial would continue. □

Example 9.5. Binary outcome example: PREVAIL II   The PREVAIL II trial randomized participants with Ebola virus disease in Liberia, Guinea, and Sierra Leone to either a control arm consisting of supportive care or a treatment arm consisting of supportive care plus the triple monoclonal antibody product ZMapp. The trial planned to have 100 participants per arm, but the epidemic ended before enrollment could be completed. The final results on the primary endpoint of 28-day mortality were $\hat{p}_C = 13/35$ and $\hat{p}_T = 8/36$, where C and T denote control and treatment arms, respectively. The Bayesian analysis used in PREVAIL II is asymptotically equivalent to a z-test of proportions. For simplicity, we assume a z-test of proportions. The treatment difference $\hat{p}_C - \hat{p}_T$ has variance $p_C(1 - p_C)/35 + p_T(1 - p_T)/36$. The *score statistic* uses the null variance estimate $\bar{p}(1 - \bar{p})(1/35 + 1/36)$. Which of the two variances should we use to compute information? If we use $p_C(1 - p_C)/35 + p_T(1 - p_T)/36$, the information is

$$I = \frac{1}{\text{var}(\hat{p}_T - \hat{p}_C)} = \frac{1}{p_C(1 - p_C)/35 + p_T(1 - p_T)/36}.$$

At the originally planned end of the trial, the information is

$$I_{\text{end}} = \frac{1}{p_C(1 - p_C)/100 + p_T(1 - p_T)/100}.$$

Unlike in the t-test setting, the parameters do not cancel out when we compute the information fraction I/I_{end}. That means we do not know the current information fraction precisely. We could estimate the information fraction by treating the estimates $\hat{p}_C$ and $\hat{p}_T$ as the true values p_C and p_T. But $\hat{p}_C$ and $\hat{p}_T$ may be poor estimates at an interim analysis, especially if p_C and p_T are small. A more attractive alternative is to approximate the information fraction using the null variance, $\bar{p}(1 - \bar{p})(1/35 + 1/36)$, of $\hat{p}_T - \hat{p}_C$. The current information and information at the originally planned end are

$$I \approx \frac{1}{\bar{p}(1 - \bar{p})(1/35 + 1/36)}; \quad I_{\text{end}} \approx \frac{1}{2\bar{p}(1 - \bar{p})/100}.$$

The information fraction t is

$$t = \frac{I}{I_{\text{end}}} = \frac{2\bar{p}(1 - \bar{p})/100}{\bar{p}(1 - \bar{p})(1/35 + 1/36)} = \frac{2/100}{1/35 + 1/36} \approx 0.355.$$

Therefore, the trial stopped with approximately 35.5% of the originally planned information. Note that we never had to actually compute $\bar{p} = (n_C\hat{p}_C + n_T\hat{p}_T)/(n_C + n_T)$ because $\bar{p}(1 - \bar{p})$ cancelled out in the numerator and denominator.

Note that another way to estimate the information fraction is to use the average sample size in the two arms. The average sample size is $(35 + 36)/2 = 35.5$. Therefore, the information fraction can be estimated by the ratio of the average sample size to the sample size at the end, $t = 35.5/100 = 0.355$. The two methods of estimating the information fraction are nearly identical because the sample sizes are nearly the same in the two arms. Either way one looks at it, the trial was stopped a little over one-third of the way through.

If this had been an interim analysis instead of a forced closure, the same boundary that applies to a t-test also applies to this test of proportions. For example, if this had been the first of three equally-spaced looks and the O'Brien-Fleming boundary were used, the z-score boundary from Table 9.3 would be approximately 3.471. Many people find it helpful to express boundaries not in terms of z-scores or B-values, but in terms of the treatment effect estimate $\hat{p}_C - \hat{p}_T$. A z-score of 3.471 is approximately equivalent to (using a score test with null variance)

$$\frac{\hat{p}_C - \hat{p}_T}{\sqrt{\bar{p}(1-\bar{p})(1/35+1/36)}} = 3.471$$

$$\hat{p}_C - \hat{p}_T = 3.471\sqrt{(21/71)(1-21/71)(1/35+1/36)} \approx 0.376.$$

That is, we would have to see a difference in proportions of 0.376 or greater to declare ZMapp+standard care superior to standard care alone at this analysis. The observed difference of $13/35 - 8/36 = 0.149$ falls well short. □

Example 9.6. Survival example: CAST Recall that the Cardiac Arrhythmia Suppression Trial (CAST) used the logrank statistic to test whether suppression of cardiac arrhythmias in patients with a prior heart attack reduces the hazard rate for sudden arrhythmic deaths and cardiac arrest. For the logrank statistic, we record the indicator O_i that the ith event came from the control arm. Let E_i and V_i denote the mean and variance of O_i computed under the null hypothesis. By the O minus E except after V principle, the estimator of the control to treatment log hazard ratio δ is asymptotically equivalent to (see Section 8.3.3)

$$\hat{\delta} = \frac{\sum_{i=1}^{d}(O_i - E_i)}{\sum V_i}.$$

The variance of $\hat{\delta}$ and its inverse, I, are

$$\text{var}(\hat{\delta}) \approx \frac{1}{\sum_{i=1}^{d} V_i}; \quad I = \sum_{i=1}^{d} V_i \approx d/4,$$

where d is the number of events at the interim analysis. Similarly, the information at the end of the trial is $D/4$, where D is the number of events at the end of the trial. Accordingly, the information fraction is

$$t \approx \frac{d/4}{D/4} = d/D.$$

At the first interim analysis, there were 22 sudden deaths and cardiac arrests. At that time, the number of events expected by trial's end was 425. Thus, the information fraction was $22/425 = 0.052$. □

Table 9.4 summarizes the information fraction in various scenarios encountered in clinical trials. In most settings, the information fraction can be approximated by the proportion of participants evaluated so far. In survival trials, the information fraction is the proportion of the total number of events that have occurred by the time of the interim analysis.

Table 9.4: Information fractions in different settings.

paired t-test after n of N	2-sample t-test after n_T, n_C of N_T, N_C	2-sample proportions after n_T, n_C of N_T, N_C	Logrank after d of D deaths
n/N	$\frac{n_T n_C (N_T + N_C)}{N_T N_C (n_T + n_C)} \approx n/N$	$\frac{n_T n_C (N_T + N_C)}{N_T N_C (n_T + n_C)} \approx n/N$	d/D

Table 9.5: Two-tailed B-value boundaries $a = a(k)$ for the O'Brien-Fleming procedure at $\alpha = 0.01, 0.05$, and 0.10. Boundaries for the z-score $Z(i/k)$ are $a(k)/(i/k)^{1/2}$.

k	$\alpha = .01$	$\alpha = .05$	$\alpha = .10$
1	2.576	1.960	1.645
2	2.580	1.977	1.678
3	2.595	2.004	1.710
4	2.609	2.024	1.733
5	2.621	2.040	1.751
6	2.631	2.053	1.765
7	2.640	2.063	1.776
8	2.648	2.072	1.786
9	2.654	2.080	1.794
10	2.660	2.087	1.801
∞	2.807	2.241	1.960

9.2.3   Revisiting O'Brien-Fleming

The Brownian motion framework allows us to see the O'Brien-Fleming procedure in a new light. The O'Brien-Fleming boundary is a constant boundary for $|B(t)|$. That is, for k equally-spaced looks, the boundary is crossed at information fraction $t_i = i/k$ if

$$|B(t_i)| > a,$$

where $a = a_k$ depends on k but not i. Equivalently, the boundary is crossed at t_i if

$$|Z(t_i)| > c_i = \frac{a}{\sqrt{t_i}}.$$

The critical value $a = a_k$ is given in Table 9.5 for a two-tailed test at level 0.01, 0.05, or 0.10.

For example, for $k = 4$ and $\alpha = 0.05$, Table 9.5 shows that $a = 2.024$. The boundary is crossed if the absolute value of the z-score exceeds $2.024/(1/4)^{1/2} = 4.048$, $2.024/(1/2)^{1/2} = 2.862$, $2.024/(3/4)^{1/2} = 2.337$, or $2.024/(4/4)^{1/2} = 2.024$ at the first, second, third, or fourth looks, respectively. Note that these boundaries can also be obtained from the $k = 4$ row of Table 9.3.

9.2.4   Alpha Spending Functions

Section 9.2.1 very briefly touched on spending functions, a major breakthrough in monitoring clinical trials. We now expand on this approach.

Remark 9.7. *Throughout this section, we consider one-tailed upper boundaries at level α. For a symmetric two-tailed test at level α, use the upper one-tailed boundary at level $\alpha/2$ and a symmetric lower boundary. This procedure is slightly conservative because $Z(t)$ could, theoretically, cross both boundaries at different information fractions, but the probability of this is infinitesimally tiny.*

We can motivate the idea of a spending function by thinking about the amount of alpha spent by a given boundary at different information fractions. For example, consider the

O'Brien-Fleming boundary with $\alpha = 0.025$ and 2 looks. By Table 9.3 or 9.5, the boundary at $t = 1/2$ is $1.977/(1/2)^{1/2} = 2.796$, so the amount of alpha spent at the first look is $1 - \Phi(2.796) = 0.0026$. The cumulative amount of alpha spent by $t = 1$ is $P\{Z(0.5) > 2.796$ or $Z(1) > 1.977\} = 0.025$. For 10 analyses, the cumulative amount of alpha spent by $t = 1/10, 2/10, \ldots, 1$ is shown as dots in Figure 9.5. As the number of equally-spaced looks increases without bound, the cumulative amount of alpha spent by information fraction t approaches the continuous curve in Figure 9.5. For arbitrary α, if the number of equally-spaced looks tends to infinity, the cumulative probability of crossing the O'Brien-Fleming boundary by information fraction t approaches

$$\alpha^*_{\text{O}-\text{F}}(t) = 2\left\{1 - \Phi\left(z_{\alpha/2}/\sqrt{t}\right)\right\}, \tag{9.8}$$

where $z_{\alpha/2}$ is the $(1-\alpha/2)$th quantile of a standard normal distribution function. This is a well-known result about Brownian motion (see, for example, page 346 of Karlin and Taylor, 1975). In Figure 9.5, $\alpha = 0.025$ and $z_{\alpha/2} = 2.241$, so (9.8) is

$$\alpha^*_{\text{O}-\text{F}}(t) = 2\left\{1 - \Phi\left(2.241/\sqrt{t}\right)\right\} \tag{9.9}$$

for a one-tailed test at $\alpha = 0.025$.

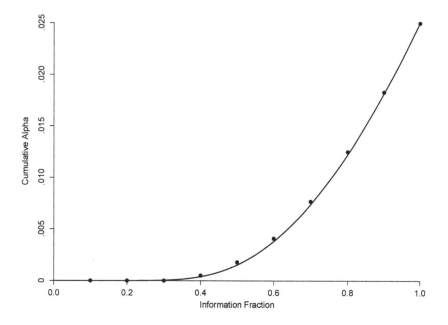

Figure 9.5: The O'Brien-Fleming-like spending function (9.8).

Note that $\alpha^*_{\text{O}-\text{F}}(t)$ is an increasing function satisfying $\alpha^*(0) = 0$ and $\alpha^*(1) = \alpha$. We call such a function an *alpha spending function* or just *spending function*. Instead of beginning with a boundary and seeing how much alpha is spent by different times, we can proceed in the opposite direction: use a spending function to construct boundaries. The subscript O-F in spending function (9.8) and (9.9) stands for O'Brien-Fleming because this spending function produces boundaries similar to those of the O'Brien-Fleming procedure when looks are equally spaced. $\alpha^*_{O-F}(t)$ spends very little alpha until t is at least $1/2$, after which the spending function rises steeply to level α at $t = 1$. This feature causes early boundaries to be very high and the final boundary to be close to what it would be with no interim monitoring.

We illustrate how to compute boundaries using spending function (9.9). Suppose that the first analysis is at information fraction $t = 0.27$. The first step in determining the boundary c_1 for $Z(0.27)$ is to determine from spending function (9.9) the amount of α spent by $t = 0.27$:

$$\alpha^*_{O-F}(0.27) = 2\{1 - \Phi(2.241/\sqrt{0.27})\} = 1.6 \times 10^{-5}.$$

As this is the first analysis, the cumulative type I error rate is simply $P\{Z(0.27) > c_1\}$. Therefore, we must determine c_1 such that

$$P\{Z(0.27) > c_1\} = 1.6 \times 10^{-5}.$$

Because $Z(0.27)$ has a standard normal distribution under the null hypothesis of no treatment effect, the first boundary is easy:

$$c_1 = \Phi^{-1}(1 - 1.6 \times 10^{-5}) \approx 4.158.$$

The z-score boundary at time 0.27 is huge! This is because spending function (9.9) spends almost no alpha by this early interim analysis. Suppose that the observed z-score at the first analysis is $Z(1) = 2.40$. Even though we would ordinarily consider such a large z-score to be strong evidence of a treatment effect, it comes nowhere close to reaching the boundary of 4.158, so we continue.

Suppose that the second analysis is at information fraction $t = 0.44$. We use spending function (9.9) to determine the cumulative type I error rate spent by time 0.44:

$$\alpha^*_{O-F}(0.44) = 2\{1 - \Phi(2.241/\sqrt{0.44})\} = 0.0007.$$

The cumulative type I error rate by the second analysis is $P(Z(0.27) > 4.158 \text{ or } Z(0.44) > c_2)$, so the boundary c_2 for $Z(0.44)$ must solve:

$$P\{Z(0.27) > 4.158 \text{ or } Z(0.44) > c_2\} = 0.0007. \tag{9.10}$$

The calculation of c_2 is not as straightforward as that of c_1 because it involves the joint distribution of $(Z(t_1), Z(t_2))$. Under the null hypothesis, $(Z(0.27), Z(0.44))$ has a bivariate normal distribution with means $(0,0)$ and variances $(1,1)$. The correlation between $Z(0.27)$ and $Z(0.44)$, and more generally, between $Z(s)$ and $Z(t)$ for $s \leq t$, can be computed using property B4 of Brownian motion (see Section 9.2.2) as follows:

$$\text{cov}\{Z(s), Z(t)\} = \text{cov}\left\{\frac{B(s)}{\sqrt{s}}, \frac{B(t)}{\sqrt{t}}\right\}$$
$$= \left(\frac{1}{\sqrt{s}}\frac{1}{\sqrt{t}}\right)\text{cov}\{B(s), B(t)\} = \left(\frac{1}{\sqrt{s}}\frac{1}{\sqrt{t}}\right)s = \sqrt{\frac{s}{t}}.$$

Therefore,

$$\boxed{\text{cov}\{Z(s), Z(t)\} = \sqrt{\frac{s}{t}}.} \tag{9.11}$$

The correlation between $Z(0.27)$ and $Z(0.44)$ is $(0.27/0.44)^{1/2} = 0.783$. We could use simulation to solve Equation (9.10) as follows. Generate 100,000 bivariate normal vectors with mean vector $(0,0)$, variances $(1,1)$, and correlation 0.783. Use a fine grid of equally-spaced candidate values for c_2; for each value, calculate the proportion $\hat{p}$ of the 100,000 vectors such that $Z(0.27) > 4.158$ or $Z(0.44) > c_2$. Choose the value c_2 such that $\hat{p}$ is closest to 0.0007. An alternative method using a clever numerical integration technique (Armitage, McPherson, and Rowe, 1969) is used in free software such as WinLD from the University of Wisconsin or the R package 'ldbounds'. Using either simulation or numerical integrations, we obtain $c_2 \approx 3.186$. Suppose that the actual z-score at the second analysis is $Z(0.44) = 2.80$. Ordinarily, such a large z-score would be very compelling, but again it does not cross the boundary of 3.186. Therefore, we continue.

Suppose that the third analysis is at $t = 0.76$. The cumulative type I error rate we can spend by time 0.76 is

$$\alpha^*_{\text{O-F}}(0.76) = 2\{1 - \Phi(2.241/\sqrt{0.76})\} = 0.0102.$$

The boundary c_3 for $Z(0.76)$ is the solution to the equation

$$P\{Z(0.27) > 4.157 \text{ or } Z(0.44) > 3.186 \text{ or } Z(0.76) > c_3\} = 0.0102. \qquad (9.12)$$

We obtain $c_3 \approx 2.330$. Suppose that the actual z-score at the third look is $Z(0.76) = 2.94$. The boundary has now been crossed because $2.94 > 2.330$. We now have statistical grounds for stopping the trial.

We have presented the *cumulative alpha formulation* of spending functions:

$$\boxed{P(Z(t_1) > c_1 \cup Z(t_2) > c_2 \cup \ldots \cup Z(t_j) > c_j) = \alpha^*(t_j).} \qquad (9.13)$$

There is an equivalent *first crossing formulation*. We can write (9.13) in terms of the probability of first crossing the boundary at different times as follows:

$$\begin{aligned} \alpha^*(t_j) &= P(\text{cross by time } t_j) \\ &= P(\text{cross by time } t_{j-1} \text{ or no cross by time } t_{j-1}, \text{but cross at time } t_j) \\ &= P(\text{cross by time } t_{j-1}) + P(\text{no cross by time } t_{j-1}, \text{but cross at time } t_j) \\ \alpha^*(t_j) &= \alpha^*(t_{j-1}) + P(Z(t_1) \leq c_1, \ldots, Z(t_{j-1}) \leq c_{j-1}, Z(t_j) > c_j). \end{aligned} \qquad (9.14)$$

Now subtract $\alpha^*(t_{j-1})$ from both sides of (9.14) to get

$$\boxed{P(Z(t_1) \leq c_1, \ldots, Z(t_{j-1}) \leq c_{j-1}, Z(t_j) > c_j) = \alpha^*(t_j) - \alpha^*(t_{j-1}).} \qquad (9.15)$$

The left side of (9.15) is the probability of first crossing the boundary at time t_j. Lan and DeMets (1983) and other articles define spending function using this first crossing formulation. The cumulative alpha formulation (9.13) and the first crossing formulation (9.15) are equivalent. They both give the same boundaries c_i, $i = 1, \ldots, k$.

Remark 9.8. *One helpful way to view a boundary c_i for $Z(t_i)$ is in terms of the one-tailed nominal p-value associated with c_i, $1 - \Phi(c_i)$. This should not be confused with the cumulative alpha spent by information fraction t_i.*

As mentioned earlier, the spending function (9.8) produces boundaries that are similar to those of the O'Brien-Fleming boundary when analyses are equally spaced in terms of information. For example, consider a trial using a one-tailed test at level $\alpha = 0.025$ with five equally spaced analyses. From Table 9.3 using two-tailed $\alpha = 0.05$, the upper z-score boundaries at the five analyses are 4.562, 3.226, 2.634, 2.281, and 2.040. It can be shown that the boundaries corresponding to spending function (9.9) at the same information fractions are 4.877, 3.357, 2.680, 2.290, and 2.031. Although the first boundary appears to be fairly different for the O'Brien-Fleming procedure and O'Brien-Fleming-like spending function (9.9), the difference in one-tailed nominal p-values corresponding to 4.562 and 4.877 is 2×10^{-6}. Likewise, the difference in nominal one-tailed p-values is very small at each analysis (see Table 9.6).

Table 9.6: Nominal one-tailed p-values corresponding to the O'Brien-Fleming procedure and the O'Brien-Fleming-like spending function $\alpha^*_{\text{O-F}}(t)$ for five equally spaced looks with one-tailed alpha of 0.025 (two-tailed alpha of 0.05).

Analysis	nominal p, O-F	nominal p, $\alpha^*_{\text{O-F}}$	|Difference|
1	2.5×10^{-6}	5.4×10^{-7}	2.0×10^{-6}
2	0.0006	0.0004	0.0002
3	0.0042	0.0037	0.0005
4	0.0113	0.0110	0.0003
5	0.0207	0.0211	0.0005

The O'Brien-Fleming-like spending function is only one choice, albeit a very popular one. There are classes of spending functions from which we may choose. Think of an alpha spending function in terms of a conditional distribution function as follows. Let T be a random variable that has nonzero probability of values in $(0, 1]$. That is, the distribution function $F(t)$ for T satisfies $F(1) - F(0) > 0$. Then the conditional distribution function of T given that $0 < T \leq 1$, namely $\{F(t) - F(0)\}/\{F(1) - F(0)\}$, is a distribution function on $(0, 1]$. Convert this to a spending function by multiplying by α:

$$\alpha^*(t) = \alpha \times \begin{cases} 0 & \text{if } t = 0 \\ \frac{F(t)-F(0)}{F(1)-F(0)} & \text{if } 0 < t \leq 1. \end{cases} \qquad (9.16)$$

If F is the exponential distribution function with parameter γ, the resulting family is the Hwang, Shi, DeCani (1990) family (also known as the *gamma family*) of spending functions

$$\alpha^*(t) = \alpha \times \begin{cases} 0 & \text{if } t = 0 \\ \frac{1-\exp(-\gamma t)}{1-\exp(-\gamma)} & \text{if } 0 < t \leq 1. \end{cases} \qquad (9.17)$$

To enrich the family, Hwang, Shi, and DeCani allow γ to be negative as well. Figure 9.6 shows some members of this family. The choice $\gamma = -4$ is close to the O'Brien-Fleming-like spending function (O-F is the dashed line). The family contains a wide array of different shapes. In fact, by taking $\gamma \to -\infty$ or $\gamma \to \infty$, we get the two extreme spending functions, $\alpha I(t = 1)$ and $\alpha I(t > 0)$, respectively, where I denotes an indicator function. The linear spending function $\alpha^*(t) = \alpha t$ results from taking the limit as $\gamma \to 0$.

Another class of spending functions is the power family (Kim and DeMets, 1987)

$$\alpha^*(t) = \alpha t^\phi, \ \phi > 0. \qquad (9.18)$$

The power family can also assume a wide range of shapes. Values of ϕ close to 0 spend almost all of the α immediately (a very bad choice!). It is best to avoid choices of ϕ less than 1. Larger values of ϕ are preferable because they conserve more of the alpha spending until the end of the trial. The two extreme spending functions, $\alpha I(t > 0)$ and $\alpha I(t = 1)$, result from taking $\phi \to 0$ or $\phi \to \infty$, respectively.

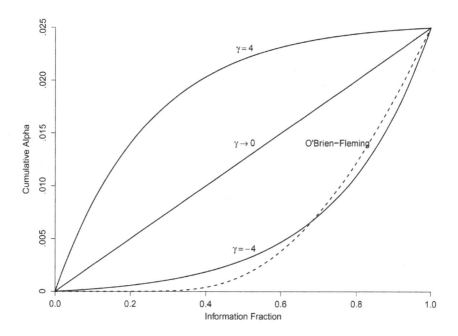

Figure 9.6: The Hwang, Shi, DeCani (1990) spending function for different values of γ, together with the O'Brien-Fleming-like spending function (dashed line).

9.2.5   Effect of Monitoring on Power

Monitoring offers the advantage of being able to stop a clinical trial early, but at the cost of some loss in power. This is easiest to see in a paired t-test setting with iid paired differences with mean μ and known variance σ^2. The most powerful one-tailed test of $\mu = 0$ versus $\mu > 0$ rejects the null hypothesis if the z-score using all N observations exceeds z_α, the $(1 - \alpha)$th quantile of a standard normal distribution (see chapter 8 of Casella and Berger, 2002). Diverting some portion of the alpha to a subset of the data necessarily decreases power. But that is exactly what happens with monitoring: we allocate some alpha to observations available at interim analyses. Therefore, power is no greater than in a trial with no monitoring. Still, power is at least as large as $P_\theta\{Z(1) > c(1)\}$, where θ and $c(1)$ are the expected value of $Z(1)$ and the group-sequential boundary at the end of the trial, respectively. This follows from the fact that the null hypothesis will be rejected if $Z(1) > c(1)$. Therefore, the following inequality holds:

$$P_\theta(Z > c(1)) \leq \text{power with monitoring} \leq P_\theta(Z > z_\alpha)$$
$$= \text{power with no monitoring.} \qquad (9.19)$$

For conservative boundaries that are high early, the boundary $c(1)$ at the end of the trial is close to z_α. Therefore, the left and right sides of (9.19) are both nearly the same. In that case, the reduction in power from monitoring is minimal.

   The EZ principle (Principle 8.1) implies that power for an unmonitored trial depends only on the expected z-score; power for a monitored trial depends only on the drift parameter θ, the expected z-score at the end of the trial. Free 'WinLD' software at the University of Wisconsin or the R package 'ldbounds' can be used to calculate the drift parameter required to have a desired level of power. We can then use the drift parameter to compute the required sample size. We illustrate the calculation for a trial with four equally-spaced analyses using the O'Brien-Fleming-like spending function. Suppose we want 85% power. The boundaries for a two-tailed test at $\alpha = 0.05$ using the O'Brien-Fleming-like spending function are ± 4.3326, ± 2.9631, ± 2.3590, and ± 2.0141. The drift parameter resulting in 85% probability of ever crossing the upper boundary is approximately 3.025. That is, for 85% power accounting for monitoring, the expected z-score should be 3.025. Contrast this value with the expected z-score of $1.96 + 1.04 = 3$ required for 85% power in a trial with no monitoring (see Chapter 8). Monitoring has very little effect on the required drift parameter.

Return to Example 8.4, in which we computed the sample size needed for 85% power to detect a 50% reduction in mortality in the Pamoja Tulinde Maishe (PALM) clinical trial of Ebola virus disease in the Democratic Republic of the Congo. The anticipated 28-day mortality probability in the control arm was 0.30. Without accounting for monitoring, we equated the expected z-score to $1.96 + 1.04$ and solved for the per-arm sample size n:

$$n = \frac{2(1.96 + 1.04)^2(0.225)(0.775)}{(0.30 - 0.15)^2} = 139.5 \approx 140.$$

The only difference to account for the above monitoring plan would be to replace $1.96 + 1.04 = 3$ by approximately 3.025:

$$n = \frac{2(3.025)^2(0.225)(0.775)}{(0.30 - 0.15)^2} = 141.83 \approx 142.$$

Thus, we need to increase the per-arm sample size by only 2 people, and the total sample size by only $2(2) = 4$ people. Because the effect on the sample size of monitoring with conservative approaches like O'Brien-Fleming is minimal, it is not unusual to ignore monitoring when computing power.

On the other hand, with the Pocock spending function, there would be a large penalty to pay for monitoring. The resulting drift parameter is 3.265. Therefore, the sample size with the Pocock spending function to achieve 85% power is

$$n = \frac{2(3.265)^2(0.225)(0.775)}{(0.30 - 0.15)^2} = 165.23 \approx 166.$$

The total sample size of $2(166) = 332$ is 18.6% larger than with no monitoring. This is another confirmation that the Pocock boundary has undesirable consequences.

9.3   Small Sample Sizes

Almost all of the monitoring boundaries we have discussed are valid only when sample sizes are large because they assume asymptotic normality of the test statistic. There are two reasons that applying z-score boundaries will be inaccurate when sample sizes are small: (1) the **marginal** distribution of the test statistic T may not be standard normal under the null hypothesis and (2) the **joint** distribution of the test statistic T over different information times may not be that of z-scores. We can eliminate the first problem by obtaining a valid nominal p-value and applying a p-value boundary instead of a z-score boundary.

We illustrate the p-value boundary approach with the 2-sample t-statistic T. Suppose that a trial in a rare disease uses a continuous endpoint analyzed using a t-statistic, and there are only five participants per arm at the first of four equally-spaced analyses. T_1 will not be approximately standard normal under the null hypothesis with only ten observations, so applying a z-score boundary to T_1 will be inaccurate. Instead, we should compute the p-value using a t-distribution with 8 degrees of freedom, and then compare to the p-value boundary associated with the given monitoring procedure. Suppose that the two-tailed O'Brien-Fleming boundary at $\alpha = 0.05$ is used, and the observed value of the t-statistic is 2.105. From Table 9.3, the z-score and p-value boundaries are 4.048 and 5×10^{-5}, respectively. The two-tailed p-value for the observed t-score of 2.105 is $2 \times \{1 - G(2.105, 8)\} = 0.068$, where $G(2.105, 8)$ is the t distribution function with 8 degrees of freedom evaluated at 2.105. Instead of comparing the observed t-score 2.105 to the z-score boundary of 4.048, compare the observed p-value 0.068 to the p-value boundary of 5×10^{-5}. In this case, both procedures would reach the same conclusion not to stop at the first analysis. In fact, with a very conservative boundary like O'Brien-Fleming, either method would work reasonably well because we almost never have enough evidence to stop very early in a trial. By the time the trial might actually be stopped, the sample size will probably be large enough to be unconcerned about the normal approximation. With less conservative boundaries, the improvement of the p-value boundary approach over the z-score boundary approach can be substantial. Chapter 8 of Proschan, Lan, and Wittes (2006) shows that the p-value boundary approach yields very little alpha inflation even if sample sizes are tiny.

Of course, there is still the potential for alpha inflation caused by the fact that assumptions underlying a statistical test are unmet. For example, in the t-test setting, the observations may not be normally distributed. A re-randomization test can be used to obtain a monitoring boundary that is guaranteed to control the type I error rate for testing the strong null hypothesis that treatment has absolutely no effect. Furthermore, a re-randomization test can be used for any type of endpoint and any randomization scheme. Pawitan and Hallstrom (1990) showed how to analyze the Cardiac Arrhythmia Suppression Trial (CAST) using a re-randomization test.

We illustrate the re-randomization approach to monitoring for a trial using spending function $\alpha^*(t)$. At the first interim analysis at information fraction t_1, we try to find c_1 such that

$$P_{\text{re}}(Z(t_1) > c_1) = \alpha^*(t_1), \tag{9.20}$$

where P_{re} denotes a probability computed by fixing the data at their observed values and using the re-randomization distribution of $Z(t_1)$. The only difference from the traditional spending function approach is that probability (9.20) is computed using the re-randomization distribution of $Z(t_1)$ instead of Brownian motion. One problem is that, because the re-randomization distribution is discrete, we usually cannot satisfy (9.20) exactly. In practice, we generate a huge number of re-randomized values of $Z(t_1)$ and evaluate a fine grid of potential values for c_1. We then find the smallest value c_1 in the grid such that the proportion of re-randomized $Z(t_1)$s that exceed c_1 is $\leq \alpha^*(t_1)$. This procedure is conservative because it ensures a type I error rate no greater than $\alpha^*(t_1)$ at the first analysis.

At information fraction t_2, generate a huge number of re-randomized values of $\{Z(t_1), Z(t_2)\}$. Evaluate a fine grid of values for c_2 and find the smallest c_2 in the grid such that the proportion of re-randomized $\{Z(t_1), Z(t_2)\}$s with $Z(t_1) > c_1$ or $Z(t_2) > c_2$ is $\leq \alpha^*(t_2)$.

More generally, compute c_i as follows. Generate a huge number of re-randomized values of $\{Z(t_1), \ldots, Z(t_i)\}$. Evaluate a fine grid of values for c_i and find the smallest c_i in the grid such that the proportion of re-randomized $\{Z(t_1), \ldots, Z(t_i)\}$s with

$$Z(t_1) > c_1 \text{ or } Z(t_2) > c_2 \text{ or } \ldots \text{ or } Z(t_i) > c_i$$

is $\leq \alpha^*(t_i)$, $i = 1, 2, \ldots, k$.

9.4   Futility Monitoring

9.4.1   What Is Futility?

Despite promising results in pre-clinical and early phase studies, about 40% of Phase III clinical trials do not show statistically significant results. It can become painfully clear midway through a trial that continuation is futile. Futility that is caused by things like poor recruitment, too much loss to follow-up, or non-adherence of participants is called *operational futility*, meaning futility caused by the operation of the trial. In other cases, futility might result from the treatment being less effective than anticipated. In that case, a null result still answers the study question.

9.4.2   Conditional Power

One very important statistical tool that can guide the decision to stop a trial for futility is *conditional power (CP)*. Conditional power is the conditional probability of reaching a statistically significant treatment benefit by the end of the trial, given current results. It can be computed only by someone who has access to data by arm. If CP is low, we are likely to observe a null result at the end. Whether that null result will still answer the trial's question depends on unconditional power, the power that was estimated before the trial began. The problem is that the original power calculation was based on assumptions about the values of nuisance parameters such as the control event probability for a trial with a binary endpoint, or the common variance for a trial with a continuous endpoint. Now that we have estimates of these nuisance parameters from the trial itself, we can revise the original power calculation. A low value for *revised power* tells us that the trial could not really answer its intended question. A low value for both conditional power and revised power signals that not only are we likely to reach a null result, but that null result will not be meaningful because the trial had insufficient power to answer its intended question. Such a circumstance cries out for stopping for futility.

We now show how to use the B-value formulation to compute conditional power. Results at the interim analysis with information fraction t are summarized by either $Z(t)$ or the B-value $B(t) = t^{1/2}Z(t)$. Given that $B(t) = b$, the probability of reaching a statistically significant result at the end (information fraction 1) is $P\{Z(1) > c \,|\, B(t) = b\}$, where c is the boundary at the end of the trial. But $Z(1) = B(1)$, so we can express conditional power as

$$
\begin{aligned}
CP = P\{B(1) > c \,|\, B(t) = b\} &= P\{B(1) - B(t) > c - B(t) \,|\, B(t) = b\} \\
&= P\{B(1) - B(t) > c - b \,|\, B(t) = b\} \\
&= P\{B(1) - B(t) > c - b\}.
\end{aligned}
\tag{9.21}
$$

The last line follows from the fact that $B(t)$ has independent increments: $B(1) - B(t)$ is independent of $B(t)$. Therefore, the probability that $B(1) - B(t) > c - b$) does not change when we condition on $B(t) = b$. Also, $B(1) - B(t)$ is normally distributed with mean $\theta(1-t)$ and variance $1-t$ by property B5 of Brownian motion (see Section 9.2.2). Now standardize $B(1) - B(t)$ by subtracting its mean and dividing by its standard deviation in Equation (9.21):

$$
\begin{aligned}
CP = P&\left\{ \frac{B(1) - B(t) - \theta(1-t)}{\sqrt{1-t}} > \frac{c - b - \theta(1-t)}{\sqrt{1-t}} \right\} \\
&= 1 - \Phi\left\{ \frac{c - b - \theta(1-t)}{\sqrt{1-t}} \right\} = \Phi\left\{ \frac{b + \theta(1-t) - c}{\sqrt{1-t}} \right\},
\end{aligned}
\tag{9.22}
$$

where $\Phi(\cdot)$ is the normal distribution function. The last step follows from the fact that $\Phi(-t) = 1 - \Phi(t)$ for any t.

The astute reader might be wondering why we did not compute conditional power by the cumulative probability of crossing the boundary, rather than just the probability of crossing the boundary at the last analysis. It would be more accurate to use the cumulative crossing probability, but for common monitoring boundaries that spend very little alpha early, (9.22) is an excellent approximation. Furthermore, the approximation remains accurate if we replace the final boundary value c by z_α (see Section 9.2.5).

Formula (9.22) shows that conditional power depends on θ, the expected z-score at the end of the trial. Recall from Chapter 8 that θ is closely related to power. If the trial was originally powered at 80%, 85%, or 90%, then θ is approximately 2.80, 3.00, or 3.24, respectively. This assumes that nuisance parameters were estimated correctly. When nuisance parameters were incorrect, then it can be helpful to recompute the expected z-score, as we will see in the next example. Another choice for the treatment effect is the empirical effect, the one observed this far. Remember that $E\{B(t)\} = \theta t$, so the empirical estimate of θ is $B(t)/t$. Conditional power computed under the empirical estimate is extremely variable and can sometimes be misleading, especially early in a trial. The primary conditional power calculation should be under the originally assumed treatment effect. The idea is that if results are so disappointing that conditional power is bleak even under what now appears to be an overly optimistic assumption, it may be time to stop the trial.

Example 9.9. Consider a trial randomizing patients with hepatitis B to a new drug (N) or the standard drug S. The primary outcome is change in the logarithm (base 10) of hepatitis B viral load from baseline to 1 week, analyzed using a t-test. The standard deviation of the change in log viral loads is expected to be approximately 2.80, so a sample size of 250 per arm gives 85% power to detect a 0.8 log difference.

At an interim analysis after 108 and 111 observations in arms S and N, the mean changes in log viral load, 1 week minus baseline, are $\bar{Y}_S = -0.30$ and $\bar{Y}_N = -0.18$, with standard deviations of change $s_S = 2.35$ and $s_N = 2.60$, respectively. The pooled variance is

$$s^2 = \frac{(108-1)s_S^2 + (111-1)s_N^2}{108 + 111 - 2} = 6.150.$$

The information fraction is approximately the average sample size divided by the average sample size at the end of the trial, $t = 109.5/250 = 0.44$. More precisely,

$$t = \frac{1/\text{var}(\hat{\delta})}{1/\text{var}(\hat{\delta}_{\text{end}})} = \frac{1/\{\sigma^2(1/108 + 1/111)\}}{1/(2\sigma^2/250)} = 0.438.$$

The z-score (t-statistic) and B-value are

$$Z(0.438) == \frac{\bar{Y}_S - \bar{Y}_N}{\sqrt{s^2(1/n_S + 1/n_N)}} = \frac{-0.30 - (-0.18)}{\sqrt{6.150(1/108 + 1/111)}} = -0.358.$$

$$B(0.438) = \sqrt{0.438}(-0.358) = -0.237.$$

Because power at the beginning of the trial was 0.85, the expected z-score at the end of the trial is approximately $\theta = 1.96 + 1.04 = 3$, so conditional power is approximately

$$CP_3 = \Phi\left(\frac{-0.237 + 3(1 - 0.438) - 1.96}{\sqrt{1 - 0.438}}\right) = \Phi(-0.682) = 0.25.$$

Conditional power is low under the originally hypothesized treatment effect. Conditional power under other assumptions about the treatment effect are even lower. Currently, the treatment effect is in the wrong direction. Assume the null hypothesis is true. Then the expected z-score at the end is $\theta = 0$ and conditional power is

$$CP_0 = \Phi\left(\frac{-0.237 + 0(1 - 0.438) - 1.96}{\sqrt{1 - 0.438}}\right) = \Phi(-2.931) = 0.002.$$

In other words, even if the true treatment effect is 0 instead of negative, the probability of reaching a statistically significant result is only 2 in a thousand. Remember, however, that the primary conditional power calculation should be under the originally hypothesized treatment effect.

$\square$

Example 9.9 raises an interesting question: What value of conditional power is too low to continue the trial? Different people have different thresholds, but as a general rule, conditional power thresholds are often 0.20 or lower. That is, serious consideration for stopping a trial might be given if conditional power, computed under the originally hypothesized treatment effect, drops below 0.20, or maybe 0.15. Conditional power is often used informally rather than as a binding rule. A binding rule of the form: stop whenever $CP \leq \gamma$, where γ is a threshold value, is called *stochastic curtailment*.

One concern about futility stopping is that power will be reduced because some of the trials that were stopped for futility might have resulted in a statistically significant result if continued to fruition. Whether that is likely depends on how aggressive the futility rule is. For example, power could be substantially reduced with an aggressive stochastic curtailment rule such as stopping if $CP \leq 0.50$. On the other hand, the rule that stops when $CP \leq 0.10$ loses very little power.

Theorem 9.10. (Lan, Simon, and Halperin, 1982) *Suppose that power for a trial with no interim monitoring is P. If the trial is monitored continuously, power using the stochastic curtailment rule that stops when $CP \leq \gamma$ is $P/(1 - \gamma)$. If the trial is monitored a finite number of times instead of continuously, power exceeds $P/(1 - \gamma)$.*

Example 9.11. PREVAIL II trial in Ebola virus disease. Recall that the PREVAIL II trial of Ebola virus disease in Western Africa compared the triple monoclonal antibody product ZMapp plus standard care to standard care alone. The primary endpoint was 28-day mortality, and the target sample size was 100 per arm, which yields approximately 87% power to detect a 50% reduction in mortality probability, from 0.40 to 0.20. Although a Bayesian analysis was used, the prior distribution was such that the usual z-test of proportions is a good approximation to the Bayesian test of treatment effect at the end of the trial.

Table 9.7: 28-day mortality in the PREVAIL II trial in Ebola virus disease in western Africa.

	Dead	Alive	
Standard care+ZMapp	8	28	36
Standard care	13	22	35
	21		71

After 71 observations, the epidemic ended with results shown in Table 9.7. An interesting question is whether results would have been statistically significant at the end of the trial. The information fraction is estimated by (see Example 9.5)

$$t = \frac{1/\{p(1 - p)(1/35 + 1/36)\}}{100/\{2p(1 - p)\}} = 0.355.$$

The overall proportion of deaths by 28 days is $\hat{p} = 21/71$, so the current z-score is

$$Z(0.355) = \frac{13/35 - 8/36}{\sqrt{(21/71)(1 - 21/71)(1/35 + 1/36)}} = 1.377.$$

The B-value is

$$B(0.355) = (0.355)^{1/2} Z(0.355) = 0.820.$$

Remember that the most important conditional power calculation assumes the originally hypothesized treatment effect. The expected z-score at the end of the trial under the original assumptions is

$$\theta = \mathrm{E}\{Z(1)\} = \frac{0.40 - 0.20}{\sqrt{2(0.30)(1 - 0.30)/100}} = 3.086.$$

Therefore, conditional power under the original assumptions is approximately

$$\Phi\left(\frac{0.820 + 3.086(1 - 0.355) - 1.96}{\sqrt{1 - 0.355}}\right) = \Phi(1.059) = 0.86.$$

If the original sample size assumptions are correct, the trial was on schedule to show a statistically significant benefit by the end.

A DSMB often wants to see conditional power computed under the empirical estimate of treatment effect as well. The current trend estimate of θ is

$$\hat{\theta} = \frac{B(t)}{t} = \frac{0.820}{t} = \frac{0.820}{0.355} = 2.310.$$

Conditional power under the empirical estimate of treatment effect is approximately

$$\Phi\left(\frac{0.820 + 2.310(1 - 0.355) - 1.96}{\sqrt{1 - 0.355}}\right) = \Phi(0.436) = 0.67.$$

We see that there is a fairly large difference between conditional power under the original and empirical estimates of θ. The problem with computing conditional power under the empirical estimate of the treatment effect is that it is highly variable. That is why we prefer to make futility decisions based on conditional power under the originally hypothesized treatment effect.

Note that we can also compute conditional power exactly. There are $100 - 36 = 64$ and $100 - 35 = 65$ remaining observations in the treatment and control arms, so the numbers Y_T and Y_C of remaining events in the treatment and control arms are binomial $(64, p_T)$ and $(65, p_C)$. Exact conditional power can be computed as

$$\sum_{y_T=0}^{64} \sum_{y_C=0}^{65} \binom{64}{y_T} \binom{65}{y_C} p_T^{y_T}(1 - p_T)^{64-y_T} p_C^{y_C}(1 - p_C)^{65-p_C} I(P \leq \alpha), \tag{9.23}$$

where $I(P \leq \alpha)$ is the indicator that the p-value from the test of proportions with $x_T + y_T$ events out of 100 people in the treatment arm and $x_C + y_C$ events out of 100 people in the control arm is less than or equal to α. Exact conditional powers are 0.82 and 0.60 under the original assumption $(p_C, p_T) = (0.40, 0.20)$ and under the empirical estimates $(\hat{p}_C, \hat{p}_T) = (13/35, 8/36)$, respectively. These CPs are somewhat lower than the asymptotic approximations of 0.86 and 0.67 reported above because the final sample size of 100 per arm is not huge. It is always a good idea to compute exact CP when using a test of proportions.

Li, Evans, Uno et al. (2009), building on the idea of Evans, Li, and Wei (2007), proposed a graphical procedure called a *predicted interval plot* that nicely supplements conditional power calculations. We apply the technique by simulating the remaining data a large number of times and computing the final confidence interval for each simulated completed trial. We then order the intervals by their point estimates of the treatment effect. Figure 9.7 shows 100 such intervals simulated using the originally hypothesized p_C and p_T (left) and the empirical estimates $\hat{p}_C$ and $\hat{p}_T$ (right). Under either of the two assumptions, a large proportion of the final confidence intervals are entirely to the right of 0 (dashed vertical line). The graph provides visual confirmation that, had this been an interim analysis instead of a forced closure of the trial, there would be no evidence of futility.   □

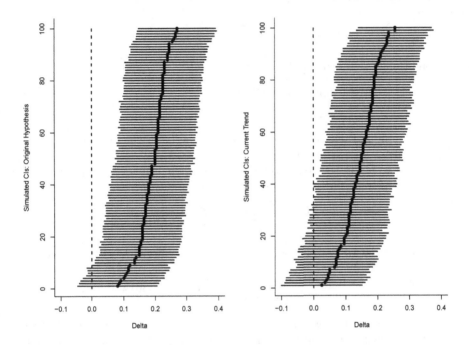

Figure 9.7: Predicted interval plot by simulating the remaining data from PREVAIL II and computing confidence intervals 100 times under two different assumptions about p_T and p_C for future data. Left: using the original assumption that $p_C = 0.40$ and $p_T = 0.20$. Right: using the empirical estimates $\hat{p}_C$ and $\hat{p}_T$ of p_C and p_T.

Example 9.12. Suppose that the PREVAIL II of Example 9.11 analyzed time to death using the logrank test instead of a test of proportions, and that they had power 0.80 to detect a control to treatment hazard ratio of 1.60. The expected z-score at the end of the trial and number of deaths for 80% power are $\theta = 2.80$ and $4(2.80^2)/\{\ln(1.60)\}^2 \approx 142$. The information fraction is estimated by the ratio of the current number of deaths to the number expected by the end of the trial, $d/D = 21/142 = 0.148$. Suppose that the value of the logrank z-score is $Z = 0.830$. The B-value is

$$B(0.148) = \sqrt{0.148}(0.830) = 0.319.$$

Conditional power is approximately

$$CP_{2.80} = \Phi\left(\frac{0.319 + 2.80(1 - 0.148) - 1.96}{\sqrt{1 - 0.148}}\right) = \Phi(0.807) = 0.79.$$

When the amount of information is so low (15% in this example), it is nearly impossible to stop for futility using conditional power. That is why conditional power is often not even computed until at least 25% of the information has accrued. □

See Example 9.14 for another example of the use of conditional power in a survival setting in the Cardiac Arrhythmia Suppression Trial (CAST).

9.4.3 Beta Spending Functions

Another approach to futility monitoring uses the same spending function approach as in Section 9.2.4, but spends type II, rather than type I, error rate (Pampallona, Tsiatis, and Kim, 2001). Such an increasing function, $\beta^*(t)$, satisfying $\beta^*(0) = 0$ and $\beta^*(1) = \beta$, is called a *beta spending function*. A beta spending function differs from an alpha spending function in only two ways: (1) the total error rate is β instead of α, and (2) the beta spending function finds lower (futility) boundaries rather than upper (efficacy) boundaries. Of course, if $\alpha^*(t)$ is any alpha spending function, then $(\beta/\alpha)\alpha^*(t)$ is a beta spending function.

We can choose a conservative beta spending function that saves most of the beta for the end of the trial or spend more aggressively to discard treatments that are not showing promise. The latter can be an attractive option in multi-arm trials for a new disease like coronavirus disease (COVID-19) for which there is an imperative to quickly find a treatment that works. The Hwang, Shih, DeCani (1990) class of spending functions (9.17) can be tailored to the desired rate of beta spending; $\gamma = -4$ produces extreme lower boundaries that are very difficult to cross early, whereas γ values close to 0 produce less extreme earlier boundaries.

One important point about beta spending functions is that the lower boundaries are considered binding. Having binding lower boundaries means that the type I error rate associated with an upper efficacy boundary is actually reduced. This is because some paths that would have crossed the upper boundary will first cross the lower boundary, causing stoppage for futility. Consequently, the upper efficacy boundary is often lowered to account for the lower boundary and still control the type I error rate. The problem with this strategy is that if a lower boundary is crossed but the trial continues, the type I error rate is no longer controlled at the desired level. This issue is not specific to beta spending functions. It arises whenever the upper boundary is adjusted downward as a result of having a binding lower boundary.

> **Remark 9.13.** *We recommend against adjusting upper (efficacy) boundaries to account for lower futility boundaries because DSMBs often regard futility boundaries as advisory rather than binding.*

9.5 Practical Aspects of Monitoring

Effective monitoring of clinical trials requires judgment in addition to statistical knowledge. Decisions can be difficult. Data and safety monitoring boards often wrestle with balancing risks and benefits of interventions. For example, in the Promoting Maternal and Infant Survival Everywhere (PROMISE) trial of interventions intended to reduce mother to child transmission of HIV, one regimen better prevented transmission, but was associated with a higher proportion of birth complications (Fowler, Qin, Fiscus et al., 2016). We offer some examples to illustrate the practical and statistical aspects of monitoring.

Example 9.14. Cardiac Arrhythmia Suppression Trial (CAST). We return to the CAST trial of Examples 4.11, 5.1, and 9.6. Recall that CAST tested whether a strategy of suppressing cardiac arrhythmias in patients with a prior heart attack would reduce the incidence of sudden death and cardiac arrest. CAST was a classic case of trying to demonstrate that a beneficial effect on a surrogate endpoint, cardiac arrhythmias, would translate into a beneficial effect on the serious clinical endpoint, sudden death/cardiac arrest. A one-tailed logrank test was to be used partly because a deleterious effect of treatment was not expected. After all, there had been substantial evidence that arrhythmias increased the risk of sudden death/cardiac arrest, and recall that CAST enrolled only participants whose arrhythmias could be suppressed. The majority of cardiologists believed that these drugs worked, and some people questioned whether a clinical trial that deprived half of the patients of antiarrhythmics was even ethical. A further argument for a one-tailed test was that even if these drugs were harmful, there would be no interest in **proving** harm; the trial would be stopped before there was enough evidence to do that. Nevertheless, on March 14, 1987, the DSMB recommended including a symmetric lower boundary on the grounds that one could never rule out harm.

The DSMB opted to start out blinded to treatment arm. They would see results by Arm X versus Arm Y without knowing which arm was which. Their rationale was that they would break the blind as soon as they saw a difference that was of concern. In the meantime, they argued, it would be helpful to think about how they would feel depending on whether the results favored treatment or placebo.

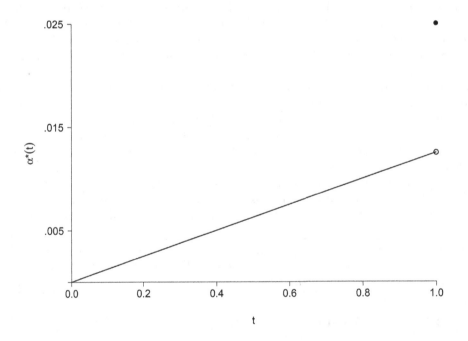

Figure 9.8: The spending function used in the Cardiac Arrhythmia Suppression Trial (CAST): $\alpha^*(t) = 0.0125t$ for $0 \leq t < 1$ and 0.025 for $t = 1$.

A linear spending function with slope 0.0125 was used until the end of the trial, at which time the remaining alpha, $0.025 - 0.0125 = 0.0125$, would be spent (Figure 9.8). The original sample size calculation was based on the anticipation of 425 events by trial's end.

The first interim analysis occurred on September 16, 1988 with 22 events. No boundary had yet been calculated because it was very early in the trial. There had been only 22 of the expected 425 events, so the information fraction was $22/425 = 0.052$. If the boundary had been in place, the alpha to spend would have been

$$\alpha^*(0.05) = 0.0125(0.05) = 0.000625.$$

The boundary would have been $\pm\Phi^{-1}(1 - 0.000625) = \pm3.22$. Interestingly, there was already a large difference between arms at the first analysis: 3 of 576 participants in Arm X and 19 of 571 participants in Arm Y had a sudden death/cardiac arrest, logrank z-score: -3.43. The DSMB argued that it was very early in the trial, and no matter which way the results went, they would not be convincing enough to stop the trial. The board remained blinded.

At the second interim analysis on April 16-17, 1989, there were 48 events. It became clear that the total number of events by trial's end had been overestimated. The new projection was that there would be approximately 300 events by the end of the trial. With this revised estimate, the **actual** information fractions at the first and second interim analyses were $22/300 = 0.07$ and $48/300 = 0.16$. To be conservative, the boundary at the second analysis was computed assuming that the boundary of 3.22 at the first analysis had actually been used. The boundary c_2 at the second interim analysis was computed by setting $c_1 = 3.22$ and determining c_2 such that the cumulative probability of crossing c_1 or c_2 at the revised information fractions 0.07 or 0.16 was $\alpha^*(0.16) = 0.0125(0.16) = 0.002$. This resulted in $c_2 = \pm2.97$.

The actual results at the second analysis were startling. There were now 13 sudden deaths/cardiac arrests in Arm X and 35 in Arm Y. The DSMB became unblinded and saw that Arm X was placebo! The logrank z-score was -3.22, crossing the lower boundary of -2.97. Suppression of cardiac arrhythmias with these drugs was actually harmful.

Was there any chance that results might reverse by the end of the trial? Conditional power can be used to answer this question. Recall from Equation (8.14) that the expected logrank z-score with D total events is approximately

$$\ln(HR)\sqrt{D/4},$$

where HR is the control to treatment hazard ratio and D is the number of events by the end of the trial. The expected z-score with a hazard ratio of 1.333 and the revised estimate of 300 events by the end is

$$\ln(1.333)\sqrt{300/4} = 2.491.$$

The current information fraction and B-value are $t = 48/300 = 0.16$ and

$$B(0.16) = (0.16)^{1/2}(-3.22) = -1.288.$$

By Formula (9.22), conditional power is

$$CP_{2.491}(0.16) = \Phi\left(\frac{-1.288 + 2.491(1 - 0.16) - 1.96}{\sqrt{1 - 0.16}}\right) = \Phi(-1.261) = 0.10. \qquad (9.24)$$

In other words, the probability that results would magically turn around and produce a statistically significant benefit by the end of the trial was very low, even when computed under the optimistic treatment benefit originally hypothesized. Given the current data, even the null hypothesis seems optimistic! Conditional power assuming the null hypothesis for future data is obtained by replacing 2.491 by 0 in Equation (9.24):

$$CP_0(0.16) = \Phi\left(\frac{-1.288 + 0(1 - 0.16) - 1.96}{\sqrt{1 - 0.16}}\right) = \Phi(-3.544) = 0.0002.$$

Prospects for a turnaround were bleak.

A natural question the DSMB had was whether there could be a labeling error. Perhaps all participants assigned to placebo were actually given active medication and vice versa. To test this theory, the study had a subset of patients return their medication to be chemically analyzed. There was no mistake. Another thought was that there might be some serious baseline imbalance such that the placebo patients were actually much healthier than the active arm patients. But baseline characteristics were balanced, as expected in a trial of that size. Furthermore, analyses adjusting for any baseline differences corroborated harmful results in patients assigned to antiarrhythmic medications. Analyses of secondary endpoints such as mortality also indicated harm, and it was not just confined to one subgroup.

There was one card left to be played. Recall that CAST did not use one specific drug. Instead, there was a titration phase during which different drugs were tried until one was found that suppressed at least 80% of arrhythmias. Consequently, some patients in the active arm were on encainide, some were on flecainide, and some were on moricizine. Could it be that harm was confined to only one or two drugs? Further analysis suggested that encainide and flecainide might be the culprits. Results for the third drug, moricizine, appeared promising.

The decision was made to enter a new phase, CAST II, randomizing patients to moricizine versus placebo. Patients previously randomized to encainide or flecainide or their placebo would be eligible to be re-randomized to either moricizine or placebo. Thus, patients previously randomized to active drug might be re-randomized to placebo and vice versa. Several other changes were made. The theory was that any harm of active medication would be confined predominantly to less sick patients, so entry criteria were modified to enroll sicker patients. Additionally, because of the experience in CAST I, an asymmetric boundary was instituted allocating $\alpha = 0.05$ for harm and $\alpha = 0.025$ for benefit. Another very important change was that there would be an initial 2-week placebo controlled phase to determine whether there was early harm in starting moricizine. In CAST I, there had been no way to tell whether too many patients were having events during the drug titration phase at the beginning of the trial because there was no matching placebo titration.

The DSMB chose to remain blinded in CAST II. On April 26, 1991, the DSMB saw 3 participants out of 577 in Arm P and 12 participants out of 572 in arm Q with events. On July 31, 1991, there were 3 events in Arm P and 15 in Arm Q. The DSMB became unblinded and learned that Arm P was placebo. Moricizine was showing harm. Conditional power calculations showed very low probability of a turnaround by the end of the trial. CAST II was terminated.

Among the many lessons learned from the Cardiac Arrhythmia Suppression Trial (CAST) are:

1. Benefit on a surrogate need not translate into benefit on the serious clinical outcome.

2. Harm can never be ruled out in advance in clinical trials. Always include a boundary for harm.

3. Benefit and harm boundaries need not be symmetric, and the total type I error rate for benefit and harm can exceed 0.05.

4. If a trial includes a drug titration phase, include a placebo titration phase to assess potential harm.

5. Blinding of a DSMB should be discouraged.

The last point deserves further explanation because some might find it controversial. We want to make clear that the DSMB in CAST was outstanding. Their extremely thoughtful and thorough reasoning were exemplary. Nonetheless, we believe that blinding a DSMB can have negative consequences. Proponents of blinding argue that it makes the DSMB more objective. The opposite is more likely to be true. When a DSMB does not know which arm is which, their preconceived ideas enter in a maximal way. When CAST began, most experts believed that suppressing arrhythmias would be beneficial. Even though the CAST DSMB attempted to imagine how they would feel if results favored treatment or if they favored placebo, the natural tendency would be to assume that results favored treatment. The DSMB stated unequivocally at the early interim analysis that, regardless of the direction of effect, results were not convincing enough to take action. Still, might that conviction have been driven in part by a belief that results were going in the right direction? We also question the argument that it is helpful to try to imagine how one would feel no matter which way the results went. Is it really helpful to divert deliberation time to pondering something that is not happening? Our conclusion is that DSMBs should be unblinded from the beginning.   □

Example 9.15. Antihypertensive and Lipid-Lowering Treatment to prevent Heart Attack Trial (ALLHAT) ALLHAT randomized 42,418 patients with hypertension and at least one other cardiovascular risk factor to one of four arms: chlorthalidone (a diuretic), doxazosin (an alpha blocker), amlodipine (a calcium channel blocker), and lisinopril (an angiotensin converting enzyme (ACE) inhibitor). Chlorthalidone served as the active control because it had a long track record and was inexpensive compared to the other drugs. This is an important consideration because hypertension disproportionately affects African Americans, a group that has historically been at an economic disadvantage. The goal of ALLHAT was to reduce blood pressure by a comparable amount in different arms to determine whether specific drugs had a more beneficial effect on the primary endpoint of nonfatal heart attack or fatal coronary heart disease (CHD).

At an interim analysis, there were many more cases of congestive heart failure (CHF) in the doxazosin arm than in the chlorthalidone arm. The z-score was -10.72! The problem was that CHF was not even a pre-specified secondary endpoint, although it was one component of cardiovascular disease (CVD), which was a pre-specified secondary endpoint. The z-score for CVD was -6.77. An even larger problem with trying to interpret the result was that chlorthalidone was a drug that was often used to treat heart failure. Perhaps the between-arm difference resulted from chlorthalidone's masking the symptoms of heart failure, making CHF more difficult to diagnose in the chlorthalidone arm. Even under the best circumstances, the diagnosis of heart failure was considered somewhat difficult and subjective.

Given the above concerns, statisticians performed the following analyses to determine whether the difference was real or a product of masking. First, they presented results on a related, but less subjective endpoint, hospitalized and fatal CHF. There was a large difference between arms on this more objective endpoint. Next, they compared baseline characteristics across the two arms for patients with CHF. If the between-arm difference was caused by masking, one would expect patients diagnosed with CHF in the chlorthalidone arm to be only the most obvious cases, so their disease would be clearly seen even though some symptoms were masked. Their baseline health would likely be worse than that of patients with CHF in the doxazosin arm. Baseline characteristics of CHF patients were similar in the two arms. Next, a random sample of 50 suspected CHF cases were reviewed by 2 members of the Endpoint Committee. If masking explained differences, then in the chlorthalidone arm, only the most obvious cases would be detected. Therefore, one would expect better agreement in the diagnosis of CHF among patients in the chlorthalidone arm. On the contrary, there was about 70% agreement in both arms. Similarly, they checked the ejection fractions (the fractions of blood pumped out by the heart), expecting to find lower ejection fractions in the chlorthalidone arm under the masking conjecture. That also did not happen. Finally, they checked the case fatality rate of patients diagnosed with CHF in the two arms. Under the masking hypothesis, the case fatality rate should be higher in the chlorthalidone arm, again because only the sickest, most obvious cases would be detected. The case fatality rate was somewhat higher in the chlorthalidone arm, but it was quite high in both arms. In the words of one DSMB member, "If you don't believe it is heart failure, call it whatever you like; whatever it is carries a high mortality rate." In the end, the doxazosin arm was dropped from the trial.

Example 9.16. The Pamoja Tulinde Maisha (PALM) trial   The Pamoja Tulinde Maisha ("together save lives" in Kiswahili) (PALM) trial randomized participants with Ebola virus disease in the Democratic Republic of the Congo to one of four interventions: (1) ZMapp, a triple monoclonal antibody, (2) Remdesivir, a direct acting antiviral, (3) MAb114, a single monoclonal antibody, or (4) REGN-EB3, a triple monoclonal antibody. The ZMapp arm was the control to which all other arms were compared with respect to the primary endpoint of death within 28 days of randomization.

When the statistical team prepared for an interim analysis, they specified an enrollment cutoff date, meaning that only participants randomized by that date would be included in the DSMB report. The idea is to allow participants to have had 28 days of follow-up plus an additional 7 days to make sure that all deaths are counted, plus additional time to prepare the DSMB report and allow the DSMB to review it. A consequence of this procedure is that, if enrollment is occurring rapidly, the number of participants analyzed at the DSMB meeting could be much smaller than the number randomized by the date of that meeting. In fact, that is exactly what happened.

At its DSMB meeting on August 9, 2019, 681 patients had been enrolled, but only 376 patients before the data cutoff date. Two arms, MAb114 and REGN-EB3, had substantially lower mortality than the other two arms, but had not yet crossed the monitoring boundary with ZMapp using the 376 patients in the DSMB report. Nonetheless, there was a serious possibility that results in the full cohort of 681 patients might cross a boundary. There was a compelling need for an updated analysis, but what analysis? One possibility is to compute, among all randomized in each arm, the proportion who had died, and compare proportions between each arm and the ZMapp control. That would incorporate data from all 681 participants, but would not reflect 28-day mortality because many participants had fewer than 28 days of follow-up. Another option is to compute rates; in each arm, divide the number of deaths by the total follow-up time, and compare rates between each arm and the ZMapp control. That makes an assumption that the rate of accumulation of deaths is constant over follow-up time, which might not hold. Another option is to compute the Kaplan-Meier estimate of the probability of death by 28 days in each arm, and compare using a normal approximation with Greenwood's variance formula (see Chapter 7).

In the setting of Ebola virus, there was an even simpler option. Sadly, almost all Ebola deaths (97%) occur within 10 days of randomization. Within each arm, we counted all deaths among all patients who had at least 10 days of follow-up. This analysis using the very accurate surrogate incorporated data from many more people. We counted the surrogate analysis as another interim analysis. The boundary for the comparison of REGN-EB3 with ZMapp was crossed, and the boundary for MAb114 versus ZMapp was very close to being crossed. The DSMB made the recommendation to discontinue randomization to the ZMapp and Remdesivir arms. They further recommended reporting final results when all people randomized by August 9, 2019 reached 28 days of follow-up. There was a small risk that the final results might drop under the boundary, but conditional power calculations showed that was quite unlikely. When the final results were in, both REGN-EB3 and MAb114 had crossed their monitoring boundaries with ZMapp.

The PALM trial overcame tremendous obstacles. It was conducted in a country beset by civil unrest; there were more than 100 warring factions, and Ebola treatment units were attacked and burned down on at least two occasions. The brave men and women in the Democratic Republic of the Congo refused to give up, rebuilding the treatment units and reopening remarkably quickly. PALM received the 2019 David A. Sackett Trial of the Year award from the Society for Clinical Trials. □

9.6 Inference after a Monitored Trial

This section attempts to briefly summarize what could easily be a book in itself, the complications of performing inference following a trial that is monitored. The trial is either stopped early or continues to fruition and reaches either a statistically significant or nonsignificant conclusion. Assume throughout this section that monitoring boundaries are strictly followed. In practice, this is not always the case, but evaluation of properties of procedures is nearly impossible without imposing this constraint.

9.6.1 Statistical Contrast between Unmonitored and Monitored Trials

With no monitoring, use of a *sufficient statistic* is paramount. Imagine randomly generating data by first generating a statistic S like $\bar{X}$ from its distribution, then generating the data from their conditional distribution given S. If this conditional distribution does not depend on the parameter, the statistic is said to be *sufficient*. Once we know S, the individual data points give us no more information about the parameter. Estimators and hypothesis tests can always be improved by using a sufficient statistic (see Casella and Berger, 2002). The same is true in the monitoring setting, but the sufficient statistic is slightly more complicated. Consider the setting of independent normal observations with unknown means μ_T and μ_C in the treatment and control arms and common, known variance σ^2. We want to estimate $\delta = \mu_T - \mu_C$. We can view either $\bar{Y}_T - \bar{Y}_C$ or the z-score $Z = (\bar{Y}_T - \bar{Y}_C)/\{\sigma^2(1/n_T + 1/n_C)\}^{1/2}$ as the sufficient statistic. In the monitoring setting, the sufficient statistic is the pair $\{\tau, Z(\tau)\}$, where τ is the random information fraction when the trial is stopped and $Z(\tau)$ is the z-score at that information fraction (see chapter 7 of Proschan, Lan, and Wittes, 2006). Equivalently, we can view $\{\tau, B(\tau)\}$ as the sufficient statistic. With no monitoring, the sufficient statistic Z is *complete*, which implies that there is at most one function of Z that is unbiased for $\mu_T - \mu_C$. The unbiased estimator with smallest variance is simply $\bar{Y}_T - \bar{Y}_C$. In the monitoring setting, the sufficient statistic is not complete, so there can be many functions of $\{\tau, Z(\tau)\}$ that are unbiased for δ, and there may not be an unbiased estimator with smallest variance.

Another problem with monitoring is that natural estimators of the treatment effect, such as the maximum likelihood estimator, are biased because of stopping on a random high. To understand this issue, suppose that $\hat{\delta}_1$ and $\hat{\delta}_2$ are two unbiased estimators of the treatment effect δ. If we flip a coin to pick which estimator to use, the randomly picked estimator will still provide an unbiased estimate of δ. But now suppose we do the following. Peak at $\hat{\delta}_1$; if it is large, report $\hat{\delta}_1$, whereas if $\hat{\delta}_1$ is small, report $\hat{\delta}_2$. We can instinctively sense that this tends to overestimate the treatment effect. Now modify the procedure as follows. If $\hat{\delta}_1$ is large, report $\hat{\delta}_1$, while if $\hat{\delta}_1$ is small, report the average of $\hat{\delta}_1$ and $\hat{\delta}_2$. Again this will tend to overestimate δ. Large values of $\hat{\delta}_1$ will be reported as is, but small values of $\hat{\delta}_1$ will be averaged with $\hat{\delta}_2$, which is likely to be larger than $\hat{\delta}_1$, given that $\hat{\delta}_1$ is small. This is exactly what happens with monitoring. If an interim result shows a strong enough treatment benefit, the trial is stopped early and the large treatment benefit is reported. On the other hand, if the interim result does not show a strong benefit, the trial continues to the end and the interim estimate is averaged with the estimate from the remaining data. It can be shown that early stopping for benefit always results in a maximum likelihood estimate of treatment effect that is biased high (see Appendix 7.7 of Proschan, Lan, and Wittes, 2006).

The problem of biased estimation goes hand in hand with an overly optimistic nominal p-value. When the treatment effect estimator is asymptotically normal, the nominal p-value for a one-tailed test that rejects for large values of $\hat{\delta}$ is $1 - \Phi(\hat{\delta}/\hat{se})$, where $\hat{se}$ is the estimated standard error of $\hat{\delta}$. Because $\hat{\delta}$ tends to overestimate δ when we stop a trial for benefit, $\hat{\delta}/\hat{se}$ also tends to be larger than it should, and the p-value $1 - \Phi(\hat{\delta}/se)$ tends to be too small. Another way to express the problem is that the null distribution of a nominal p-value for a continuous test statistic is no longer uniformly distributed on $(0, 1)$, as it would be in the setting of no interim monitoring.

9.6.2   Defining a P-Value after a Monitored Trial

How can we define a p-value that has better properties than the nominal p-value? In the nonmonitoring setting, a p-value is the probability of a result at least as extreme, in the direction of the alternative hypothesis, as the observed result. In the monitoring setting, there is no unique way to define 'at least as extreme.' For example, consider a trial with primary endpoint death by 28 days after randomization. At the third of four equally-spaced analyses, the boundary is crossed and the difference in proportions is $\hat{p}_C - \hat{p}_T = 0.10$. The observed stopping time is $\tau_{\text{obs}} = 0.75$. With the *maximum likelihood estimator (MLE) ordering*, all that matters is the value of the MLE at the time the trial is stopped. In this case, the p-value using the MLE ordering is

$$P\{\hat{p}_C(\tau) - \hat{p}_T(\tau) \geq 0.10\} = P\left[\cup_{i=1}^{4}(\{\tau = t_i\} \cap \{\hat{p}_C(t_i) - \hat{p}_T(t_i) \geq 0.10\})\right] \qquad (9.25)$$

where $\hat{p}_C(t_i)$ and $\hat{p}_T(t_i)$ are the proportions of people in the control and treatment arms who have died by 28 days by information fraction t_i, $t_i = 0.25, 0.50, 0.75$, or 1. Even though we stopped at $t = 0.75$, Formula (9.25) shows that we have to compute a probability that includes the future possibility, $\{\tau = 1\} \cap \{\hat{p}_C(1) - \hat{p}_T(1) \geq 0.10\}$. It seems odd that a p-value would include probabilities of things that might happen in the future. Why should our evaluation of the evidence so far depend on what we intend to do in the future? In this example, the only future look is at information fraction 1, but suppose we had stopped at $t = 0.50$. Then we would need to include two future events, one at $t = 0.75$ and the other at $t = 1$. For all we know, had the trial continued, the look that was originally scheduled at $t = 0.75$ might have actually occurred at $t = 0.82$. This is one of the unsettling consequences of having a p-value depend on future plans.

The same issue arises if we order outcomes by the z-score at the random time that the trial was stopped. In our original example above, suppose that the observed z-score when the trial was stopped at $\tau = 0.75$ was 2.65. The one-tailed p-value using the *z-score ordering* is

$$P\{Z(\tau) \geq 2.65\} = P\left[\cup_{i=1}^{4}\{\tau = t_i\} \cap \{Z(t_i) > 2.65\}\right].$$

Again the p-value includes the probability of the future event $\{\tau = 1\} \cap \{Z(1) \geq 2.65\}$.

The *stagewise ordering* considers only outcomes up to and including the stage of the given analysis. The one-tailed *stagewise p-value* is the probability of stopping for benefit earlier than the current stage plus the probability of not stopping earlier, but obtaining at least as large a z-score at the current analysis. In the above example, the stagewise p-value is

$$p = P(\text{cross before } t=0.75) + P(\text{no cross before } t = 0.75, \text{ but } Z(0.75) \geq 2.65)$$
$$= P[\{Z(0.25) > c_1\} \cup \{Z(0.50) > c_2\} \cup \{Z(0.75) \geq 2.65\}]. \tag{9.26}$$

Thus, the stagewise p-value is the null cumulative probability of crossing by time 0.75 if we use boundaries c_1, c_2, and 2.65 at information fractions 0.25, 0.50, and 0.75, respectively. Assume that we used the O'Brien-Fleming-like spending function. The boundaries at $t = 0.025, 0.50$, and 0.75 are 4.3326, 2.9631, and 2.3590, respectively. The one-tailed stagewise p-value is 0.0048, and the two-tailed p-value using symmetric boundaries is $2(0.0048) = 0.0096$.

The stagewise p-value has the following desirable properties: (1) the p-value is uniformly distributed if H_0 is true, (2) the p-value is α or less if and only if the boundary has been crossed, (3) the p-value depends only on current and past results, not on how many future looks are planned and when they will occur, and (4) if the trial is stopped at the first look with data D, the p-value is the same as it would be for a trial with no monitoring that yielded the same data D. Although the MLE, z-score, and stagewise ordering all have property (1), the stagewise ordering is the only one satisfying properties (2),(3), and (4). For these reasons, we believe that the stagewise ordering should be used to compute p-values.

We can also compute a p-value for nonzero null hypotheses. Return to the above example in which we stopped the trial at the third look with $Z(0.75) = 2.65$. Suppose we want to conduct a one-tailed test of the null hypothesis that the mean θ of the z-score at the planned end of the trial is 3.0. That is, we want to test $H_0 : \theta = 3$ versus $H_1 : \theta > 3$. To calculate the p-value, compute the probability of outcomes at least as extreme as the observed one, but under the assumption that $\theta = 3$:

$$P_{\theta=3}(\{Z(0.25) > 4.3326\} \cup \{Z(0.50) > 2.9631\} \cup \{Z(0.75) > 2.6500\}). \tag{9.27}$$

The p-value is 0.4893. In other words, the one-tailed p-value for testing $\theta = 3$ versus $\theta > 3$ is 0.4893.

9.6.3   Defining a Confidence Interval after a Monitored Trial

We can also compute a confidence interval for the drift parameter θ by inverting two one-tailed tests. Find the value θ_0 such that the p-value for testing $H_0 : \theta = \theta_0$ versus $H_1 : \theta > \theta_0$ is 0.025. The null hypothesis is rejected if the p-value (9.27) is less than 0.025. The p-value is an increasing function of θ_0, so the set of values θ_0 that are not rejected by the test is an interval of the form (L, ∞). We find that the one-tailed p-value for testing $H_0 : \theta = 0.7435$ versus the alternative $H_1 : \theta > 0.7435$ is 0.025. Therefore, the set of θ_0 for which the test is not rejected is $(0.7435, \infty)$. Likewise, we can test $H_0 : \theta = \theta_0$ versus $H_1 : \theta < \theta_0$. The p-value is one minus Expression (9.27), so the null hypothesis is rejected if Expression (9.27) is > 0.975. The set of values θ_0 that are rejected by this test is an interval of the form $(-\infty, U)$. In this case, $U = 5.3039$. The two-tailed confidence interval for the drift parameter θ consists of values θ_0 that are not rejected by either test, namely $(0.7435, 5.3039)$.

Of course, we are usually interested in computing a confidence interval for the natural parameter δ rather than the drift parameter. The natural and drift parameters are related by

$$\theta = \frac{\delta}{\widehat{se}(\hat{\delta})}; \quad \delta = \theta \, \widehat{se}(\hat{\delta}),$$

so the final step is multiplying the confidence limits for θ by $\widehat{se}(\hat{\delta})$ to get a confidence interval for δ. For instance, suppose that the z-test was of the control minus treatment proportions who died within 28 days, and the proportions after 200 and 204 patients in the control and treatment arms were $\hat{p}_C = 0.38$ and $\hat{p}_T = 0.20$, respectively. The approximate confidence interval for $p_C - p_T$ would be

$$\left(0.7435\sqrt{\frac{(0.38)(1-0.38)}{200} + \frac{(0.20)(1-0.20)}{204}}, 5.3039\sqrt{\frac{(0.38)(1-0.38)}{200} + \frac{(0.20)(1-0.20)}{204}} \right)$$

$$= (0.033, 0.235).$$

9.6.4   Correcting Bias after a Monitored Trial

We have seen how to obtain a confidence interval for δ, but how do we estimate δ after a monitored trial stops? We begin by estimating the drift parameter θ and then transform to estimate the natural parameter. In the nonmonitoring setting, the estimator $\hat{\theta}$ is in the middle of any confidence interval for θ, whether the confidence level is 90, 95, 99%, etc. If this were true in the monitoring setting, we could just take the center of the 95% confidence interval for θ to be our estimate of the drift parameter. In the present example, we would get $\hat{\theta} = (0.7435 + 5.3039)/2 = 3.0237$. However, the middle of a 99% confidence interval is slightly different: $(0.0173 + 6.0186)/2 = 3.018$. If we use a confidence level converging to 0, the confidence interval becomes narrower and narrower, becoming a single point in the limit. That single point is the *median point estimator* proposed by Kim (1989). We can approximate the median point estimator by using the midpoint of the 0.01%, confidence interval $(3.031, 3.031)$. This results in $\hat{\theta} = 3.031$. Note that an equivalent formulation of the median point estimator for θ is that it is the value θ_0 such that the p-value (9.27) is 0.50. Convert the median point estimator of θ to the median point estimator of $\delta = p_C - p_T$ by multiplying by the estimated standard error of $\hat{p}_C - \hat{p}_T$:

$$3.031\sqrt{\frac{(0.38)(1 - 0.38)}{200} + \frac{(0.20)(1 - 0.20)}{204}} = 0.134.$$

9.7   Bayesian Monitoring

We give a very brief overview of Bayesian methods in monitoring clinical trials. An excellent, accessible introduction to the contrast between Bayesian and frequentist approaches to clinical trials is Berger and Berry (1988). References specific to Bayesian monitoring include Freedman and Spiegelhalter (1989), Rosner (2005) in the context of survival trials, and Berry, et al. (2010) in adaptive clinical trials. Lee and Chu (2012) provide an overview of actual clinical trials analyzed using Bayesian methodology.

Bayesian statisticians use different criteria than frequentists for monitoring clinical trials. They specify a *prior distribution* reflecting their uncertainty about the treatment effect and then update that distribution after seeing data at an interim analysis. The updated, or *posterior distribution* for the treatment effect can be used to make stopping decisions. One simple example is to calculate the posterior probability that the treatment effect is greater than δ_0, where δ_0 might be 0 or some other number. If the criterion for early stopping is that the posterior probability of treatment being more effective than control is at least 0.95, then the same multiplicity problem that confronts the frequentist also confronts the Bayesian. The probability of falsely declaring a treatment benefit may be unacceptably high. Accordingly, most Bayesians use a more stringent criterion for declaring benefit at an interim analysis than at the planned end of the trial. For instance, a Bayesian analog of the Haybittle-Peto procedure is to stop at an interim analysis if the posterior probability that the treatment is superior to control is at least 0.999. The criterion at the end of the trial might be a posterior probability of 0.975 or greater.

Another approach to Bayesian monitoring uses *predictive probability* rather than posterior probability. Predictive probability also uses the posterior distribution of δ given the data, but then we calculate the probability that the trial will reach the efficacy criterion at the end of the trial, given the data at the interim analysis. The efficacy criterion at the end is ordinarily a Bayesian one, but it need not be. For example, one could compute the probability of reaching a statistically significant result at the end using a frequentist hypothesis test, given the data at the interim analysis. This frequentist/Bayesian hybrid is called *predictive power*. It can be thought of as conditional power averaged over the posterior distribution of δ. Equivalently, we can average over the posterior density $\pi(\theta \mid Z(t))$ of θ given the z-score $Z(t)$, where θ is the drift parameter:

$$PP(t) = \int CP_\theta(t)\pi(\theta \mid Z(t))d\theta.$$

Predictive power using a given threshold tends to result in earlier stopping than conditional power using the same threshold with unpromising interim results. This is because (1) $Z(t)$ will be low and (2) the posterior distribution of θ given $Z(t)$ will be negatively affected. With conditional power, only item (1) occurs.

An advantage of Bayesian thinking is that estimates and *credible intervals* for the parameter following a clinical trial are effortless. For a 95% credible interval, one simply finds lower and upper limits (L, U) such that the posterior probability that $\delta < L$ and the posterior probability that $\delta > H$ are both 0.025. That way, the posterior probability that $\delta \in [L, U]$ is 0.95. Bayesians interpret credible intervals differently from the way frequentists interpret confidence intervals. Frequentists are taught that only the endpoints of the confidence interval are random, so once the confidence interval is computed and $L = l$ and $U = u$ are fixed, it makes no sense to say that there is 95% probability that $\delta \in (l, u)$. To a Bayesian, the endpoints (l, u) are still fixed constants after the data are observed, but it **does** make sense to say that there is 95% probability that $\delta \in [l, u]$. Furthermore, the Bayesian need not struggle with what constitutes 'at least as extreme' as the observed outcome. Only the outcome actually observed matters. Another advantage is that even if we do not strictly adhere to the monitoring boundary (e.g., a boundary is crossed, but the trial continues), posterior probabilities given the interim data are sensible and easy to compute. Nonetheless, even Bayesians are concerned about having an unacceptably high false positive probability, and that probability cannot be calculated if one does not adhere to boundaries.

Example 9.17. PREVAIL II Recall the PREVAIL II trial for the treatment of Ebola virus in Western Africa. The trial compared ZMapp plus standard care with standard care alone with respect to 28-day mortality. A Bayesian design was selected partly because Bayesian methodology seamlessly facilitates inference following a trial with the potential for adaptations. The prior distribution for the probability of death by 28 days in a given arm was uniform $(0, 1)$. This choice was made based on the following considerations. First, the probability of death by 28 days was thought to be close to 0.5 but mortality varied by region and times, so there was substantial uncertainty. Second, the uniform distribution is quickly overwhelmed by trial data, so the prior distribution does not have undue influence on conclusions. Third, the uniform prior is a beta distribution with parameters $\alpha = 1$ and $\beta = 1$, and the beta family is a *conjugate prior* for the binomial, meaning that the posterior distribution is also beta (see Example 1.6).

If p is the probability of death by 28 days in an arm, the posterior distribution after observing x deaths out of n people is beta with parameters $\alpha + x$ and $\beta + n - x$. It is as if the prior distribution corresponds to prior data on $\alpha + \beta$ people, of whom α died by 28 days. When we combine the prior data with the observed data from the trial, there are $\alpha + x$ deaths and $\beta + n - x$ survivors. With $\alpha = 1$ and $\beta = 1$, the prior data consists of only two observations, one of which is a death. The posterior distribution is beta with parameters $1 + x$ and $1 + n - x$. At the time the trial stopped because the epidemic ended, 13 out of 35 people died by day 28 in the standard care arm (S) and 8 of 36 people died in the ZMapp plus standard care arm (Z). Accordingly, the posterior probability distributions are beta $(1 + 13, 1 + 35 - 13) = (14, 23)$ and $(1 + 8, 1 + 36 - 8) = (9, 29)$ in arms S and Z. Let p_S and p_Z denote the probability of death in arms S and Z. One can determine the posterior distribution of $p_Z - p_S$ analytically (see Proschan, Dodd, and Price, 2016) or through simulation. For the latter approach, simulate p_S and p_Z independently from beta $(14, 23)$ and beta $(9, 29)$ distributions, compute $p_Z - p_S$, and repeat a huge number of times. The mean of the posterior distribution is -0.14. The 0.025 and 0.975 percentiles of the simulated differences, namely $(-0.34, 0.06)$, form the 95% credible interval for $p_Z - p_S$. We can also compute the posterior probability that the true mortality probability is lower in arm Z using the proportion of simulated $p_Z - p_S$ that are negative. We can perform similar calculations for the ratio, p_Z/p_S.

Given that the trial ended early, the predictive probability of success at the planned end of the trial with 100 people per arm is of interest. Arm Z would be declared beneficial at the end if the posterior probability that $p_Z < p_S$ was at least 0.975. It turns out that this criterion is equivalent to adding a death to arm S and a survival to arm Z, and declaring benefit if the a one-tailed p-value using Fisher's exact test is 0.025 or less (see Proschan, Dodd, and Price, 2016). Therefore, one could estimate the predictive probability of success as follows:

1. Simulate p_S and p_Z from beta $(14, 23)$ and beta $(9, 29)$ distributions.

2. Simulate the numbers of deaths x_S and x_Z for the remaining $100 - 35 = 65$ and $100 - 36 = 64$ observations in arms S and Z using binomial $(65, p_S)$ and binomial $(64, p_Z)$ distributions.

3. Add one death to Arm S and one survival to Arm Z, so that there are $13 + x_S + 1$ out of 101 observations in Arm S and $8 + x_Z$ deaths out of 101 observations in arm Z.

4. Compute the one-tailed p-value for Fisher's exact and record whether it is less than 0.025.

5. Repeat the above steps a huge number of times and calculate the proportion of times the p-value in step 4 is 0.025 or less.

Implementation of this algorithm resulted in a predictive power of 0.53. Recall from Example 9.11 that exact conditional power under the current trend was 0.60. Why is predictive power lower than CP under the current trend? The criterion at the end of the trial for predictive power is a little different than for conditional power. For predictive power, the posterior probability that $p_T < p_C$ must be at least 0.975 at the end, whereas for conditional power, the p-value must be < 0.025 at the end. Still, this difference has little effect; using the same p-value < 0.025 criterion for both methods at the end changes predictive power very little, from 0.53 to 0.54. The real explanation for why predictive power is several points lower than conditional power under the current trend is as follows. The prior distribution of p_T and p_C is of independent uniforms on $(0, 1)$, so the prior expected difference, $E(p_C - p_T)$, is 0. The posterior estimate of $p_C - p_T$ lies between the prior estimate of 0 and the empirical estimate, $\hat{p}_C - \hat{p}_T$. Because the posterior estimate is not as optimistic as the empirical estimate, predictive power is lower than conditional power under the empirical estimate. If the empirical estimate of treatment effect had been in the opposite direction (i.e., $\hat{p}_C - \hat{p}_T < 0$), predictive power would have been larger than conditional power under the empirical estimate. This has an important ramification. Suppose we use a fixed futility threshold of, say, 0.20 for either predictive power or conditional power under the empirical estimate. When results are most suggestive of futility (i.e., $\hat{p}_C - \hat{p}_T < 0$), using the predictive power threshold makes it harder to stop than using the same conditional power threshold.

Exercises

1. Why is Pocock's boundary not commonly used in clinical trials?

2. Which of the classical monitoring boundaries, Haybittle-Peto, O'Brien-Fleming, or Pocock, is valid regardless of the joint distribution of z-scores over time?

3. Do you think a data and safety monitoring board should start out blinded and break the blind only after they see a sufficiently large difference? Defend your answer.

4. In a trial with a continuous endpoint analyzed using a t-test, what is the information fraction if the final sample size is 300 patients and the current sample sizes are 88 and 83 patients in the treatment and control arms?

5. Consider a trial with primary endpoint mortality, analyzed using a logrank test. The trial expects 4,000 patients and 200 deaths by the end. At an interim analysis, there are 506 and 515 patients in the treatment and control arms. There have been 38 and 48 deaths in the treatment and control arm thus far. What is the information fraction?

6. Consider a trial with a continuous endpoint analyzed using a t-test. Suppose that the ratio of the treatment to control sample sizes remains the same throughout. Show that the information fraction, defined by $\{\mathrm{var}(\hat{\delta})\}^{-1}/\{\mathrm{var}(\hat{\delta}_{\mathrm{end}})\}^{-1}$, reduces to the ratio of the interim to final sample size.

7. Let $B(t)$ be Brownian motion. Supply the "why" for the two missing steps of the following proof that $\mathrm{var}\{B(1) - B(t)\} = 1 - t$:

$$
\begin{aligned}
1 &= \mathrm{var}\{B(1)\} \quad (\text{because } B(1) = Z(1)) \\
&= \mathrm{var}[B(t) + \{B(1) - B(t)\}] \quad (\text{added and subtracted the} \\
&\quad \times \text{ same thing, } B(t)) \\
&= \mathrm{var}\{B(t)\} + \mathrm{var}\{B(1) - B(t)\} \quad (\textbf{Why?}) \\
&= t + \mathrm{var}\{B(1) - B(t)\} \quad (\textbf{Why?}) \\
1 - t &= \mathrm{var}\{B(1) - B(t)\} \quad (\text{subtracted } t \text{ from both sides}). \quad (9.28)
\end{aligned}
$$

8. In Example 9.12, calculate conditional power under the assumption that the control to treatment hazard ratio is 1.30.

9. Consider a trial that was originally powered at 85% for a two-tailed test at $\alpha = 0.05$. If the z-score at information fraction 0.5 is 0, what is the approximate conditional power under the original hypothesis?

10. Consider a trial with two-tailed $\alpha = 0.01$ and four equally-spaced looks.

    (a) Use Table 9.5 to compute the O'Brien-Fleming boundary.

    (b) Using software such as WinLD, compute the spending function analog to the O'Brien-Fleming boundary. Do you get the same boundary as in part a)?

(c) Now repeat the spending function boundary but change the third analysis time from 0.75 to 0.85. Did the boundaries at 0.25 and 0.50 change?

(d) What do think will happen to the final (fourth) boundary if you change the information time of the third analysis from 0.75 to 0.999? Now see if you were correct.

11. Consider a clinical trial with three equally-spaced looks and 90% power for a two-tailed test at $\alpha = 0.05$.

(a) Compute the drift parameter for the Pocock-like spending function. If a t-test is used and the sample size is large, approximately how much larger will the sample size need to be with monitoring compared to with no monitoring?

(b) Repeat part (a), but using the O'Brien-Fleming-like spending function.

12. Explain why power for the O'Brien-Fleming procedure is almost the same as for a trial with no interim monitoring.

13. Consider a trial that generates symmetric upper and lower boundaries, each at level 0.025, using the linear spending function $\alpha^*(t) = 0.025t$. The first two interim analyses are at information fractions 0.20 and 0.50. The z-score at $t = 0.50$ is 3.5, so the trial is stopped for efficacy.

(a) Compute the empirical estimate $B(0.50)/0.50$ of the drift parameter. Is this empirical estimate unbiased?

(b) Estimate the drift parameter θ using Kim's method using the stagewise ordering.

(c) Suppose that the trial analyzed a survival endpoint using the logrank test. Had it not stopped early, it would have continued until 150 events. Convert the estimate of θ in part (b) to an estimate of the hazard ratio.

(d) Under the assumptions of part (c), compute a 95% confidence interval for the hazard ratio.

9.8   Summary

1. Clinical trials are monitored for efficacy and safety by an independent committee of experts, the Data and Safety Monitoring Board (DSMB), which makes recommendations to the sponsor about whether to continue or stop the trial, or make any modifications.

2. Efficacy boundaries control the familywise error rate from multiple interim analyses.

(a) The most popular boundaries are high early, allowing the final boundary to be close to what it would be with no monitoring. Such boundaries have almost no reduction in power compared to no monitoring.

(b) The modified Haybittle-Peto boundary, based on the Bonferroni inequality, works regardless of the joint distribution of the test statistic over time.

(c) A very popular method is the Lan-DeMets alpha spending function approach, which does not require pre-specification of the number or timing of looks.

3. The information fraction t is the proportion of the trial completed, which is the ratio of interim to final sample sizes for most trials, and the ratio of interim to final number of events for survival trials.

4. When sample sizes are large, the B-value $B(t) = \sqrt{t}\, Z(t)$ has approximately the same joint distribution over time as Brownian motion with drift θ, where θ is the expected z-score at the end of the trial ($\theta = 0$ under the null hypothesis and $\theta = 2.80$, 3.00, and 3.24 under alternative hypotheses for 80, 85, and 90% power).

5. If the sample size is too small to rely on Brownian motion, boundaries can be based on the re-randomization distribution of the test statistic over time.

6. Futility monitoring is designed to eliminate poorly performing treatments that have little chance to show benefit by the end of the trial.

   (a) Useful tools for futility analysis are conditional power, revised unconditional power, predicted interval plots, and beta spending functions.

   (b) Stopping for futility has the potential to increase the type II error rate because a trial stopped because of a disappointing trend might have reversed and resulted in a statistically significant benefit if continued to fruition.

7. Estimation and p-values at the end of a trial that uses group-sequential monitoring are complicated by several factors:

   (a) The sufficient statistic is a pair, the stopping time and the z-score when the trial stopped. Accordingly, the likelihood ratio is not a monotone function of the z-score like it is with no monitoring.

   (b) The maximum likelihood estimator of treatment effect is biased in a trial using group-sequential monitoring.

   (c) There are multiple ways to order the sample space following a monitored trial, including by (1) the MLE, (2) the z-score, (3) the likelihood ratio, and (4) the stage at which the trial was stopped.

8. Bayesian monitoring has some philosophical advantages and easily facilitates estimation following a monitored trial.

Chapter 10

M&Ms: Multiplicity and Missing Data

10.1 Introduction

Two of the most important topics in clinical trials are multiplicity and missing data. Both affect the interpretation of the strength of evidence of a treatment effect. Multiple comparisons at level α are more likely to result in at least one claim of benefit even if there is no true benefit. For example, we expect to see one false claim of benefit if we perform twenty tests, even when all hypotheses are truly null. Missing data compromises the integrity of a trial in a different way. Randomization and comparison of randomized groups are at the heart of any clinical trial. Missing data interfere with the ability to compare randomized arms. The nonmissing data in different arms are **not** protected by randomization. Some treatments may have intolerable effects that cause people to withdraw from the trial, while other treatments or placebo may be easy to tolerate, resulting in very little missing data. The nonmissing people in the treatment arm can be very different from the nonmissing people in the control arm. Clinical trialists want to ensure that any claims of treatment benefit can be trusted. For these reasons, they tend to prefer conservative approaches to handling multiplicity and missing data.

10.2 Multiple Comparisons

10.2.1 The Debate

Multiple comparison adjustment is one of the thorniest issues in clinical trials. Some people argue that we should maximize the amount of information we get out of a clinical trial by answering as many questions as possible. But key to the frequentist reasoning in clinical trials is the idea that chance provides a poor explanation for statistically significant results. That no longer holds with multiple comparisons. Consider an extreme example in which 100 doses of a drug are compared to placebo, and the manufacturer will claim benefit if any dose is statistically significantly better than the placebo at one-tailed alpha of 0.05. Suppose that the drug truly has no benefit at any dose. The number of false claims of treatment benefit has a binomial distribution with $n = 100$ and probability parameter $p = 0.05$. On average, we expect to see $100(0.05) = 5$ false claims of benefit. It is extremely likely that at least one false declaration will be made: the probability of making no false declarations is

$$P(0 \text{ false declarations}) = \prod_{i=1}^{100} P(\text{comparison } i \text{ is not statistically significant})$$

$$= \prod_{i=1}^{100} (1 - 0.05) = (0.95)^{100} = 0.006. \qquad (10.1)$$

In other words, the probability of rejecting at least one true null hypothesis, called the *familywise error rate (FWER)*, is $1 - P(0$ false declarations of benefit$) = 1 - 0.006 = 0.994$. There is a strong argument for adjusting the level of evidence required for each comparison to guarantee some desired FWER. But there is a counter-argument. If these comparisons had been made in separate trials, no one would be demanding that the investigators adjust for all past and future comparisons (Rothman, 1990). So which argument is right, the one supporting always adjusting or the one supporting never adjusting for multiple comparisons?

Most people choose a middle ground between always adjusting and never adjusting for multiple comparisons. Important considerations guiding the decision are

1. whether the trial is intended to definitively answer several questions,

2. the degree of multiplicity,

3. whether the questions belong to a related family or are completely separate, and

4. whether there is an appearance of trying to gain from the multiplicity

(Proschan and Waclawiw, 2000). Concerning the first point, a phase II trial might choose not to adjust for multiple comparisons because the intent is to determine whether the evidence is promising enough for a definitive phase III trial. A phase III trial, on the other hand, typically would adjust for multiple comparisons. Consistent with item 2, the greater the number of comparisons, the more obliged we feel to make some sort of adjustment. After all, even with no adjustment, the FWER can be no greater than $2(0.05) = 0.10$ with two comparisons at level 0.05 each. That may be considered an acceptable FWER. On the other hand, the FWER with 4 comparisons at 0.05 each might be close to 0.20. That probably would not be considered acceptable. A trial answering a family of related questions gives the air of definitiveness and calls for a multiple comparison adjustment. In contrast, factorial trials might answer multiple unrelated questions. For example, the Women's Angiographic Vitamin and Estrogen (WAVE) factorial trial evaluated the effects of two very different interventions, hormone replacement therapy and antioxidant vitamins, on progression of heart disease in postmenopausal women with heart disease. In fact, the two components were originally planned as two separate trials and were combined to conserve resources. The separate trials argument of Rothman is compelling for WAVE and many other factorial trials.

Item number 4 above has generated some controversy (Dixon and Pennello, 2001; Proschan and Waclawiw, 2001) but is very important. For example, a pharmaceutical company comparing three doses of their drug to a placebo would be reluctant to make each comparison using $\alpha = 0.05$ and declare benefit if any dose was statistically significantly better than placebo. The company might be accused of trying to 'game the system' by getting three 'bites at the apple' instead of one. Regulatory agencies want a low probability of approving an ineffective treatment, so they would be unlikely to endorse unadjusted comparisons at level 0.05 in this setting.

Remark 10.1. *A multiplicity adjustment is not needed when a claim of benefit requires all hypotheses in a family to be rejected instead of at least one.*

Remark 10.1 applies to the setting of a combination drug such as two different blood pressure medications combined in one pill. To be approved, a combination drug must prove superiority over each of its constituents. Separate null hypotheses H_0 : combination drug is no better than constituent i, $i = 1, \ldots, k$ are tested with no adjustment for multiple comparisons. The probability of falsely rejecting **all** null hypotheses is α or less if each test uses level α.

10.2.2 Control of Familywise Error Rate

There are two different levels of control of the familywise error rate, *weak control* and *strong control*. We explain these concepts in the context of an early multiple comparison procedure suggested by Fisher.

Example 10.2. Fisher's LSD Consider all pairwise comparisons of means among four arms, (A,B,C,D). The six null hypotheses are $H_{0AB} : \mu_A = \mu_B$, $H_{0AC} : \mu_A = \mu_C$, $H_{0AD} : \mu_A = \mu_D$, $H_{0BC} : \mu_B = \mu_C$, $H_{0BD} : \mu_B = \mu_D$, and $H_{0CD} : \mu_C = \mu_D$. Conducting pairwise t-tests at level α would lead to an inflated FWER under the *global null hypothesis* H_0 in which all pairwise nulls are true. Equivalently, H_0 is that $\mu_A = \mu_B = \mu_C = \mu_D$. One method offering some protection against the alpha inflation problem is to first simultaneously compare all arms using an F-test. If the F-statistic is not statistically significant at level α, no pairs of means are declared different. If the F-statistic is statistically significant at level α, then each pairwise comparison is made using a t-test at the same level, α. This is called *Fisher's least significant difference (LSD)* procedure. If the global null hypothesis is true, the FWER of Fisher's LSD procedure is no greater than α because the F-statistic must be statistically significant, and the probability of that is α. Therefore, Fisher's LSD procedure protects the FWER under the global null hypothesis.

Even though Fisher's LSD controls the FWER when the global null is true, it does not protect against making at least one false declaration of treatment benefit under all configurations of treatment means. For example, suppose that $\mu_A = \mu_B = \mu_C$, but μ_D is very far away from the other three. This is depicted by Figure 10.1, in which horizontal distance represents magnitude of the difference between population means.

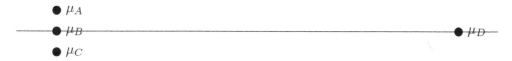

Figure 10.1: Configuration of population means that inflates the FWER for Fisher's LSD procedure.

The F-statistic is virtually guaranteed to be statistically significant at level α because μ_D is so far from the other population means. Because all pairwise comparisons are now made at level α, the probability of falsely declaring at least one pairwise difference among arms A, B, and C is substantially greater than α. For this reason, control of the FWER under the global null hypothesis is called *weak control of the FWER*. □

Incidentally, there is a more stringent method called the *Newman-Keuls procedure*. Newman-Keuls rejects a given pairwise comparison (i, j) if and only if its pairwise t-statistic is significant, the F-statistics for all triplets containing i and j are significant, the F-statistics for all quadruplets containing i and j are significant, $\ldots$, the F-statistic for comparing all k means is significant, all at level α. Even this more stringent procedure does not strongly control the type I error rate (see Exercise 8 and its hint).

Example 10.3. Bonferroni Now consider a different setting in which each of three arms, D, E, and F, is compared to the same control arm, C. Three null hypotheses, $H_{0CD} : \mu_C =$

μ_D, $H_{0CE} : \mu_C = \mu_E$, and $H_{0CF} : \mu_C = \mu_F$, are tested using a *Bonferroni correction* in which we divide α by the number of comparisons. Thus, we use level $\alpha/3$ for each of the three comparisons. Let $R(C, D)$ denote that H_{0CD} is rejected at level $\alpha/3$, and similarly for other pairwise comparisons with arm C. Under the global null hypothesis, the FWER is protected because

$$\begin{aligned} P_0\{R(C,D) \cup R(C,E) \cup R(C,F)\} &\leq P\{R(C,D)\} + R(C,E) + R(C,F) \\ &= 3(\alpha/3) = \alpha. \end{aligned} \qquad (10.2)$$

This Bonferroni method controls the FWER not just under the global null hypothesis $H_0 = H_{0CD} \cap H_{0CE} \cap H_{0CF} = \{(\mu_C, \mu_D, \mu_E, \mu_F) : \mu_C = \mu_D = \mu_E = \mu_F\}$, but under all other scenarios where one or more nulls is true. For example, suppose that two means equal the control mean. Without loss of generality, assume that $\mu_C = \mu_D = \mu_E$, but $\mu_C \neq \mu_F$. Now only two type I errors are possible. The probability of making at least one false declaration of a pairwise difference with control under this configuration of means is

$$\begin{aligned} P_0\{R(C,D) \cup R(C,E)\} &\leq P\{R(C,D)\} + R(C,E) \\ &= 2(\alpha/3) < \alpha. \end{aligned} \qquad (10.3)$$

Similarly, suppose exactly one mean equals the control mean. Without loss of generality, assume that $\mu_C = \mu_D$, $\mu_C \neq \mu_E$, $\mu_C \neq \mu_F$. The probability of a type I error is $P\{R(C,D)\} = \alpha/3$. We have shown that, regardless of how many null hypotheses are true, the probability of falsely rejecting at least one true null is controlled at level α. A procedure that controls the FWER not just under the global null hypothesis, but under any configuration such that one or more null hypotheses is true, is said to provide *strong control of the FWER*.   □

10.2.3   Showing Strong Control by Enumeration

In many settings, we can do what we did in Example 10.3, namely enumerate all possibilities to prove strong control of the FWER. The following example is another illustration of this method.

Example 10.4. Gatekeeping procedure Consider the comparison of a low dose and high dose of a drug to placebo. The two null hypotheses are $H_{0L} : \mu_L = \mu_0$, $H_{0H} : \mu_H = \mu_0$, where μ_0, μ_L, and μ_H are the population means in the placebo, low-dose, and high-dose arms. The manufacturer is confident that the high dose will have the strongest effect, but the low dose should also be effective compared to placebo. They first compare the high dose to placebo at level 0.05. If that comparison is not statistically significant, they discontinue testing and declare no comparison statistically significant. On the other hand, if the comparison of the high dose to placebo is statistically significant at $\alpha = 0.05$, they declare that comparison statistically significant and compare the low dose to placebo at level 0.05. This is known as a *gatekeeping procedure*. The high dose versus the placebo comparison is the 'gate' that, if opened (by virtue of rejection of H_{0H}), allows passage to the comparison of the low dose to placebo.

   To see that the procedure strongly controls the FWER, consider the separate possibilities. If $\mu_H = \mu_0$, the FWER is controlled regardless of the value of μ_L because, to declare any comparison statistically significant, we must first reject H_{0H}, which has probability 0.05. On the other hand, if $\mu_H \neq \mu_0$, then at most type I error is possible, namely rejecting H_{0L} when $\mu_L = \mu_0$. But this event has probability 0.05 because a level α test is used for H_{0L}. Thus, regardless of the true values of μ_0, μ_L, and μ_H, the FWER is 0.05 or less.   □

10.2.4 Intuition Behind Multiple Comparison Procedures

A clever, *sequentially rejective Bonferroni* procedure proposed by Holm (1979) also strongly controls the FWER and is uniformly more powerful than the usual Bonferroni method. Suppose there are k comparisons, and $p_{(1)} < p_{(2)} < \ldots < p_{(k)}$ are the ordered p-values. First compare $p_{(1)}$ to α/k. If $p_{(1)} > \alpha/k$, declare no comparison statistically significant. On the other hand, if $p_{(1)} \leq \alpha/k$, declare that comparison statistically significant and compare $p_{(2)}$ to $\alpha/(k-1)$. If $p_{(2)} > \alpha/(k-1)$, declare no further comparisons statistically significant. On the other hand, if $p_{(2)} \leq \alpha/(k-1)$, declare that comparison statistically significant and compare $p_{(3)}$ to $\alpha/(k-2)$, and so on. The intuition behind the procedure is simple: if $p_{(1)} \leq \alpha/k$, then we either made a type I error on that comparison or we did not. If we did, then in terms of FWER, it does not matter what happens next because we have already made at least one type I error. On the other hand, if we did not already make a type I error with the comparison corresponding to $p_{(1)}$, then that null hypothesis must be false. But that means at most $k-1$ hypotheses are true, so we could have used $\alpha/(k-1)$ for all comparisons. Likewise, for the comparison involving $p_{(2)}$, if we have already made at least one type I error on the hypothesis associated with $p_{(1)}$ or $p_{(2)}$, then it does not matter what happens next. If we have not already made at least one type I error, then at most $k-2$ null hypotheses are true. In the latter case, we could have used Bonferroni $\alpha/(k-2)$ for all comparisons, and so on.

Example 10.5. Holm's sequentially rejective Bonferroni Return to Example 10.3 comparing arms D, E, and F to C. Suppose that the p-values for testing the three null hypotheses, H_{0CD}, H_{0CE}, and H_{0CF} are 0.07, 0.015, and 0.022, respectively. Because the smallest p-value is 0.015, which is $\leq 0.05/3 = 0.017$, we reject null hypothesis H_{0CE}. We then compare the second smallest p-value, 0.022, to $0.05/2 = 0.025$. Because $0.022 \leq 0.025$, we reject null hypothesis H_{0CF} and compare the largest of the three p-values, 0.07, to 0.05. Because $0.07 > 0.05$, we fail to reject H_{0CD}. Note that with the usual Bonferroni procedure, only H_{0CE} could be rejected because only its p-value is $\leq 0.05/3 = 0.017$. $\qquad\square$

Holm's sequentially rejective Bonferroni procedure is a special case of a powerful idea of transferring alpha from rejected null hypotheses to other hypotheses (Bretz et al, 2011). It is a graphical technique that succinctly summarizes what would be cumbersome to describe in words. Before any testing begins, we specify an initial set, $\alpha_1, \ldots, \alpha_k$, $\sum_{i=1}^{k} \alpha_i = \alpha$, of significance levels for the k hypothesis tests. The hypotheses are denoted as nodes (usually circles or rectangles), and the associated alpha levels are specified inside the nodes. We also pre-specify and denote by arrows how to transfer alpha from that comparison if it is statistically significant.

Example 10.6. Graphical alpha transfer Return to the comparison of arms D, E, and F to control arm C in Example 10.5. That example used Holm's procedure, but we now illustrate that the same answer results from the graphical alpha transfer procedure depicted in Figure 10.2. The 0.05 overall alpha is initially divided equally (0.05/3) among the three comparisons with control. After rejection of a comparison, its alpha level is transferred equally among the two remaining arms. To show that conclusions do not depend on order of testing, we consider both a succinct order and a clumsy order. The succinct order is to begin with the smallest p-value, 0.015 associated with H_{0CE}. As in Example 10.5, we reject H_{0CE} because $0.015 \leq 0.05/3$. We then transfer half of its 0.05/3 to H_{0CD} and half to H_{0CF}. That is, we add $(1/2)(0.05/3) = 0.05/6$ to the current alpha levels for H_{0CD} and H_{0CF}. The new alpha level for H_{0CD} and H_{0CF} becomes $0.05/3 + 0.05/6 = 0.05/2 = 0.025$. Look next at the second smallest p-value, 0.022 associated with H_{0CF}. We reject H_{0CF} because $0.022 \leq 0.025$. We now transfer its alpha level to the remaining comparison, H_{0CD}.

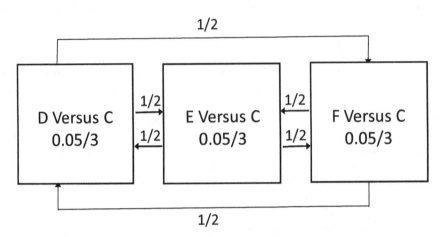

Figure 10.2: The alpha transfer principle applied to comparisons of arms D, E, and F to control arm C. The arrows and their associated numbers indicate the direction and proportion of alpha to be transferred if the given comparison is statistically significant.

This comparison is now made at level $0.05/2 + 0.05/2 = 0.05$. Because $0.07 > 0.05$, we fail to reject H_{0CD}.

The clumsier order begins with the largest p-value, 0.07 associated with H_{0CD}. H_{0CD} is not rejected and none of its $0.05/3$ is transferred to the other two comparisons. Suppose we examine the second largest p-value next, 0.022 associated with H_{0CF}. H_{0CF} is not rejected because $0.022 > 0.05/3$. None of the $0.05/3$ associated with H_{0CF} is transferred. Now examine the smallest p-value, 0.015 associated with H_{0CE}. Reject H_{0CE} because $0.015 \leq 0.05/3$. We then transfer one-half of the $0.05/3$ associated with H_{0CE} to each of H_{0CD} and H_{0CF}. That is, we add $(1/2)(0.05/3) = 0.05/6$ to $0.05/3$ to get $0.05/2$. We can now re-test H_{0CD} using level $0.05/2$. Again it is not statistically significant, so none of its $0.05/2$ is transferred to the last comparison, H_{0CF}. We test H_{0CF} at $0.05/2$ because of the transfer of $(1/2)(0.05/3)$ from the rejection of H_{0CE}. The p-value of 0.015 for H_{0CF} is $\leq 0.05/2$, so we can now transfer $0.05/2$ from H_{0CF} to the current alpha level of $0.05/2$ for H_{0CD}. In other words, we can now re-test H_{0CD} at level $0.05/2 + 0.05/2 = 0.05$. It does not reach statistical significance, and no more alpha can be transferred. We reach the same conclusion as with the succinct order: hypotheses H_{0CD} and H_{0CF} are rejected.   □

Example 10.6 shows that order of testing does not affect results. Still, some orders are more efficient in terms of number of steps. The shortcut method is as follows. Let α_i, $i = 1, \ldots, k$ be the initial allocation of type I error rate across the k hypotheses, with $\sum_{i=1}^{k} \leq \alpha$. Denote by π_{ij} the proportion of alpha transferred from hypothesis i to hypothesis j if hypothesis i is rejected, with $\pi_{ii} = 0$ and $\sum_j \pi_{ij} \leq 1$.

1. Let j be the index of the comparison with the smallest 'relative' p-value, p_i/α_i.

2. If $p_j \leq \alpha_j$, reject H_j; otherwise stop.

3. Update the graph as follows:

   (a) Delete node j and do the following:

      i. For each remaining H_m, replace α_m by $\alpha_m + \alpha_j \pi_{jm}$.

      ii. For each remaining distinct pair (H_m, H_r), replace π_{mr} by $(\pi_{mr} + \pi_{mj}\pi_{jr})/(1 - \pi_{mj}\pi_{jm})$.

4. If there is at least one hypothesis left in the graph, return to step 1; otherwise stop.

Theorem 10.7. *(Bretz et al., 2011) The preceding steps define a shortcut to a procedure that strongly controls the FWER.*

10.2.5 Independent Comparisons

We briefly discuss a method developed for independent comparisons that only weakly controls the FWER. The reason for this diversion is that it was the impetus for a procedure that does strongly control the FWER in many settings and is quite powerful. Simes (1986) proposed the following method for independent test statistics. Let $p_{(1)} < p_{(2)} < \cdots < p_{(k)}$ denote the ordered p-values. Reject the global null hypothesis if $p_{(j)} \leq (j/k)\alpha$ for any $j = 1, \ldots, k$. Simes recognized that the method cannot be used to reliably identify the specific hypotheses that are false.

Here is a slight simplification of an example Hommel (1988) gave to show the extent of inflation of the FWER of the Simes procedure under configurations other than the global null. Suppose that $k = 1000$ and 501 of the 1000 null hypotheses are true, while the remaining 499 are so false that the corresponding p-values are infinitesimally close to 0. Then the smallest 499 p-values are nearly guaranteed to correspond to the false hypotheses. Among the 501 true nulls, the smallest p-value cutoff using the Simes procedure will be $(500/1000)\alpha = \alpha/2$.

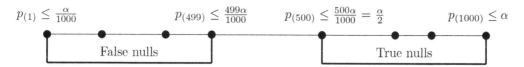

Figure 10.3: Simes procedure for 1000 null hypotheses, 499 of which are so false that their p-values are virtually guaranteed to be the smallest 499 of the 1000 p-values.

If the test of any of the 501 true null hypotheses is statistically significant at level $\alpha/2$, then at least type I error will be made. Consequently, the FWER is at least

$$1 - (1 - \alpha/2)^{501}.$$

When $\alpha = 0.05$, the FWER is 0.999997 instead of 0.05.

    We will see shortly how the closure principle described in Section 10.2.6 led to an improvement of the Simes procedure.

10.2.6 Closure Principle

Consider hypotheses $H_{01}, \ldots, H_{0k}$. Suppose there is an α level test for each hypothesis that can be written as an intersection of one or more of $H_{01}, \ldots, H_{0k}$. The closure principle rejects H_{0j} if and only if every intersection hypothesis containing H_{0j} is rejected by its α level test.

Theorem 10.8. *(Marcus, Peritz, and Gabriel, 1976) The closure principle strongly controls the FWER for the family $H_{01}, \ldots, H_{0k}$.*

To see why Theorem 10.8 holds, let H_{0i}, $i \in I$, be the set of true null hypotheses, where I is a set of indices. To reject any of the true null hypotheses, we must reject $\cap_{i \in I} H_{0i}$ using its alpha level test. Because this has probability α or less, the closure principle strongly controls the FWER. $\square$

The closure principle can be used to show that the sequentially rejective Bonferroni method strongly controls the type I error rate. In fact, the sequentially rejective Bonferroni procedure is equivalent to rejecting H_{0j} if and only if every intersection of i null hypotheses that include index j is rejected using a level α/i test, $i = 1, \ldots, k$.

Hommel (1988) used the closure principle to strengthen the Simes (1986) method for independent test statistics. Hommel's modification strongly controls the FWER whenever the unmodified Simes procedure weakly controls the FWER. In particular Hommel's modification strongly controls the FWER when the test statistics are independent. Hochberg (1988) simplified the modified Simes procedure while maintaining strong control as follows. Apply Holm's procedure in reverse order. Begin with $p_{(k)}$, the largest p-value rather than the smallest. If $p_{(k)} \leq \alpha$, declare all comparisons statistically significant. On the other hand, if $p_{(k)} > \alpha$, declare that comparison not statistically significant and compare the second largest p-value, $p_{(k-1)}$, to $\alpha/2$. If $p_{(k-1)} \leq \alpha/2$, declare the comparisons associated with $p_{(1)}, \ldots, p_{(k-1)}$ all statistically significant. On the other hand, if $p_{(k-1)} > \alpha/2$, declare that comparison not statistically significant and compare the third largest p-value, $p_{(k-2)}$, to $\alpha/3$, and so on. *Hochberg's procedure* is also called the *Benjamini-Hochberg procedure* when used in the context of controlling a different kind of error rate called the *false discovery rate (FDR)*. The procedure has been shown to strongly control the FWER under independence and, more generally, for a fairly broad class of multivariate distributions (Sarkar, 1998).

The sequence of α levels associated with $p_{(1)}, \ldots, p_{(k)}$ is the same with the Holm and Hochberg procedures. The difference is that Holm begins with the smallest p-value, while Hochberg begins with the largest p-value (Figure 10.4).

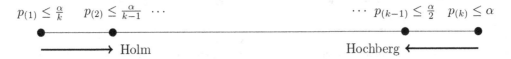

$$p_{(1)} \leq \tfrac{\alpha}{k} \qquad p_{(2)} \leq \tfrac{\alpha}{k-1} \quad \cdots \qquad\qquad\qquad \cdots \ p_{(k-1)} \leq \tfrac{\alpha}{2} \quad p_{(k)} \leq \alpha$$

Holm $\longrightarrow$ Hochberg $\longleftarrow$

Figure 10.4: Hochberg and Holm procedures.

The set of hypotheses rejected by Hochberg's procedure always contains those rejected by Holm's procedure. To see this, suppose that Holm's method declares $p_{(1)}, \ldots, p_{(j)}$ statistically significant, but not $p_{(j+1)}$ (and, therefore, not $p_{(j+1)}, \ldots, p_{(k)}$). Even if Hochberg finds no $p_{(m)}$ statistically significant for $m \geq j+1$, it will still declare $p_{(j)}$ statistically significant because Holm's method did, and both methods use the same alpha levels. Also, once Hochberg's procedure finds one p-value statistically significant, all hypotheses with smaller p-values are automatically rejected. Therefore, Hochberg's procedure declares $p_{(1)}, \ldots, p_{(j)}$ statistically significant. Thus, any hypothesis rejected by Holm's procedure is rejected by Hochberg's procedure. Consequently, Hochberg's method is always at least as powerful as Holm's method.

The closure method is so deceptively simple that it can be misinterpreted. For example, return to Example 10.2 involving pairwise comparisons of the means of arms A, B, C, and D. The closure method appears to imply that the Newman-Keuls procedure, described immediately following Example 10.2, strongly controls the type I error rate, but it does not (see Exercise 8). The problem is that Newman-Keuls does not consider **every** intersection. For example, consider the closure method for testing H_{0AB}. Denote by H_{0ABC} the hypothesis that $\mu_A = \mu_B = \mu_C$, and similarly for H_{0ABD} and H_{ABCD}. The Newman-Keuls procedure requires rejection of (1) H_{0AB}, (2) H_{0ABC}, (3) H_{0ABD}, and (4) H_{0ABCD} by their

α level tests. Conspicuously absent from this list is a test of $H_{0AB} \cap H_{0CD}$. The closure method requires the p-value for the test of $H_{0AB} \cap H_{0CD}$ to be significant at level α for every configuration of means such that $\mu_A = \mu_B$ and $\mu_C = \mu_D$. One such configuration is $\mu_A = \mu_B = \mu_1$ and $\mu_C = \mu_D = \mu_2$, where $|\mu_1 - \mu_2|$ is huge (see the hint in Exercise 8).

Example 10.9. Return to Example 10.5 comparing arms D, E, and F to control arm C. Change the p-values for testing the three null hypotheses, H_{0CD}, H_{0CE}, and H_{0CF} to 0.07, 0.019, and 0.022, respectively. To apply Hochberg's method, begin by comparing the largest p-value, 0.07, to 0.05. Because $0.07 > 0.05$, we do not declare arm D's mean different from arm C's. Next, compare the second largest p-value, 0.022, to $0.05/2 = 0.025$. Because the second smallest p-value is ≤ 0.025, we declare all remaining comparisons statistically significant. In other words, we declare the means in each of arms E and F different from the mean in arm C. If we had applied Holm's sequentially rejective Bonferonni method instead, we would have stopped at the first step with no null hypotheses rejected because the smallest p-value, 0.019, is larger than $0.05/3$. $\qquad\square$

Example 10.10. Primary and secondary endpoints with monitoring: Hung, Wang, and O'Neill (2007) There is often keen interest in both a primary and secondary endpoint in a clinical trial. For example, in a vaccine trial for coronavirus disease caused by SARS-CoV-2, (COVID-19), prevention of disease may be of primary interest, but prevention of serious disease is an important secondary endpoint. In a treatment trial of patients hospitalized with COVID-19, progression to ventilation or death may be the primary endpoint, but death is certainly an important secondary endpoint. Monitoring boundaries are usually used for the primary, but not the secondary, endpoint. Can the closure principle be used to show that, having rejected the null hypothesis for the primary endpoint at an interim analysis, we can use full level alpha for the secondary endpoint at that same time? Hung, Wang, and O'Neill, R. (2007) show that this strategy can inflate the type I error rate. The problem is that the look time for the secondary endpoint is not pre-specified, but is a random variable. Furthermore, that random time is very informative about the treatment effect for the secondary endpoint because the primary and secondary endpoints are almost always quite correlated. Theorem 10.8 would require a valid, level α test of the secondary endpoint irrespective of the primary endpoint. Testing the secondary endpoint at a random time that is informative about its result is not a valid, level α procedure. The situation is analogous to monitoring a single endpoint over time, but using outcome results to decide when future looks occur. Such data-driven look times are known to inflate the type I error rate, although not substantially for commonly used spending functions (Proschan, Follmann, and Waclawiw, 1992).

If we had pre-specified a valid boundary for the secondary endpoint and pretended that that boundary was used at each previous interim analysis, the type I error rate would have been controlled because that is a valid, level α procedure for the secondary endpoint irrespective of the primary endpoint. Tamhane, Mehta, and Liu (2010) give analytic results and use numerical integration to conclude that use of O'Brien-Fleming and Pocock boundaries for the primary and secondary endpoints, respectively, has favorable properties. Spending function analogs can also be used. For example, suppose that the z-statistic for the primary endpoint crosses the O'Brien-Fleming-like spending function boundary. For the secondary endpoint, we compute the current Pocock-like spending function boundary by pretending that the secondary endpoint was monitored at each previous analysis. $\qquad\square$

10.3   Dunnett Procedure and Conditioning Technique

Consider the comparison of multiple treatments to the same control arm in a trial with a continuous outcome. For simplicity, assume that sample sizes are large enough to treat the common within-arm variance as known. We can express the probability of at least one type I error under the global null hypothesis with a very useful conditioning trick that produces conditionally iid random variables. After all, the only reason that the pairwise z-statistics

$$Z_i = \frac{\bar{Y}_i - \bar{Y}_0}{\sqrt{2\sigma^2/n}} \tag{10.4}$$

are dependent is that the same control sample mean $\bar{Y}_0$ appears in (10.4) for each i. Conditioning on $\bar{Y}_0 = y_0$ makes $\bar{Y}_0$ a constant and makes

$$Z_i = \frac{\bar{Y}_i - y_0}{\sqrt{2\sigma^2/n}}, \; i = 1, \ldots, k$$

iid normal random variables with null mean and variance

$$\mathrm{E}_0(Z_i \,|\, \bar{Y}_0 = y_0) = \frac{\mu_0 - y_0}{\sqrt{2\sigma^2/n}}; \quad \mathrm{var}_0(Z_i \,|\, \bar{Y}_0 = y_0) = \frac{\sigma^2/n}{2\sigma^2/n} = 1/2.$$

Consider a one-tailed test rejecting the null hypothesis when $Z_i > c$. We can determine c to control the FWER as follows. Conditional on $\bar{Y}_0 = y_0$, the probability of 0 type I errors is

$$P(0 \text{ errors} \,|\, \bar{Y}_0 = y_0) = \prod_{i=1}^{k} P\left\{ N\left(\frac{\mu_0 - y_0}{\sqrt{2\sigma^2/n}}, 1/2 \right) \leq c \right\}$$

$$= \Phi^k \left\{ \frac{c - \frac{\mu_0 - y_0}{\sqrt{2\sigma^2/n}}}{\sqrt{1/2}} \right\} = \Phi^k \left\{ \sqrt{2}\,c - \frac{\mu_0 - y_0}{\sigma/\sqrt{n}} \right\}. \tag{10.5}$$

We now 'uncondition' on $\bar{Y}_0$ by integrating over its distribution to find the probability of 0 errors under the global null:

$$P(0 \text{ errors}) = E[P(0 \text{ errors} \,|\, \bar{Y}_0)] = \int_{-\infty}^{\infty} \Phi^k \left\{ \sqrt{2}\,c - \frac{\mu_0 - y_0}{\sigma/\sqrt{n}} \right\} f(y_0) dy_0,$$

where $f(y_0)$ is the normal density function with null mean $E_0(\bar{Y}_0) = \mu_0$ and variance $\mathrm{var}(\bar{Y}_0) = \sigma^2/n$. Using the change of variable $z = (y_0 - \mu_0)/(\sigma/\sqrt{n})$, we get

$$P(0 \text{ errors}) = \int_{-\infty}^{\infty} \Phi^k \left\{ \sqrt{2}\,c + z \right\} \phi(z) dz, \tag{10.6}$$

where ϕ is the standard normal density function. We then equate (10.6) to $1 - \alpha$ and solve for c. This same technique of conditioning on the control mean to create independent statistics works for equicorrelated multivariate normal observations (see Exercise 13).

Table 10.1 shows critical values c and the corresponding two-tailed p-value p to control the two-tailed FWER at 0.05 for the Dunnett procedure. For example, with 4 active arms compared to a control, declare mean i different from the control mean if $|Z_i| \geq 2.442$ (or equivalently, $p_i \leq 0.015$).

There is also a sequentially rejective version of the Dunnett procedure that we illustrate for 3 active arms compared to a control. First compare the smallest p-value, $p_{(1)}$, to 0.019; if $p_{(1)} > 0.019$, declare no differences with control and stop. If $p_{(1)} \leq 0.019$, declare that arm different from control and compare the second smallest p-value, $p_{(2)}$, to 0.027. If $p_{(2)} > 0.027$, declare no further differences with control and stop. If $p_{(2)} \leq 0.027$, declare that arm different from control and compare the largest p-value, $p_{(3)}$, to 0.05.

Table 10.1: Critical values for the absolute value of the z-score or two-tailed p-value for a large-sample, two-tailed Dunnett procedure at level 0.05.

k	1	2	3	4	5	6
Z-boundary	1.960	2.212	2.349	2.442	2.511	2.567
Two-tailed p-value boundary	0.050	0.027	0.019	0.015	0.012	0.010

10.4 Missing Data

10.4.1 Definitions and Example

Missing data interfere with the ability to compare randomized arms in a clinical trial. If Mother Nature randomly selected which observations to cover up, then there would be no problem with analyzing only nonmissing data in each arm. When the probability that outcomes are missing does not depend on their values, data are said to be *missing completely at random (MCAR)*. (Rubin, 1976; Little and Rubin, 2019). In making this definition more precise, we follow the ubiquitous but unfortunate convention of letting $M = 1$ denote a nonmissing observation. Let $\boldsymbol{Y}$ denote the set of outcomes in the trial and $\boldsymbol{M}$ the set of 'missing' indicators. Data are *MCAR* if $P(\boldsymbol{M} = \boldsymbol{m} \mid \boldsymbol{Y} = \boldsymbol{y})$ does not depend on $\boldsymbol{y}$. Under this assumption, there is no bias introduced from ignoring missing observations. The MCAR assumption is extremely unlikely to hold in clinical trials. For example, a patient may drop out of a trial because they feel too sick to continue. In a trial of interventions to treat substance abuse, a participant who stops attending scheduled drug tests may be doing so because they know that they will test positive. There are numerous explanations for why the probability of a missing observation might depend on the value of the observation. When data are not MCAR, ignoring missing data can lead to serious bias.

Example 10.11. Consider a trial involving weight loss interventions, and let $X_0, \ldots, X_5, Y$ denote weights at baseline and monthly thereafter until the primary outcome at month 6, Y. Given that observations on different people are independent, we focus on a single individual. Let $M = 1$ denote that Y is observed for that person and, for simplicity, assume that $X_0, \ldots, X_5$ are always observed. It is likely that $P(M = 1 \mid Y = y)$ is smaller for larger values of y. That is, patients who gain weight are less likely to have an observed primary outcome than those who lose weight. They may feel guilty or ashamed that they gained weight. Therefore, the data are not likely to be MCAR.

Even though the data are not MCAR, there are observed data $\boldsymbol{X} = (X_0, \ldots, X_5)$ that can give us good information about Y and whether Y is likely to be observed. Thus, even though $P(M = m \mid Y = y)$ depends on $\boldsymbol{y}$, it may be that

$$P(M = m \mid \boldsymbol{X} = \boldsymbol{x}, Y = y) = P(M = m \mid \boldsymbol{X} = \boldsymbol{x}). \tag{10.7}$$

This *missing at random (MAR)* condition says that, given the observed data $\boldsymbol{x}$, the value of the outcome gives no additional information about whether it will be observed. An equivalent way to express MAR (Exercise 9) is that, given the observed data $\boldsymbol{x}$, whether the primary outcome is missing gives no additional information about its value:

$$f(y \mid \boldsymbol{X} = \boldsymbol{x}, M = m) = g(y \mid \boldsymbol{X} = \boldsymbol{x}). \tag{10.8}$$

where f and g are conditional probability mass (or density) functions. MAR is more realistic than MCAR. Under MAR, two people with the same observed data $\boldsymbol{x}$ are expected to have similar Y values even if one of the two people's Y value is missing. □

Note that in the definition of MAR, X can include post-randomization variables. In Example 10.11, X included follow-up weights. As usual, we have to be very careful about post-randomization variables in clinical trials. We do not want to adjust treatment effects for these variables because treatment can affect not only the primary outcome, but other variables as well. In Example 10.11, 'adjusting' for post-randomization weights makes no sense because that would adjust away most differences in weight at 6 months (the primary outcome). However, using post-randomization covariates to predict what the missing observations would have been is a very reasonable strategy.

10.4.2   Methods for Data That Are MAR

There are different methods of analyzing data that are MAR, some of which use only baseline data because of the concern raised at the end of Section 10.4 about using post-randomization variables. The drawback of using only baseline data is that it may not adequately predict an outcome and whether that outcome will be missing. Nonetheless, we begin with methods for missing data that use only baseline variables.

A straightforward example is when the outcome Y is continuous and $X_1, \ldots, X_p$ are p baseline covariates. Assume that Y follows the linear model $Y = \beta_0 + \beta_1 X_1 + \ldots + \ldots + \beta_p X_p + \epsilon$, where ϵ is a normally distributed error with mean 0 and variance σ^2. This includes the analysis of covariance (ANCOVA) model in which one of the covariates is the baseline value of the outcome variable. Suppose that patients 1 and 2 have the same baseline values $(x_1, \ldots, x_p)$ for all covariates. For example, both patients are females, aged 35, and have systolic blood pressure 134. The only difference is that the outcome is missing for patient 1 and present for patient 2. Suppose that the linear model is correct and the baseline covariates perfectly predict who will have missing data. In that case, we do not get additional information about whether an observation will be missing by looking at post-randomization data. Then the conditional density of Y given $X = x$ is the same for patients 1 and 2. That is, equation (10.8) holds and the data are MAR. It is as if Mother Nature randomly picked, among participants with the same baseline variables, which ones would have observed and which would have missing data. Under these strong assumptions, excluding patient 1 creates no bias. One way to view things is that patient 2 adequately represents the missing patient 1. We do not believe this method would work well in Example 10.11. It is very unlikely that baseline weight predicts whether the 6-month outcome will be missing so well that follow-up weights do not give additional information.

Another method, the *propensity score*, explicitly models the probability of being observed as a function of baseline covariates. For example, we could use logistic regression with outcome M_i, the indicator that the primary outcome for participant i is observed, and baseline variables x as predictors:

$$\ln\left\{ \frac{P(M=1)}{1 - P(M=1)} \right\} = \beta^T x; \quad P(M=1) = \frac{\exp(\beta^T x)}{1 + \exp(\beta^T x)}.$$

The predicted probability of having an observed outcome is the *propensity* for being observed. A common method partitions participants according to quintiles of propensity scores. Although there may be large differences in outcomes of participants in different quintiles, differences within each quintile would be expected to be smaller because the propensity to be missing is similar for those within a given quintile. Within a quintile, missing and nonmissing observations should be comparable. It is as if Mother Nature randomly picked, among patients with similar propensity for having an observed value, which ones would be observed, and which would not.

Compute the estimated treatment effect $\hat{\theta}_i$ and its variance estimate V_i using the nonmissing observations within quintile i. For example, for a difference in means, compute

$\hat{\theta}_i = \bar{Y}_{Ti} - \bar{Y}_{Ci}$, the treatment-to-control difference in sample means for nonmissing observations in stratum i. The variance estimate V_i could be $\hat{s}_i^2(1/n_{Ti} + 1/n_{Ci})$, where $\hat{s}_i^2$ is the pooled variance in the ith stratum. Other variance estimates could be used as well, such as the one used with Welch's unequal variance t-test. We then compute the stratified treatment effect estimator and its estimated standard error ($\widehat{\text{se}}$):

$$\hat{\theta} = \frac{\sum_{i=1}^{5}(1/V_i)\hat{\theta}_i}{\sum_{i=1}^{5}(1/V_i)}; \quad \widehat{\text{se}}(\hat{\theta}) = \frac{1}{\sqrt{\sum(1/V_i)}}.$$

An alternative to the quintile approach is to include the propensity score as a continuous covariate in the model used to estimate the treatment effect. Only a single degree of freedom is lost instead of multiple degrees of freedom if all baseline variables comprising the propensity score are included as covariates. This parsimony is important in a small clinical trial.

As noted above, baseline data are not likely to accurately predict whether the outcome is missing or the value of the outcome. Post-randomization data, such as the follow-up weights in Example 10.11, ought to improve these predictions. But we have warned of the potential perils of adjusting for post-randomization covariates, so what should we do? One approach is to incorporate interim values into the outcome itself. Consider Example 10.11. We could use, as primary outcome, the slope relating a participant's weight to time from randomization. Compute a slope for each participant and average those slopes over all people in each arm. The treatment effect estimate is the difference in average slopes in the treatment and control arms. This is appealing in at least two ways. First, a slope would be expected to have a smaller variance than a single value. Second, we can compute a slope even with only 2 observations for a given person. If the MAR assumption is correct, the slope method will not introduce bias. The concern that a person who is doing poorly might not show up for the final weight measurement is automatically accounted for; the poor performance will already be reflected in that person's slope for interim weights.

A downside of the simple slope method is that the precision of a slope estimate with two observations is smaller than that of a person with no missing data. Therefore, it seems preferable to give less weight to people with fewer observed values. A more sophisticated slope analysis that gives less weight to people with fewer measurements is a *mixed model*. Let Y_{ij} be the jth observation on person i, and let z_i be the treatment indicator for participant i (0 for control, 1 for treatment). One possible mixed model is

$$Y_{ij} = \beta_0 + \beta_1 t_{ij} + \beta_2 z_i + \beta_3 z_i t_{ij} + b_{0i} + b_{1i} t_{ij} z_i + \epsilon_{ij}.$$

Here, β_0 and β_1 are the mean intercept and slope in the control arm, while β_2 and β_3 are the mean treatment minus control difference in intercept and slope, respectively. The random effects b_{0i} and b_{1i} are participant-specific deviations in intercept and slope. That is, b_{0i} is the baseline value for participant i minus the mean baseline value in the population for that arm, while b_{1i} is the slope for participant i minus the mean slope in the population for that arm. The ϵ_{ij} are random errors, assumed independent of (b_{0i}, b_{1i}). Also, random effects for different people are independent. Under the model,

$$E(Y_{ij}) = \begin{cases} \beta_0 + \beta_1 t_{ij} & \text{if } z_i = 0 \text{ (control)} \\ \beta_0 + \beta_2 + (\beta_1 + \beta_3)t_{ij} & \text{if } z_i = 1 \text{ (treatment)}. \end{cases}$$

The mixed model is a more principled way to do a slope analysis than simply using a t-test on the average slopes in each arm. The mixed model gives higher weight to slopes of people with more observed data. However, a person with twice as many observed values as another does not get twice the weight. Instead, the weights depend on the degree of within-participant variability. If the within-person variability is small, the correlation between observations on the same person is high; in that case, the person with twice as many observed values could receive much less than twice the weight. Conversely, if the within-person variability is large, the observations within a person may be close to independent; in that case, the person with twice the many observations may indeed receive nearly twice the weight.

Other principled methods of dealing with missing data are based on likelihoods. One such method is the *expectation-maximization (EM) algorithm*. Begin by filling in missing values with arbitrary initial guesses. Now that the dataset has been 'completed', compute the maximum likelihood estimate of the parameter vector θ_0. This is the 'maximization' step. Using $\hat{\theta}_0$, update the missing values by substituting their expected values (the 'expectation' step). With the updated completed dataset, compute the new maximum likelihood estimate $\hat{\theta}_1$ of θ. Continue this expectation and maximization process until successive estimates of θ are within a small tolerance of each other.

The expectation step of the EM algorithm repeatedly fills in (*imputed*) the missing values. A much more basic imputation method, *single imputation*, fills in missing data only once. For example, one might impute the mean of the group to which the patient is assigned (*mean imputation*). Treating such an observation as if it were an actual observation can be anti-conservative. To see this, consider the most extreme case possible of only one nonmissing observation in each arm. If the difference between the treatment and control observation favors the treatment, then imputing the mean in each respective arm will (1) artificially inflate the sample size in each arm and (2) make the within-arm variance 0. The difference in means will be infinitely many estimated standard errors away from 0, so the p-value will be 0. Clearly, this greatly overestimates the level of evidence in favor of the treatment. Even in less extreme settings, pretending that the imputed value is an actual value can artificially increase the sample size and decrease the standard error of the treatment effect estimate. The combined effect can greatly overstate the level of evidence of a treatment effect.

Another single imputation method that is usually ill-advised and criticized (see, e.g., Kenward and Molenberghs, 2009) is known as *last observation carried forward (LOCF)*. If the end of study outcome is missing, the last observed measurement for that person is used. In some cases, this may involve carrying forward a very remote observation, such as the baseline value. When there are numerous measurements throughout a trial, the method may be reasonable. Consider the Dietary Approaches to Stop Hypertension (DASH) trial comparing three diets to lower blood pressure for people whose baseline blood pressure was in the upper portion of the normal range. Some participants became hypertensive (diastolic blood pressure $\geq$ 90 or systolic blood pressure $\geq$ 140) and were prescribed medication. The end of study measurement is likely to be lower than it would have without medication. Blood pressure measurements were frequent throughout the trial, so a measurement just prior to being put on medication arguably better reflects what the participant's final measurement would have been.

An interesting twist on last observation carried forward is *last rank carried forward* (O'Brien, Zhang, and Bailey, 2005). Suppose patient A is missing the outcome, and the last nonmissing observation for patient A is at study visit i. Rank all participants at visit i and let P_A be the percentile of participant A. Impute rank p_A for participant A for the outcome value.

Yet another method is known as *hot-deck imputation* (Ford, 1983). For each patient with missing outcome data, identify a group of patients with similar baseline characteristics that have nonmissing outcome data. Randomly pick one and impute that patient's outcome value. One advantage of this method over imputing the same fixed number for each patient with missing data is that it incorporates variability through random selection among the group with similar baseline characteristics. A disadvantage is that two different people performing the same analysis may get different answers.

A more appealing imputation method is called *multiple imputation* (Rubin, 1978). Missing observations are imputed m times, creating m completed datasets. Rubin adopts a Bayesian perspective, so missing data are imputed using their *posterior predictive distribution*. This involves first computing the posterior distribution for parameters given the observed data, then using those parameters to sample missing data from their distribution. Nonetheless, the method can be used in frequentist settings whenever imputation includes some variability. For example, multiple imputation could be used in the context of hot deck imputation. For the ith completed dataset, the estimate $\hat{\theta}_i = \hat{\theta}(x_{\text{obs}}, x_{\text{mis}}^i)$ of treatment effect and its variance estimate V_i are computed the usual way, treating the imputed values as if they were actual observations. For example, consider the comparison of two means with variance assumed to be equal in the two arms. Suppose that n patients are assigned to each treatment, but some have missing outcomes. After the ith imputation using a model, there are n observations per arm, and the estimated variance of the treatment effect estimate $\hat{\theta}_i$ is $2s_i^2/n$, where s_i^2 is the usual pooled variance estimate used in the t-statistic.

The overall estimate of treatment effect is

$$\bar{\theta} = (1/m) \sum_{i=1}^{m} \hat{\theta}_i.$$

The estimated variance of $\bar{\theta}$ is

$$\text{var}(\bar{\theta}) = \bar{V} + (1 + 1/m)B,$$

where

$$\bar{V} = (1/m) \sum_{i=1}^{n} V_i \text{ and } B = \left(\frac{1}{m-1}\right) \sum_{i=1}^{m} (\hat{\theta}_i - \bar{\theta})^2$$

are known as the within- and between-imputation variances, respectively.

A t-test is used on $\bar{\theta}/\sqrt{\text{var}(\bar{\theta})}$, where the degrees of freedom are

$$(m-1) \left\{ 1 + \frac{\bar{V}}{(1+1/m)B} \right\}^2.$$

10.4.3 Sensitivity Analyses

The methods we have covered thus far assume that data are missing at random (MAR). This assumption is not as naive as missing completely at random (MCAR), but still might not be realistic. We will never be able to verify the MAR assumption because the data needed to do so are missing! Furthermore, clinical trialists tend to be conservative, meaning that they prefer statistical analyses that require strong evidence to declare a statistically significant benefit of treatment over control. One way to achieve this in a superiority trial is to impute in a way that brings the two treatments closer together. This section considers such conservative imputation schemes in the context of a trial with a binary outcome that indicates worsening of disease. Although such methods are considered ad hoc and unprincipled, they can be persuasive. The goal is to demonstrate that results would have maintained statistical significance even if the missing data could magically be observed.

An extremely conservative imputation scheme was suggested by Wittes, Lakatos, and Probstfield (1989). Missing observations in the control (resp., treatment) arms are imputed as 0s (resp., 1s) and are treated as actual observations in the z-statistic comparing proportions. Unless the amount of missing data is minuscule, this method severely punishes investigators for missing data. The idea is that if investigators know that there will be such a price to pay, they will take every measure to avoid missing data. That means sending visit reminders, contacting those who miss visits, and making sure that patients know the importance of maintaining follow-up even if they stop taking their medication. Still, the Wittes, Lakatos, and Probstfield penalty is seldom used because it virtually guarantees a non-significant result unless there is almost no missing data.

A less extreme penalty is to impute observations according to the observed proportion of events in the opposite arm or the observed proportion of events across both arms (Proschan, McMahon, Shih, et al., 2001). After imputing the event proportions for missing data in the two arms, use an ordinary test of proportions treating all observations as if they were observed. We illustrate the procedure in the following example.

Example 10.12. The Asymptomatic Cardiac Ischemia Pilot (ACIP) study randomized patients with myocardial ischemia to one of three arms (Knatterud et al., 1994). We focus on two of those arms, which we call treatment and control. Patients in the control arm are given medication when they experience heart-related chest pain (angina), while patients in the treatment arm receive either angioplasty or bypass surgery, at the discretion of the cardiac surgeon. The primary endpoint is absence of ischemia 12 weeks following randomization.

Table 10.2: Data in two arms of the Asymptomatic Cardiac Ischemia Pilot (ACIP) trial.

	Control	Treatment	Total
# Randomized	204	212	416
# Observed	193	192	385
# Missing	11	20	31
# Ischemia-free	75	105	180

Data from these two arms of ACIP are shown in Table 10.2. The two-tailed p-value using only the observed data is 0.002. A Wittes, Lakatos, and Probstfield worst-case analysis that assumes all patients with missing outcomes in the treatment arm have ischemia and all patients with missing outcomes in the control arm are ischemia-free yields a two-tailed p-value of 0.132. This demonstrates that even when the proportion with missing data is fairly low, the Wittes, Lakatos, and Probstfield method is extremely conservative. If the opposite arm variant of Proschan, McMahon, Shih et al. (2001) is used, the proportions free of ischemia among the 11 missing observations in the control arm and the 20 missing observations in the treatment arm are assumed to be $105/192$ and $75/193$, respectively. Therefore, the proportions free of ischemia in the control and treatment arms are imputed as

$$\{75 + 11(105/192)\}/204 = 0.397 \text{ and } \{105 + 20(75/193)\}/212 = 0.532.$$

Treating these as ordinary proportions based on 204 and 212 patients yields a z-score of 2.756 and a two-tailed p-value of 0.006.

Rather than imputing a single value for the proportion of patients free of ischemia among missing data in a given arm, we can treat this proportion as a random variable and compute conditional power for the full dataset, observed plus missing, given the observed data. Under opposite arm imputation, the numbers (X, Y) of ischemia-free patients among the 11 and 20 missing observations in the control and treatment arms are treated as binomial $(11, 105/192)$

and binomial $(20, 75/193)$, respectively. The probability that the imputed pair is (x, y) is

$$f(x,y) = \binom{11}{x} \left(\frac{105}{192}\right)^x \left(1 - \frac{105}{192}\right)^{11-x} \binom{20}{y} \left(\frac{75}{193}\right)^y \left(1 - \frac{75}{193}\right)^{20-y}. \qquad (10.9)$$

Conditional power is then

$$CP = \sum_{x=0}^{11} \sum_{y=0}^{20} f(x,y) I \left\{ \frac{(75+x)/204 - (105+y)/212}{\sqrt{\hat{p}(x,y)\{1 - \hat{p}(x,y)\}/(1/204 + 1/212)}} \leq -1.96 \right\} = 0.999.$$

There is a 99.9% probability that, if all data had been observed, the result would have been statistically significant, even under a relatively pessimistic opposite arm imputation. This bolsters our confidence that treatment is beneficial.

A similar idea uses a *tipping point analysis* to determine under what assumptions about missing data the results no longer remain statistically significant. One possible tipping point analysis assumes that the event probability among patients in the control (resp., treatment) arm with missing data is $\lambda \hat{p}_T + (1 - \lambda)\hat{p}_C$ (resp., $\lambda \hat{p}_C + (1 - \lambda)\hat{p}_T$), where $\lambda \in [0, 1)$. For example, $\lambda = 0.10$ means that the event probability among missing patients in a given arm moves 10% of the way toward the observed event probability in the opposite arm. Note that $\lambda = 1$ corresponds to opposite arm imputation. One can then determine how large λ must be to change the outcome from statistically significant to not statistically significant or vice versa. If an unrealistically large value of λ is required to change the outcome, we can be confident that the same conclusion would have been reached if we were able to observe the missing data. Tipping point analyses also indicate how the estimate of treatment effect changes under different assumptions.

Exercises:

1. Explain the rationale for making a multiple comparison adjustment in clinical trials.

2. Why do missing data threaten the validity of a clinical trial?

3. Suppose that a 7-arm trial compares each pair of arms using $\alpha = 0.05$, and the global null hypothesis is true.

    (a) What is the expected number of p-values that are 0.05 or less?

    (b) If the Bonferroni method is used to adjust for multiple comparisons, what type I error rate should be used for each comparison?

4. What is the difference between missing completely at random (MCAR) and missing at random (MAR)?

5. In the Pamoja Tulinde Maishe (PALM) trial in patients with Ebola virus disease in the Democratic Republic of the Congo, patients were randomized to ZMapp, Remdesivir, monoclonal antibody 114, or Regeneron REGN-EB3. ZMapp was the control arm to which each of the other 3 treatments was compared. The mortality rate was expected to be about 40% for this disease for which no treatments had been shown superior to standard care. Would you have used a multiple comparison adjustment for the 3 comparisons with control? Explain your reasoning.

6. The first Adaptive COVID-19 trial (ACTT-1) of hospitalized patients with coronavirus disease (COVID-19) randomized patients to Remdesivir plus standard care or placebo plus standard care to determine the effect on the primary endpoint of time to recovery.

Mortality was a secondary outcome. Patients entered the trial in one of four disease severity levels. In one of the 4 baseline severity levels, there were 25 and 9 deaths in the placebo plus standard care and Remdesivir plus standard care arms, respectively. Do you think results in that subgroup should be considered definitive? Explain your reasoning.

7. *Platform trials* compare products from different manufacturers to a control. Given that a manufacturer can choose whether to join a platform trial or conduct their own two-arm trial comparing their product to control, do you think that a multiple comparison adjustment should be used in the platform trial? Justify your answer.

8. The *Newman-Keuls procedure* comparing means among arms A, B, C, and D declares means μ_A and μ_B different if and only if all of the following are statistically significant: (1) the t-test of H_{0AB}, (2) the F-test of H_{0ABC}, (3) the F-test of H_{0ABD}, and (4) the F-test of H_{ABCD}. A similar rule is applied to each of the 6 pairwise comparisons. Show that the Newman-Keuls procedure does not strongly control the FWER for all pairwise comparisons of means. **Hint:** Consider the following configuration of means, where horizontal separation indicates differences in means.

$$\bullet\ \mu_A \qquad\qquad\qquad\qquad\qquad\qquad\qquad\qquad \bullet\ \mu_C$$

$$\bullet\ \mu_B \qquad\qquad\qquad\qquad\qquad\qquad\qquad\qquad \bullet\ \mu_D$$

9. Show that conditions (10.7) and (10.8) are equivalent. For simplicity, assume that Y is discrete.

10. Let $Y_1, \ldots, Y_n$ be iid normal with unknown mean μ and variance 1, and suppose that Y_n is missing. This exercise uses the EM algorithm to estimate μ, starting with $\hat{\mu}_0 = 0$ and imputing the value $\hat{\mu}_0$ for Y_n.

    (a) Write an expression for the new estimate, $\hat{\mu}_1$, of μ.

    (b) Imputing the new value, $\hat{\mu}_1$, for Y_n, compute the new estimate, $\hat{\mu}_2$, of μ.

    (c) Imputing the new value, $\hat{\mu}_2$, for Y_n, compute the new estimate, $\hat{\mu}_3$, of μ.

    (d) Deduce an expression for the estimate $\hat{\mu}_k$ after k steps.

    (e) Show that $\lim_{k \to \infty} \hat{\mu}_k = \bar{Y}_{n-1}$, the mean of the $n - 1$ nonmissing observations.

11. ↑ Now suppose that the baseline value X_i for patient i is highly correlated with that patient's outcome value, Y_i, $i = 1, \ldots, n$, and that the (X, Y) pairs are as shown in Table 10.3.

Table 10.3: Baseline value X_i is highly correlated with the outcome Y_i.

Patient	1	2	3	4	5	6	7	8	9	10	11
X	120	111	136	140	115	129	142	120	140	115	125
Y	132	123	144	136	125	138	145	135	150	131	

    (a) Use linear regression on the observed pairs, $(X_1, Y_1), \ldots, (X_{10}, Y_{10})$. What are the intercept, slope, and their standard errors?

    (b) Now use the linear regression to impute a value for Y_{11}. What is the imputed value for Y_{11}?

(c) With the imputed value for Y_{11}, redo the regression you did in part (a), but including 11 pairs instead of 10.

(d) Did the intercept and slope change from part (a) to part (c)? Did their standard errors change?

(e) What do you think would have happened to estimates and standard deviations if there had been 5 missing observations instead of 1?

12. Consider the use of the Bonferroni p-value threshold, α/k, when the test statistics for the k comparisons are independent. Assume that the global null hypothesis is true.

(a) What is the distribution of the number of type I errors?

(b) The *law of small numbers* states that when $n \to \infty$ and $p_n \to 0$ such that $np_n \to \lambda$, the binomial probability mass function

$$f_n(x) = \binom{n}{x} p_n^x (1 - p_n)^{n-x}, \quad x = 0, 1, \dots, n$$

converges to the Poisson probability mass function $g(x) = \exp(-\lambda)\lambda^x/x!$, $x = 0, 1, 2, \dots$. Use this result to find the approximate probability of x type I errors using the Bonferroni procedure with independent comparisons.

(c) Use the result in part (b) to compute the approximate probability of at least 1 type I error using the Bonferroni with independent test statistics.

(d) Is the Bonferroni method very conservative with a large number of independent comparisons?

13. ↑ Suppose that the test statistics $Z_1, \dots, Z_k$ in Exercise 12 are not independent. Instead, under the global null hypothesis, they have a multivariate normal distribution for which each Z_i is marginally standard normal and $\text{cor}(Z_i, Z_j) = \rho$, $i \neq j$. Then the joint distribution of $Z_1, \dots, Z_n$ is that of

$$Z_i = X + Y_i,$$

where X and $Y_1, \dots, Y_n$ are independent random variables.

(a) Find the variances σ_X^2 and σ_Y^2 of X and Y_i such that $\text{var}(Z_i) = 1$ and $\text{cov}(Z_i, Z_j) = \rho$.

(b) Use the conditioning trick to show that the probability of 0 type I errors for a one-tailed test at level 0.05 test is

$$\int_{-\infty}^{\infty} \left\{ \Phi\left(\frac{1.645 - \sqrt{\rho}\,x}{\sqrt{1 - \rho}} \right) \right\}^k \phi(x)\,dx$$

under the null hypothesis.

10.5   Summary

1. Multiple comparisons increase the familywise error rate (FWER), the probability of at least one false positive positive finding.

2. Considerations for deciding whether to adjust for multiple comparisons include relatedness and number of questions asked, whether there is controversy requiring a definitive answer, and whether multiplicity appears to give an unfair advantage to the user.

3. Weak error rate control means that the FWER is α or less under the global null hypothesis that all null hypotheses are true, whereas strong control means that the FWER is α or less regardless of which null hypotheses are true.

4. The oldest multiple adjustment method, the Bonferroni procedure, requires a p-value less than α/k for each of k comparisons. The Bonferroni method:

    (a) strongly controls the FWER;

    (b) works well when the test statistics are independent, even if k is large;

    (c) can be overly conservative with moderately positively correlated statistics, especially if k is large;

    (d) is always less powerful than Holm's sequentially rejective Bonferroni method, which also strongly controls the FWER.

5. The closure principle can be used to show strong control of the FWER.

6. The graphical method of Bretz et al. (2011) is extremely useful for succinctly representing a procedure that strongly controls the FWER.

7. Missing data break the randomized arms and are a threat to the validity of a clinical trial.

8. The first step with missing data is to compare baseline characteristics of patients with missing versus nonmissing data, and compare baseline characteristics of patients with missing data in different arms.

9. Data are virtually never missing completely at random (MCAR), so analyzing only observed data is ill-advised.

10. Imputation methods can be used in two different ways: (a) to try to accurately predict values of missing observations or (b) as a conservative sensitivity analysis to see whether conclusions are robust (e.g., a tipping point analysis).

11. Single imputation methods like last observation carried forward are usually poor choices, whereas likelihood-based methods such as the EM algorithm and multiple imputation generally perform well.

Chapter 11

Adaptive Methods

11.1 Introduction

This chapter covers one of the richest and most controversial topics in clinical trials, *adaptive methods.* These are pre-specified methods allowing design changes to be made on the basis of accumulating data from a clinical trial. Some changes are well-accepted, like minor modifications to entry criteria or allowing early stopping based on crossing a monitoring boundary. Other changes are more objectionable, such as changing the primary endpoint or primary analysis method. Remember that adaptations that seem to offer the greatest advantages are potentially the most dangerous. For example, response-adaptive randomization (RAR) is very alluring, but has disadvantages as well. Likewise, it may seem very appealing to examine data by arm to see whether there are any outliers before deciding whether to use a t-test or a Wilcoxon rank sum test. Such a strategy of checking for assumption violations and changing the analysis accordingly is often encouraged in non-randomized studies, but not in clinical trials. Making changes after examining data could inflate the probability of a false declaration of treatment benefit. It is better to specify robust methods (such as a Wilcoxon test) upfront. Remember that clinical trialists are a skeptical lot; they believe in pre-specifying everything and not making major changes. Therefore, even valid adaptive methods might be viewed unfavorably. In most cases, we recommend the use of adaptive methods that divulge virtually no information about the treatment effect. More extreme adaptations tend to generate more controversy than benefit.

A helpful dichotomy for adaptive methods is whether they occur before or after breaking the treatment blind. Adaptations based on the observed treatment effect clearly require unblinding. We will spend a considerable amount of time on adaptive methods made before breaking the treatment blind. They offer advantages without appreciable disadvantages. For instance, consider the above example involving a potential outlier. We could examine data without breaking the blind to see whether one observation is extreme relative to the others. If there is an outlier, we could use a Wilcoxon test in conjunction with a re-randomization test. There are other examples when blinded adaptations can improve power or offer other advantages. Adaptations made before breaking the blind are generally considered pristine.

11.2 Adaptive Sample Size Based on Nuisance Parameters

One of the more common adaptive methods involves sample size re-calculation. As described in Chapter 8, sample size calculation often requires estimation of a nuisance parameter. For

DOI: 10.1201/9781315164090-11

example, with a two-sample t-test applied to normally distributed data, the nuisance parameter is the common, within-arm variance σ^2. For a test of proportions, either the control probability or the overall probability of event can be considered the nuisance parameter. In either case, a preliminary estimate n_0 of sample size per arm is made based on a prior guess of the value of the nuisance parameter. After some fraction (often half) of the originally planned sample size has been evaluated for the primary outcome, the nuisance parameter is re-estimated using trial data. The revised estimate is substituted in the sample size formula to produce the final sample size.

11.2.1   Continuous Outcomes

We begin with a continuous, normally distributed outcome analyzed using either a one-sample or two-sample t-test in a paired or unpaired setting. The nuisance parameter in the paired (resp., unpaired) setting is the variance of paired differences (resp., the common, within-arm variance). The corresponding estimates are the sample variances of paired differences or the pooled variance estimator, respectively. Because the sample mean and variance of iid normal observations with finite variance are statistically independent (see, for example, theorem 5.3.1 of Casella and Berger, 2002), information used in the sample size recalculation gives no information about the treatment effect.

Stein's Method

The fact that the sample mean and variance are independent is the basis for one of the oldest methods of sample size recalculation (Stein, 1945). Although Stein's method is seldom used today, we give a detailed exposition of this instructive method. Stein considered a general linear model, but for simplicity, we focus on means.

Consider a one-sample t-test of paired differences. Let D_i be the difference between treatment and control for pair i, $i = 1, \ldots, n$. Assume that the D_i are iid $N(\delta, \sigma^2)$, and we are testing $H_0 : \delta = 0$ versus $H_1 : \delta > 0$. The nuisance parameter is the variance, $\sigma^2 = \mathrm{var}(D_i)$. Use a prior estimate σ_0^2 to calculate the planned sample size n_0. After n_1 (often, but not always, $n_1 = n_0/2$) of the planned n_0 observations, compute the sample variance $S_{n_1}^2$. Use $S_{n_1}^2$ to recompute the required sample size $n = n(S_{n_1}^2)$. At the end of the trial, use a one-sample t-test, but with $S_{n_1}^2$ instead of S_n^2 in the denominator. That is, use

$$T = \frac{\bar{D}_n}{\sqrt{S_{n_1}^2/n}} = \frac{\sqrt{n}\bar{D}_n}{S_{n_1}}. \tag{11.1}$$

We will show that $T - n^{1/2}\delta/S_{n_1}$ has a t-distribution with $n_1 - 1$ degrees of freedom. The first step is to show that, even though n is random, $n^{1/2}(\bar{D}_n - \delta)/\sigma$ has a standard normal distribution and is independent of $S_{n_1}^2$. To see this, note that once we condition on $S_{n_1}^2$, n becomes a fixed integer and $n^{1/2}(\bar{D}_n - \delta)/\sigma \sim N(0,1)$. Since $n^{1/2}(\bar{D}_n - \delta)/\sigma$ has the same conditional distribution regardless of the value of S_{n_1}, $n^{1/2}(\bar{D}_n - \delta)/\sigma$ and S_{n_1} are independent.

The next step is to show that $T - n^{1/2}\delta/S_{n_1}$ can be written as the ratio of a $N(0,1)$ random variable and $\{\chi_{n_1-1}^2/(n_1-1)\}^{1/2}$, where $\chi_{n_1-1}^2$ is a chi-square random variable with $n_1 - 1$ degrees of freedom and independent of the $N(0,1)$ variable:

$$T - \frac{\sqrt{n}\delta}{S_{n_1}} = \frac{\frac{\sqrt{n}}{\sigma}(\bar{D}_n - \delta)}{\sqrt{S_{n_1}^2/\sigma^2}} = \frac{N(0,1)}{\sqrt{\chi_{n_1-1}^2/(n_1-1)}} \sim G_{n_1-1}, \tag{11.2}$$

where G_{n_1-1} is the central t-distribution with $n_1 - 1$ degrees of freedom. This completes the proof that $T - n^{1/2}\delta/S_{n_1}$ has a t-distribution with $n_1 - 1$ degrees of freedom.

The above proof is valid regardless of the sample size rule $n = n(S_{n_1}^2)$. It is now time to determine n to have power at least $1 - \beta$ regardless of the true variance σ^2. We reject the null hypothesis if $T \geq t_{n_1-1,\alpha}$, where $t_{n_1-1,\alpha} = G_{n_1-1}^{-1}(1 - \alpha)$ is the $(1 - \alpha)$th quantile of a t-distribution with $n_1 - 1$ degrees of freedom. After the first stage, S_{n_1} is a fixed constant. Choose n such that

$$n \geq \frac{(t_{n_1-1,\alpha} + t_{n_1-1,\beta})^2 S_{n_1}^2}{\delta^2}. \tag{11.3}$$

Formula (11.3) is identical to sample size formula (8.10) except that $z_\alpha + z_\beta$ is replaced by $t_{n_1-1,\alpha} + t_{n_1-1,\beta}$ and σ^2 is replaced by $S_{n_1}^2$. Note that Formula (11.3) is equivalent to

$$t_{n_1-1,\alpha} - \frac{\sqrt{n}\delta}{S_{n_1}} \leq -t_{n_1-1,\beta}. \tag{11.4}$$

The following steps show that choosing n to satisfy Formula (11.3) ensures power at least $1 - \beta$ when the true mean is $\delta > 0$:

$$
\begin{aligned}
P(T \geq t_{n_1-1,\alpha}) &= P\left(T - \frac{\sqrt{n}\delta}{S_{n_1}} \geq t_{n_1-1,\alpha} - \frac{\sqrt{n}\delta}{S_{n_1}}\right) \\
&\geq P\left(T - \frac{\sqrt{n}\delta}{S_{n_1}} \geq -t_{n_1-1,\beta}\right) \text{ from Equation (11.4)} \\
&= 1 - G_{n_1-1}(-t_{n_1-1,\beta}) \text{ from Equation (11.2)} \\
&= G_{n_1-1}(t_{n_1-1,\beta}) \text{ by symmetry of the t-density about 0} \\
&= 1 - \beta. \tag{11.5}
\end{aligned}
$$

This proves that Stein's procedure has power at least $1 - \beta$, regardless of the true variance σ^2.

A similar approach can be used with the two-sample t-test. The first n_1 observations per arm are used to estimate the final per-arm sample size n. Let $S_{n_1}^2$ be the observed value of the pooled variance with n_1 observations per arm. The final t-statistic is

$$T = \frac{\bar{Y}_{T,n} - \bar{Y}_{C,n}}{\sqrt{2S_{n_1}^2/n}}, \tag{11.6}$$

which is referred to a t-distribution with $2(n_1 - 1)$ degrees of freedom. To achieve power at least $1 - \beta$ to detect a mean difference of δ, make

$$n \geq \frac{2S_{n_1}^2(t_{2(n_1-1),\alpha} + t_{2(n_1-1),\beta})^2}{\delta^2}. \tag{11.7}$$

Formula (11.7) is identical to formula (8.4) except that $z_\alpha + z_\beta$ is replaced by $t_{2(n_1-1),\alpha} + t_{2(n_1-1),\beta}$ and σ^2 is replaced by $S_{n_1}^2$. The procedure can be easily modified to account for unequal sample sizes in the two arms, as the following example shows.

Example 11.1. Consider a trial comparing two treatments to lower blood pressure. The primary outcome Y is the change in systolic blood pressure from baseline to end of study. We want 90% power to detect a difference of 3 mm Hg. Before the trial begins, the standard deviation of change is anticipated to be 8. The initial sample size n_0 is approximately

$$n_0 = \frac{2(8^2)(1.96 + 1.28)^2}{3^2} \approx 150$$

per arm, where we have rounded up. After 73 and 77 observations in the two arms, the sample standard deviations are 7.2 and 7.5, respectively. The pooled variance is

$$\frac{(73 - 1)(7.2)^2 + (77 - 1)(7.5)^2}{(73 - 1) + (77 - 1)} = 54.1046,$$

with $(73 - 1) + (77 - 1) = 148$ degrees of freedom. The 0.975th and 0.90th quantiles of the t-distribution with 148 degrees of freedom are 1.9761 and 1.2873, respectively. The revised sample size estimate is

$$n \geq \frac{2(54.1046)(1.9761 + 1.2873)^2}{3^2} \approx 129$$

per arm, rounding up as always in sample size calculations. Therefore, the revised sample size is smaller than the originally anticipated 150 per arm.

Even though our new target is 129 per arm at the end of the trial, we end up with 132 and 128 in the control and treatment arms, respectively. The final sample means are $\bar{Y}_{C,132} = 0.3$ and $\bar{Y}_{T,128} = -1.6$, and the final sample variances are $S_{C,132}^2 = 8.5^2$ and $S_{T,128}^2 = 9.0^2$. Stein's t-statistic ignores these final variance estimates and uses the interim pooled variance of 54.1046. We find that

$$T = \frac{0.3 - (-1.6)}{\sqrt{54.1046(1/132 + 1/128)}} = 2.0823,$$

with 148 degrees of freedom. The two-tailed p-value is 0.039. We reject the null hypothesis and declare a bigger reduction in blood pressure in the treatment arm than in the control arm.   □

Under the assumptions underlying the t-test, namely iid normal observations with finite variance, Stein's procedure works amazingly well. In fact, Zucker et al. (1999) show that Stein's method beats even the unattainable procedure of using the true variance σ^2 to form a z-score at the end of a two-stage design! Denne and Jennison (2000) show how to incorporate interim monitoring into Stein's method.

A big problem with Stein's procedure is the possibility of temporal trends. If the true variance increases over time, the first stage sample variance $S_{n_1}^2$ could underestimate the true average variance over time. That happened in Example 11.1: the final variances were 8.5^2 and 9.0^2, whereas the interim variances were 7.2^2 and 7.5^2. If these numbers reflect a change in the true variance σ^2 over time, the type I error rate of Stein's procedure can be substantially inflated. A less serious problem is that there is a perceived loss of efficiency in not using all observations to estimate σ^2. For these reasons, Stein's method is rarely, if ever, used in modern clinical trials.

Wittes and Brittain (1990) and Birkett and Day (1994)

Wittes and Brittain (1990) proposed recalculating the sample size but then using the ordinary t-statistic at the end of the trial:

$$T = \frac{\bar{Y}_{T,n} - \bar{Y}_{C,n}}{\sqrt{2S_n^2/n}},$$

where S_n^2 is the usual pooled variance estimate with n observations per arm. They called the observations used to recalculate sample size an *internal pilot study* and considered *restricted designs* in which the sample size cannot be decreased. Birkett and Day (1994) extended this work by considering an *unrestricted design* allowing the sample size to increase or decrease.

Example 11.2. Return to Example 11.1. Recall that the final sample means were $\bar{Y}_{C,132} = 0.3$ and $\bar{Y}_{T,128} = -1.6$, and the final sample variances were $s_{C,132}^2 = 8.5^2$ and $s_{T,128}^2 = 9.0^2$. Stein's procedure ignored these final variances, but the Wittes-Brittain approach uses them in the t-statistic. The pooled variance is

$$\frac{(132 - 1)(8.5)^2 + (128 - 1)(9.0)^2}{(132 - 1) + (128 - 1)} = 76.5572.$$

Therefore, the naive t-statistic is

$$T = \frac{0.3 - (-1.6)}{\sqrt{76.5572(1/132 + 1/128)}} = 1.7505,$$

with $132 + 128 - 2 = 258$ degrees of freedom. The two-tailed p-value is 0.081. The variance increased from the first stage to the second, so the statistically significant result in Example 11.1 may have been a false positive. The naive t-statistic ameliorates the problem by including the second stage observations in the final variance estimate. □

There are two potential problems with the naive t-test. First, the t-statistic at the end does not have an exact t-distribution. Second, the final variance estimate tends to slightly underestimate the true variance. This is proven rigorously in Wittes et al. (1999). We offer a somewhat more heuristic explanation here. Note that the final variance estimate is very close to a weighted combination

$$WS_1^2 + (1 - W)S_2^2, \tag{11.8}$$

of the variance estimates S_1^2 and S_2^2 in the first and second stages, where $W \approx n_1/(n_1+n_2)$. If W were fixed in advance, then (11.8) would be an unbiased estimate of σ^2. But $W = W(S_1^2)$ depends on S_1^2. Large S_1^2 indicates that our pre-specified variance estimate was too small, so we must increase n_2 to achieve the desired power. Increasing n_2 decreases W, so the weight attached to S_1^2 in (11.8) is large when S_1^2 is small and small when S_1^2 is large, causing (11.8) to be underestimated. Nonetheless, it can be shown that the final estimate of variance is only a slight underestimate. In fact, the absolute value of the difference between $E(S_1^2)$ and σ^2 is less than the standard error of S_1^2 (see Wittes et al., 1999).

Wittes and Britain (1990) show by simulation that, even though the final t-statistic does not really have a t-distribution and the final variance is a slight underestimate, the naive strategy of referring the final t-statistic to a t distribution with $n - 1$ degrees of freedom results in minimal inflation of the type I error rate and can improve power relative to the fixed sample size procedure. Multiple subsequent articles (Birkett and Day, 1994; Wittes et al., 1999) have evaluated power and verified that the naive procedure has type I error rate very close to the intended level. Coffey and Muller (1999) show how to extend formulas and results to more general linear models.

A disadvantage of the naive method is that a sum of squares decomposition formula can be used to deduce the interim treatment effect estimate. For simplicity, assume equal sample size n_1 in the two arms at the interim analysis. Even a blinded investigator can compute the *lumped variance*, $\hat{\sigma}_L^2$, of all $2n_1$ observations. The pooled variance $\hat{\sigma}_P^2 = (s_T^2 + s_C^2)/2$ is used to recompute sample size. A well-known analysis of variance decomposition formula states that the total sum of squares, $\sum_i \sum_j (y_{ij} - \bar{y})^2$, is the treatment sum of squares, $(n_1/2)(\bar{y}_T - \bar{y}_C)^2$, plus the residual sum of squares, $\sum_i (y_{Ti} - \bar{y}_T)^2 + \sum_i (y_{Ci} - \bar{y}_C)^2$. Note that the total sum of squares is $(2n_1 - 1)\hat{\sigma}_L^2$ and the residual sum of squares is $2(n_1 - 1)\hat{\sigma}_P^2$. Thus,

$$(2n_1 - 1)\hat{\sigma}_L^2 = (n_1/2)(\bar{y}_T - \bar{y}_C)^2 + 2(n_1 - 1)\hat{\sigma}_P^2.$$

Therefore, knowledge of $\hat{\sigma}_L^2$ and $\hat{\sigma}_P^2$ reveals the squared treatment effect estimate $(\bar{y}_T - \bar{y}_C)^2$. Knowledge of the treatment effect can introduce bias into randomized clinical trials. For example, staff might give additional care to placebo patients to compensate them for not receiving the treatment. For this reason, substantial attention has focused on blinded sample size recalculation, the topic of the next section.

Blinded Method

We have seen that unblinded sample size recalculation can give information about the treatment effect, which can compromise the integrity of the trial. *Blinded sample size recalculation* (Gould and Shih, 1992) gives effectively no information about the treatment effect.

The simplest blinded method uses the *lumped variance* of all observations at the interim analysis to estimate σ^2. At the end of the trial, apply the 'naive' t-test that treats the final sample size as if it were fixed in advance, At first blush, the lumped variance estimate seems problematic. A huge treatment effect will cause a large separation between the two arms and an inflated variance estimate (Figure 11.1).

Figure 11.1: A huge treatment effect causes a large separation of data in the two arms, resulting in an inflated blinded estimate of variance.

The large variance causes us to increase the sample size. But if the variance inflation is caused by a much larger than expected treatment effect, the last thing we need to do is increase the sample size!

The theoretical concern about drastically overestimating the variance does not materialize in real clinical trials because huge treatment effects are very rare. For typical treatment effects, the variance inflation is quite small. To see this, let $E = \delta/\sigma$ be the *effect size*, the treatment difference expressed in terms of the number of standard deviations. Let Z be the treatment indicator for a generic patient. Then

$$
\begin{aligned}
\operatorname{var}(Y) &= \operatorname{E}\{\operatorname{var}(Y \mid Z)\} + \operatorname{var}\{\operatorname{E}(Y \mid Z)\} \\
&= \operatorname{E}(\sigma^2) + \operatorname{var}\{\mu_C + (\mu_T - \mu_C)Z\} \\
&= \sigma^2 + (\mu_T - \mu_C)^2(1/2)(1/2) = \sigma^2 + E^2\sigma^2/4 \\
&= \sigma^2(1 + E^2/4).
\end{aligned}
\tag{11.9}
$$

Even a large effect size of $E = 1/2$ translates to a lumped variance of $1.0625\sigma^2$, only a 6% inflation of the variance and 3% inflation of the standard deviation. A more typical effect size of $E = 1/3$ results in approximately a 3% inflation of variance and 1% inflation of the standard deviation.

The only difference in execution of blinded, versus unblinded, estimation is that the final sample size calculation is based on the lumped variance. In Example 11.1, suppose that the lumped variance at the interim analysis had been $8.5^2 = 72.25$. The approximate per-arm sample size for 90% power would have been calculated as

$$
\frac{2(72.25)(1.96 + 1.28)^2}{3^2} = 169.
$$

At the end of the trial with 169 per arm, the naive t-test would be used with $(169 - 1) + (169 - 1) = 338$ degrees of freedom.

11.2.2   Binary Outcomes

For trials with a binary outcome, the nuisance parameter can be thought of as either the probability of event in the control arm or the overall event probability across both arms. The control probability seems most reasonable because it is the event rate in the absence of the new treatment. Therefore, it seems natural to start by computing the event proportion $\hat{p}_{C1}$ in the control arm at an interim analysis with n_1 observations and treating it as if it were the true control probability p_C. The next step would be to apply the specified relative reduction in event rate (e.g., 25%) due to treatment to compute p_T. The final step would use sample size Formula (8.12) to compute the sample size. But there is a problem with this strategy: $\hat{p}_{C1}$ is correlated with the interim treatment effect estimate, $\hat{p}_{C1} - \hat{p}_{T1}$:

$$\text{cov}(\hat{p}_{C1}, \hat{p}_{T_1} - \hat{p}_{C1}) = \text{cov}(\hat{p}_{C1}, \hat{p}_{T1}) - \text{cov}(\hat{p}_{C1}, \hat{p}_{C1})$$
$$= 0 - \text{var}(\hat{p}_{C1})$$
$$= p_C(1 - p_C)/n_1. \tag{11.10}$$

Therefore, the control event proportion is actually giving us some information about the estimated treatment effect, even if the null hypothesis is true. This can inflate the type I error rate. In contrast, the overall event proportion at the interim analysis is uncorrelated with the interim treatment effect estimate under the null hypothesis $H_0 : p_T = p_C = p$:

$$\text{cov}\left\{(\hat{p}_{T1} + \hat{p}_{C1})/2, \hat{p}_{T_1} - \hat{p}_{C1}\right\}$$

$$= (1/2)\left\{\text{cov}(\hat{p}_{T_1}, \hat{p}_{T1}) - \text{cov}(\hat{p}_{T1}, \hat{p}_{C1}) + \text{cov}(\hat{p}_{C1}, \hat{p}_{T1}) - \text{cov}(\hat{p}_{C1}, \hat{p}_{C1})\right\}$$
$$= (1/2)\left\{\text{var}(\hat{p}_{T1}) - 0 + 0 - \text{var}(\hat{p}_{C1})\right\}$$
$$= (1/2)\left\{p_T(1 - p_T)/n_1 - p_C(1 - p_C)/n_1\right\}$$
$$= (1/2)\left\{p(1 - p)/n_1 - p(1 - p)/n_1\right\}$$
$$= 0. \tag{11.11}$$

An important point is that $(\hat{p}_{T1} + \hat{p}_{C1})$ and $(\hat{p}_{T1} - \hat{p}_{C1})$ are uncorrelated only under the null hypothesis. Still, from a superiority testing standpoint, the null behavior of a test statistic is what determines the type I error rate. Lack of correlation suggests that the overall event proportion gives almost no information about the estimated treatment effect. We say "almost no information" instead of "no information" because lack of correlation is not the same as statistical independence. For example, if the overall proportion is 0 or 1, we know that the difference in proportions is 0. Nonetheless, $(\hat{p}_{T1} + \hat{p}_{C1})$ and $(\hat{p}_{T1} - \hat{p}_{C1})$ have an approximate bivariate normal distribution if n_1 is large, and for the bivariate normal, lack of correlation **does** imply independence. For these reasons, blinded estimation using the overall event proportion is preferred in clinical trials.

Gould (1992) showed how to recalculate sample size on the basis of blinded data when the treatment effect is expressed in terms of the difference, ratio, or odds ratio of probabilities of events in the two arms. Suppose we want to detect power $1 - \beta$ to detect a relative risk R. After n_1 observations per arm, compute the overall event proportion $\hat{p} = (\hat{p}_{T1} + \hat{p}_{C1})/2$ and treat it as if it were $(p_T + p_C)/2$. Equate

$$(p_T + p_C)/2 = \hat{p}_1$$
$$p_T/p_C = R \tag{11.12}$$

and solve for p_T and p_C. From the second equation, $p_T = Rp_C$. Substituting this value into the first equation and solving yields

$$p_C = \frac{2\hat{p}_1}{R+1}, \quad p_T = \frac{2R\hat{p}_1}{R+1}. \tag{11.13}$$

Example 11.3. In Example 8.4, we computed the sample size for a trial of Ebola virus disease in which the primary outcome was 28-day mortality. The control event probability was anticipated to be 0.30, and investigators wanted 85% power to detect a 50% reduction in the treatment arm. The per-arm sample size was estimated as

$$n_0 = \frac{2(1.96 + 1.04)^2(0.225)(1 - 0.225)}{(0.30 - 0.15)^2} = 139.5 \approx 140.$$

Suppose that, at the planned halfway point with $n_1 = 70$ patients per arm, the observed event proportion in all participants was $\hat{p}_1 = 0.20$. Applying Equation (11.13) with $R = 0.5$ and $\hat{p}_1 = 0.20$ yields

$$p_C = \frac{2(0.20)}{0.5 + 1} = 4/15, \quad p_T = \frac{2(0.5)(0.20)}{0.5 + 1} = 2/15.$$

The new estimate of sample size per arm is

$$n_1 = \frac{2(1.96 + 1.04)^2(0.20)(1 - 0.20)}{(4/15 - 2/15)^2} = 162.$$

We would increase the sample size from 140 per arm to 162/arm.

Gould (1992) also discussed the idea of incorporating prior information about event probabilities using a beta-binomial procedure like that described in Section 1.2.4.

11.3   Adaptive Sample Size Based on Treatment Effect

11.3.1   Introduction and Notation

In rare cases like emerging infectious diseases, clinical trials are undertaken when there is virtually no information on the size of the treatment effect. For example, early in the COVID-19 (coronavirus disease caused by SARS-COV-2) pandemic, nothing was known about the effect of potential interventions like the antiviral drug Remdesivir or the corticosteroid Dexamethasone. Lack of knowledge hampers sample size calculations. But remember from Chapter 8 that the treatment effect is very different from nuisance parameters in the sense that nuisance parameters must be accurately **estimated**, whereas the treatment effect can be **specified** as the smallest meaningful effect. Even if we do not know how large an effect to expect, we can calculate the sample size based on the smallest effect worth detecting. When no information is available about either the likely effect or the smallest meaningful effect, we might pursue methods that use interim data to estimate the treatment effect and change the sample size accordingly. We emphasize that the proportion of trials requiring these methods is very small. This is fortunate, as these methods can generate substantial controversy. There is a growing consensus that in settings with very little prior information, the best strategy is to specify a very large sample size and use standard group-sequential monitoring to stop early, if warranted.

The most common adaptive sample size methods based on the treatment effect are two-stage procedures. An initial per-arm sample size n_0 (fixed) for the trial is determined based on pre-trial estimates of nuisance parameters and the treatment effect. After observing n_1 observations per arm (fixed), we compute either a z-score Z_1 or a p-value P_1 and use it to determine the second stage sample size n_2. For simplicity, we take the first stage to be half of the planned trial, $n_1 = n_0/2$. Because the second stage sample size n_2 depends on results in the first stage, it is random. Results in stage 2 are summarized by a z-score Z_2 or a p-value P_2. At the end of the trial, we combine the two z-scores or p-values using a *z-score combination function or p-value combination function* to make inferences about the treatment effect. Throughout Section 11.3, we assume a one-tailed test for which large z-scores indicate an effective treatment.

We begin in Section 11.3.2 with a brief review of methods of combining evidence from two stages in a non-adaptive setting. We show in Section 11.3.3 the key result that z-scores (Z_1, Z_2) and p-values (P_1, P_2) from the two stages have the same null distribution in an adaptive sample size setting as in the non-adaptive setting. Therefore, rejection regions that have level alpha in a non-adaptive setting maintain level alpha in an adaptive setting in which the second stage sample size depends on data from the first stage. We use this result to understand numerous adaptive methods proposed in the literature.

Table 11.3 summarizes our notation and assumptions used throughout Section 11.3.

Table 11.1: Notation used throughout Section 11.3

Term	Explanation/Assumption
Testing scenario	one-tailed; large z-scores indicate treatment is beneficial
n_0	fixed, initial per-arm sample size based on pre-trial estimates
n_1	fixed per-arm sample size in stage 1 (internal pilot); we assume $n_1 = n_0/2$
n_2	random per-arm sample stage in stage 2
$n = n_1 + n_2$	random final sample size
(Z_1, Z)	z-scores for data in stage i only, $i = 1, 2$
(P_1, P_2)	p-values for data in stage i only, $i = 1, 2$

11.3.2 Non-adaptive Two-Stage Setting

Combining Z-Scores

It is helpful to think first about a non-adaptive setting with two equal stages of size $n_0/2$ per arm. Consider a continuous, normally distributed outcome with common, known variance σ^2, so that data within the treatment and control arms are iid $N(\mu_T, \sigma^2)$ and iid $N(\mu_C, \sigma^2)$, respectively. We are interested in testing $H_0 : \mu_T - \mu_C = 0$ versus the alternative $H_1 : \mu_T - \mu_C > 0$. Let $\bar{Y}_{Ti}$ and $\bar{Y}_{Ci}$ be the sample means in the treatment and control arms for the $n_0/2$ observations per arm in stage i, $i = 1, 2$. The z-score Z_i from stage i is

$$Z_i = \frac{\bar{Y}_{Ti} - \bar{Y}_{Ci}}{\sqrt{2\sigma^2/(n_0/2)}}, \quad i = 1, 2.$$

(Z_1, Z_2) are iid $N(0,1)$ under H_0. Also, the usual cumulative z-score at the end with n_0 observations per arm is

$$Z = \frac{\bar{Y}_T - \bar{Y}_C}{\sqrt{2\sigma^2/n_0}} = \left(\frac{1}{\sqrt{2}}\right) \left(\frac{\bar{Y}_{T1} - \bar{Y}_{C1}}{\sqrt{2\sigma^2/(n_0/2)}} + \frac{\bar{Y}_{T2} - \bar{Y}_{C2}}{\sqrt{2\sigma^2/(n_0/2)}}\right)$$

$$= \frac{Z_1 + Z_2}{\sqrt{2}} = f(Z_1 + Z_2). \tag{11.14}$$

Thus, the cumulative z-score at the end of the trial can be written as a *z-score combination function*, $f(Z_1, Z_2)$, of the stagewise z-scores. Also, the rejection region $Z \geq z_\alpha$ can be written as a two-dimensional region for the stagewise z-scores:

$$R = \left\{ (z_1, z_2) \in \Re^2 : \frac{z_1 + z_2}{\sqrt{2}} \geq z_\alpha \right\}. \tag{11.15}$$

In the more realistic setting of unknown σ^2, we must estimate it and use t-statistics instead of z-statistics. Still, when sample sizes are large, the cumulative t-statistic at the end, with z-statistics replaced by t-statistics that use sample variances in place of σ^2, has approximately the same distribution as (11.14). Similarly, rejection region (11.15) yields type I error rate approximately α if z-statistics are replaced by t-statistics.

Z-score combination function (11.14) is just one of many choices. Another z-score combination function is

$$f(Z_1, Z_2) = Z_1^2 + Z_2^2, \tag{11.16}$$

which has a chi-squared distribution with 2 degrees of freedom under the null hypothesis.

Combining P-values

A different method of synthesizing results from the two stages can be used when σ^2 is unknown. Compute the (one-tailed) p-value P_i from the usual t-statistic T_i applied to data from stage i, $i = 1, 2$. Let $G_{n_0-2}(t)$ be the t-distribution function with $n_0 - 2$ degrees of freedom. Then $U_i = G_{n_0-2}(T_i)$ is uniformly distributed because

$$P(U_i \leq u) = P\{G_{n_0-2}(T_i) \leq u\} = P\{T_i \leq G_{n_0-2}^{-1}(u)\} = G_{n_0-2}\{G_{n_0-2}^{-1}(u)\} = u.$$

These steps can be repeated for any continuous distribution function, so the one-tailed p-value is uniformly distributed for any test statistic with a continuous distribution. Because U_i is uniform under H_0, so is the one-tailed p-value from stage i, $P_i = 1 - G_{n_0-2}(T_i) = 1 - U_i$. Furthermore, P_1 and P_2 are independent. We can combine the two independent p-values using a *p-value combination function* $g(P_1, P_2)$.

Fisher's method combines the two independent p-values by $-2\ln(P_1 P_2)$ (Fisher, 1925). Under H_0, $-2\ln(P_i)$ has an exponential distribution with parameter $1/2$ because

$$P\{-2\ln(P_i) \leq x\} = P\{P_i \geq e^{-x/2}\} = 1 - \exp(-x/2).$$

The exponential distribution with parameter $1/2$ is also the chi-squared distribution with 2 degrees of freedom, so Fisher's p-value combination function,

$$Y = -2\ln(P_1 P_2) = \{-2\ln(P_1)\} + \{-2\ln(P_2)\},$$

is the sum of two independent chi-squared random variables, each with 2 degrees of freedom. Accordingly, Y has a chi-squared distribution with $2 + 2 = 4$ degrees of freedom under the null hypothesis. We use this fact to compute an overall p-value combining the two independent p-values. For example, if two p-values are 0.03 and 0.01, then $Y = -2\ln\{(0.03)(0.01)\} = 16.2235$, and the overall p-value is $1 - F_4(16.2235) = 0.0027$, where $F_4(\cdot)$ is the chi-squared distribution function with 4 degrees of freedom. We reject the null hypothesis if the overall p-value is α or less. Alternatively, we reject H_0 if $Y \geq \chi^2_{4,\alpha}$, where $\chi^2_{4,\alpha}$ is the $(1 - \alpha)$th quantile of a chi-squared distribution with 4 degrees of freedom. The two-dimensional rejection region R for the two p-values is

$$\{(p_1, p_2) \in (0, 1) \times (0, 1) : -2\ln(p_1 p_2) \geq \chi^2_{4,\alpha}\}. \tag{11.17}$$

The above example concerned the comparison of treatment and control means for a continuous outcome, but the conclusions apply asymptotically to many other settings. For example, the z-test of proportions is asymptotically equivalent to (11.14), where Z_i are the z-scores for the tests of proportions restricted to the data in stage i, $i = 1, 2$. More generally, Chapter 9 showed that the null joint distribution of $B(t) = \sqrt{t}Z(t)$ over t is approximately that of standard Brownian motion, where $Z(t)$ is the z-score for all data by information fraction t. Brownian motion has independent increments, so

$$Z_1 = \frac{B(1/2)}{\sqrt{1/2}} \quad \text{and} \quad Z_2 = \frac{B(1) - B(1/2)}{\sqrt{1/2}}$$

are iid standard normal deviates. Similarly, one-tailed p-values $P_i = 1 - \Phi(Z_i)$ are iid uniforms under the null hypothesis. Rejection regions such as (11.15) and (11.17) maintain level α asymptotically to many settings, including tests of proportions, Wald and score statistics in modeling contexts, and log hazard ratios in survival settings like the logrank test and the Cox proportional hazards model.

11.3.3 Adaptation Principle

The fundamental fact about two-stage adaptive methods based on the treatment effect is summarized in the following adaptation principle.

Principle 11.4. Adaptation Principle

1. *Suppose that the null distribution of first and second stage z-scores (Z_1, Z_2) in a fixed sample size setting is iid $N(0, 1)$. Then the same is true if the second stage sample size $n_2 = n_2(Z_1)$ depends on Z_1.*

2. *Suppose that the null distribution of first and second stage p-values (P_1, P_2) in a fixed sample size setting is iid $\text{Unif}(0, 1)$. Then the same is true if $n_2 = n_2(P_1)$ depends on P_1.*

Consequently, any level α rejection region R for (Z_1, Z_2) or (P_1, P_2) in a fixed sample size setting maintains level α in an adaptive sample size setting.

The proof is actually very easy. For example, in the case of p-values, suppose that $n_2 = n_2(P_1)$ is some function of P_1. Given $P_1 = p_1$, $n_2 = n_2(p_1)$ becomes a fixed constant. The n_2 observations in the second stage are iid continuous observations, so the second stage p-value P_2 has a uniform distribution under H_0. Thus, under H_0, P_1 is uniform and $P_2 \mid P_1$ is also uniform, even if the second stage sample size is changed. Because the conditional distribution of P_2 given $P_1 = p_1$ is the same (namely uniform) for all values of p_1, P_1 and P_2 are independent and each is uniformly distributed. This completes the proof for p-values. The proof for z-scores is not difficult and is left to Exercise 6.

The adaptation principle does not apply under the alternative hypothesis. In that case, the conditional distribution of Z_2 given Z_1, and of P_2 given P_1, will depend on the second stage sample size.

11.3.4 Bauer-Köhne (1994)

Bauer and Köhne (1994) applied Fisher's combination of p-values, $Y = -2\ln(P_1 P_2)$, to the adaptive setting. The adaptation principle ensures that the null distribution of Y is chi-squared with 4 degrees of freedom even when the second stage sample size is changed on the basis of P_1. The only requirements are that, in the nonadaptive setting and under the null hypothesis,

1. each p-value has a uniform distribution and

2. P_1 and P_2 are independent.

Therefore, the following adaptive procedure of Bauer and Köhne maintains level α.

1. After computing the first stage p-value p_1, decide the second stage sample size n_2 using **any** sample size rule $n_2(p_1)$.

2. After computing the second stage p-value p_2, reject the null hypothesis if $-2\ln(P_1 P_2) \geq \chi^2_{4,\alpha}$, where $\chi^2_{4,\alpha}$ is the $(1-\alpha)$th quantile of a chi-squared distribution with 4 degrees of freedom.

Notice that if $-2\ln(p_1) \geq \chi^2_{4,\alpha}$, there is no need for a second stage; regardless of p_2, $-2\ln(p_1 p_2) \geq \chi^2_{4,\alpha}$. Therefore, the Bauer-Köhne procedure can be described as follows. Reject the null hypothesis

$$
\begin{cases}
\text{in stage 1 if} & -2\ln(P_1) \geq \chi^2_{4,\alpha} \\
\text{in stage 2 if} & -2\ln(P_1) < \chi^2_{4,\alpha} \text{ and } -2\ln(P_1 P_2) \geq \chi^2_{4,\alpha}.
\end{cases} \tag{11.18}
$$

Bauer and Köhne further modified the procedure by allowing a different critical value at stage 1. Reject the null hypothesis

$$
\begin{cases}
\text{in stage 1 if} & -2\ln(P_1) \geq c_1 \\
\text{in stage 2 if} & -2\ln(P_1) < c_1 \text{ and } -2\ln(P_1 P_2) \geq c_2,
\end{cases} \tag{11.19}
$$

where c_1 and c_2 are selected such that

$$
\begin{aligned}
\alpha &= P(Y_1 \geq c_1) + P(Y_1 < c_1 \cap Y_1 + Y_2 \geq c_2) \\
&= \exp(-c_1/2) + \int_0^{c_1} P(Y_2 \geq c_2 - y_1)(1/2)\exp(-y_1/2)dy_1 \\
&= \exp(-c_1/2) + \int_0^{c_1} \exp\{-(c_2 - y_1)/2\}(1/2)\exp(-y_1/2)dy_1 \\
&= \exp(-c_1/2) + \exp(-c_2)\{\exp(c_1/2) - 1\}.
\end{aligned} \tag{11.20}
$$

Fisher's combination procedure is just one *p-value combination function*. Any p-value combination function procedure that is valid for fixed sample sizes remains valid in the adaptive sample size setting.

11.3.5   Proschan and Hunsberger (1995)

Proschan and Hunsberger (1995) approached adaptive sample size calculation from a different perspective. Their first step was to determine the maximum type I error rate resulting from adaptively changing the sample size while maintaining the conventional criterion for statistical significance at the end of the trial. Consider a t-test with sample sizes large enough to treat the variance as known, so the final t-statistic becomes a z-statistic with $n = n_1 + n_2$ observations per arm:

$$
Z = \frac{\sqrt{n_1}\, Z_1 + \sqrt{n_2}\, Z_2}{\sqrt{n_1 + n_2}}. \tag{11.21}
$$

Suppose that one naively uses the conventional criterion for statistical significance, $Z > z_\alpha$, as if the sample size had been fixed in advance. Note that the adaptation principle does **not** apply because the weight attached to Z_2 in (11.21) is not fixed. To maximize the type I error rate, Proschan and Hunsberger determined the second stage sample size $n_2 = n_2(Z_1)$ that maximizes the conditional type I error rate given that $Z = z_1$. They showed that the maximum type I error rate approaches

$$
\alpha_{\max} = \alpha + \frac{e^{-z_\alpha^2/2}}{4}. \tag{11.22}
$$

For a one-tailed test using $\alpha = 0.05$ or 0.025, the maximum type I error rate is 0.1146 or 0.0616, respectively. In other words, the type I error rate can be more than doubled if we naively change the sample size based on the treatment effect and apply the usual z-statistic and its critical value at the end.

To fix this problem, Proschan and Hunsberger changed the critical value at the end to make the conditional type I error some number $A(Z_1)$, where the function $A(Z_1)$ is preselected to make the overall type I error rate equal to α. This is accomplished by restricting A to the class of functions satisfying

$$\int_{-\infty}^{\infty} A(z_1)\phi(z_1)dz_1 = \alpha. \tag{11.23}$$

A function $A(z_1)$, $0 \le A(z_1) \le 1$ satisfying (11.23) is called a *conditional error function*. The left side of (11.23) is the conditional type I error rate averaged over the standard normal density function $\phi(z_1)$ for Z_1. This average conditional error rate is the unconditional type I error rate, so condition (11.23) ensures type I error rate α. To satisfy (11.23), we must use the following critical value c for the final z-score (11.21):

$$c = \frac{\sqrt{n_1}\, z_1 + \sqrt{n_2}\, z_A}{\sqrt{n_1 + n_2}}, \tag{11.24}$$

where z_A is the $\{1 - A(z_1)\}$th quantile of the standard normal distribution.

In summary, Proschan and Hunsberger described their procedure as follows:

1. Pre-specify a function $A(z_1)$ dictating the conditional type I error rate to use after observing $Z_1 = z_1$, where $A(z_1)$ satisfies (11.23).

2. After observing $Z_1 = z_1$, determine the second stage per-arm sample size using **any** sample size rule $n_2 = n_2(z_1)$.

3. After observing the n_2 observations per arm in stage 2, compute the final z-score Z using (11.21), and reject the null hypothesis if $Z \ge c$, where c is given by (11.24).

In practice, σ^2 is unknown, and the ordinary t-statistic with $n_1 + n_2$ observations is used in lieu of (11.21).

Proschan and Hunsberger used a sample size rule $n_2 = n_2(z_1)$ that achieves a desired conditional power $1 - \beta$ under an alternative hypothesis in which the between-arm difference in means is δ. They found that n_2 satisfies

$$\mathrm{E}(Z_2 \,|\, Z_1 = z_1, \delta) = z_A + z_\beta \tag{11.25}$$

$$\frac{\delta}{\sqrt{2\sigma^2/n_2}} = z_A + z_\beta, \tag{11.26}$$

where z_A and z_β are the $\{1 - A(z_1)\}$th and $(1 - \beta)$th quantiles of the standard normal distribution, respectively. Note the similarity between Equation (11.25) and the key sample size equation (8.2) from Chapter 8, and similarly between (11.26) and (8.3). Equation (11.25) is identical to (8.2), except that it is applied to data from the second stage only and uses alpha level $A(z_1)$. The same comment applies to the comparison between (11.25) and (8.3). It is readily seen that the condition $Z \ge c$ is equivalent to $Z_2 \ge A(z_1)$. Therefore, the Proschan and Hunsberger procedure is equivalent to the following steps (Chi and Liu, 1999):

1. Pre-specify a function $A(z_1)$ relating the observed first-stage z-score z_1 to the alpha level to be used in stage 2.

2. After observing $Z_1 = z_1$, determine the second stage per-arm sample using **any** sample size rule $n_2 = n_2(z_1)$.

3. Perform a z-test on the **second stage data only**, but use alpha level $A(z_1)$.

It turns out that the conditional error approach is just another way to view a z-score combination method. For example, consider the z-score combination function

$$Z = \frac{Z_1 + Z_2}{\sqrt{2}}. \tag{11.27}$$

The null hypothesis will be rejected if $(Z_1 + Z_2)/\sqrt{2} > z_\alpha$, where z_α is the $(1 - \alpha)$th quantile of the standard normal distribution. Once we observe $Z_1 = z_1$, the only remaining randomness lies in Z_2. The test will be statistically significant precisely when

$$\frac{z_1 + Z_2}{\sqrt{2}} \geq z_\alpha, \text{ which is equivalent to } Z_2 \geq \sqrt{2}\, z_\alpha - z_1. \tag{11.28}$$

In other words, the conditional type I error rate is $P\left(Z_2 \geq \sqrt{2}\, z_\alpha - z_1\right)$, which corresponds to conditional error function

$$A(z_1) = 1 - \Phi\left(\sqrt{2}\, z_\alpha - z_1\right). \tag{11.29}$$

The same connection holds for any z-score combination function $T(Z_1, Z_2)$ that is increasing in each argument for fixed value of the other argument. Suppose c_α is a constant such that $P\{T(Z_1, Z_2) \geq c_\alpha\} = \alpha$. Given $Z_1 = z_1$, the null hypothesis will be rejected if $T(z_1, Z_2) > c_\alpha$ which corresponds to a region of the form $Z_2 \geq b$ (or $Z_2 > b$) for some number $b = b(z_1)$. The conditional type I error rate is $A(z_1) = P\{Z_2 \geq b(z_1)\}$.

Also, z-score combination functions are equivalent to p-value combination functions because the p-value P_i and z-score Z_i in stage i are 1-1 transformations of each other:

$$P_i = 1 - \Phi(Z_i); \quad Z_i = \Phi^{-1}(1 - P_i).$$

Chen, DeMets, and Lan (2004)

Chen, DeMets, and Lan (2004) devised an appealing method of increasing the sample size when results are not as strong as expected, but still promising. Consider a trial with a single interim analysis solely to determine whether to increase the final sample size. Define the interim result to be promising if conditional power computed under the current trend estimate of treatment effect is at least 0.5. In terms of the monitoring and B-value framework of Chapter 9, promising means the following.

$$\text{Promising}: CP_{\theta = B(t)/t}(t) \geq 0.50. \tag{11.30}$$

Under this circumstance, increasing the sample size actually *decreases* the conditional type I error rate given $Z_1 = z_1$. Therefore, the overall type I error rate can only decrease by increasing the sample size when the interim result is promising. The specific rule for deciding how much to increase the sample size is irrelevant.

To see that increasing the sample size decreases the conditional type I error rate when the interim result is promising, write the current trend estimate $B(t)/t$ as $z/\sqrt{t}$, where z is the interim z-score. Substituting $z/\sqrt{t}$ for θ and z_α for c into Equation (9.22) shows that (11.30) is equivalent to $z \geq z_\alpha\sqrt{t}$. If we do not change the sample size, the conditional type I error rate is obtained from conditional power formula (9.22) by substituting 0 for θ and z_α for c. This yields

$$CP_0 = \Phi\{x(t)\}, \tag{11.31}$$

where

$$x(t) = \left(\frac{z\sqrt{t} - z_\alpha}{\sqrt{1-t}}\right).$$

The derivative of $x(t)$ is easily seen to be positive for $z > z_\alpha\sqrt{t}$, so $x(t)$ is increasing in t. If we now decide to increase the sample size, the current information fraction t decreases, as do $x(t)$ and the conditional error rate, (11.31). This shows that increasing the sample size when the interim result is promising decreases the conditional type I error rate.

Chen, DeMets, and Lan (2004) also prove that the type I error rate is controlled with two analyses when early stopping for futility or efficacy are allowed. Begin by specifying a spending function $\alpha^*(t)$ and an initial guess of the sample size. Let t_{orig} be the information fraction of the interim analysis relative to the originally planned sample size. For example, if the interim analysis is after half of the originally planned sample size, then $t_{orig} = 1/2$. Let c_1 and c_2 be the boundaries at the interim and final analyses if the sample size is unchanged. That is c_1 and c_2 satisfy

$$P_0\{Z(t_{orig}) > c_1\} = \alpha^*(t_{orig}); \quad P_0\{Z(t_{orig}) \leq c_1 \cap Z(1) > c_2\} = \alpha^*(1) - \alpha^*(t_{orig}), \tag{11.32}$$

where P_0 denotes probabilities computed under the null hypothesis. Note that $\{Z(t_{orig}), Z(1)\}$ are bivariate normal with 0 means, unit variances, and correlation $\sqrt{t_{orig}}$. If $Z(t_{orig}) > c_1$, the trial is stopped for efficacy. If $Z(t_{orig}) \leq c_1$ and (11.30) holds, we can increase the sample size by an arbitrary amount. The final critical value is exactly the same whether or not the sample size is increased, namely the c_2 satisfying (11.32).

Chen, Lan, and DeMets (2004) also explain how to extend the procedure to more than two analyses. In that case, conditional power is defined as the probability of rejecting the null hypothesis at at least one of the future analyses. Although they do not prove control of the type I error rate, their simulation results suggest good error rate control with more than two analyses.

Müller and Schäfer (2004): Conditional Error Principle

Müller and Schäfer (2004) develop a very general method, called the *conditional error principle*, to alter the design of a trial. At an interim analysis, let x be the observed value of the test statistic X. Define the conditional rejection probability (CRP) of the original design as the conditional probability of rejecting the null hypothesis at at least one of the remaining analyses, given $X = x$.

Principle 11.5. *Changing the design of a clinical trial cannot inflate the type I error rate as long as the CRP of the new design is less than or equal to the CRP of the original design.*

The proof is quite simple. The overall error rates of the original and new designs are $\int CRP_{orig}(x)f(x)dx$ and $\int CRP_{new}(x)f(x)dx$, where $f(x)$ is the density or probability mass function for X. If the original design has type I error rate α and the CRP of the new design is less than or equal to the CRP of the original design, then the new design has type I error rate

$$\int CRP_{new}(x)f(x)dx \leq \int CRP_{orig}f(x)dx = \alpha.$$

Therefore, the type I error rate is controlled at level α. The procedure can be adapted to settings in which computation of the CRP is complicated by nuisance parameters (Gutjahr, Brannath, and Bauer, 2011).

One of the simpler applications of the conditional error principle is to change the number of interim analyses in response to a statistic that is close to a monitoring boundary. For instance, suppose that the original plan was to use the O'Brien-like spending function with one interim analysis at the halfway point and a final analysis. Suppose that the actual information time of the first analysis is $t_1 = 0.47$, so the z-score boundary is $c_1 = 3.0679$. Suppose that the observed z-score is $Z(0.47) = 2.80$. As a result of the z-score being close to its boundary, the DSMB decides to insert another analysis at planned information fraction 0.75. It is known that the type I error rate can be increased with data-driven look times, although the inflation is small for the common spending functions. Nonetheless, if we want to ensure no inflation of the type I error rate, we can use the conditional error principle as detailed below.

First, calculate the CRP under the original design. The boundary at the end of the originally designed trial is 1.9661. The CRP of the original design is conditional power, $CP_0(0.47)$, computed under the null hypothesis and using final boundary 1.9661. Substituting 1.9661 for c, 0 for θ, and $2.80\sqrt{0.47}$ for b in conditional power formula (9.22), we obtain

$$CRP_{\text{orig}} = P_0\{Z(1) > 1.9661 \,|\, Z_1(0.47) = 2.80\}$$

$$= CP_0(0.47) = 1 - \Phi\left(\frac{1.9661 - \sqrt{0.47}(2.80)}{\sqrt{1 - 0.47}}\right)$$

$$= 0.4745. \tag{11.33}$$

We must now specify z-score boundaries for the two remaining analyses for the new design to make the CRP of the new design 0.4745. There are infinitely many ways to do this, and we can choose **any** of them. One way is to pretend that the original design also had a planned look at $t = 0.75$. In that case, the z-score boundaries at $t = 0.75$ and $t = 1$ would have been 2.3535 and 2.0135, respectively. For the new design, we can retain the boundary 2.3535 at $t = 0.75$ and determine the final boundary such that the CRP is 0.4745. This leads to

$$0.4745 = P_0\left(Z(0.75) > 2.3535 \cup Z(1) > d \,|\, Z(0.47) = 2.80\right)$$

$$= P_0\left\{B(0.75) > 2.3535\sqrt{0.75} \cup B(1) > d \,|\, B(0.47) = 2.80\sqrt{0.47}\right\}$$

$$= P_0\{B(0.75) > 2.0382 \cup B(1) > d \,|\, B(0.47) = 1.9196\}$$

$$= P_0\left(\frac{B(0.75) - B(0.47)}{\sqrt{0.75 - 0.47}} > \frac{2.0382 - 1.9196}{\sqrt{0.75 - 0.47}} \cup \frac{B(1) - B(0.47)}{\sqrt{1 - 0.47}} > \frac{d - 1.9196}{\sqrt{1 - 0.47}}\right.$$

$$\left. \left|\, B(0.47) = 1.9196\right.\right)$$

$$= P_0\left(\frac{B(0.75) - B(0.47)}{\sqrt{0.75 - 0.47}} > 0.2241 \cup \frac{B(1) - B(0.47)}{\sqrt{1 - 0.47}} > \frac{d - 1.9196}{\sqrt{1 - 0.47}}\right). \tag{11.34}$$

The last step follows from the independent increments property of Brownian motion. Specifically, the variables

$$\{B(t) - B(0.47), \ t \geq 0.47\}, \tag{11.35}$$

are independent of $B(0.47)$, so we can ignore the conditioning event $B(0.47) = 1.9196$ when calculating probabilities involving the set (11.35). In fact, if we define a new time scale u and a new process

$$B'(u) = B(u + 0.47) - B(0.47), \ u \geq 0,$$

it is not difficult to show that $B'(u)$ is also a Brownian motion. Times $t = 0.75$ and $t = 1$ on the original time scale correspond to times $u = 0.75 - 0.47 = 0.28$ and $u = 1 - 0.47 = 0.53$ on the new time scale. Therefore, (11.34) becomes

$$P_0 \left(Z'(0.28) > 0.2241 \cup Z'(0.53) > \frac{d - 1.9196}{\sqrt{0.53}} \right), \tag{11.36}$$

where $Z'(u)$ has the same joint distributions as a z-process, namely multivariate normal with zero means, unit variances, and covariances given by (9.11). Equate (11.36) to 0.4745 and solve for d to find $d = 2.309$. That is, the final z-score boundary for this implementation of the conditional error principle is 2.309.

We paid a high price for being able to add an unplanned look with this implementation of the conditional error principle. Remember that there are infinitely many boundaries that satisfy the CRP requirement (11.33), so we can evaluate different boundaries and pick one with more favorable properties. For instance, instead of using the boundary 2.3535 at $t = 0.75$, we could have maintained the same ratio, $2.3535/2.0135 = 1.1689$ of z-score boundaries at $t = 0.75$ and $t = 1$ that would have occurred if the study had originally been designed with 3 analyses at information times $(0.47, 0.75, 1)$. It can be shown that the boundaries for the new design at $t = 0.75$ and $t = 1$ that maintain ratio 1.1689 and result in a CRP of 0.4745 are 2.484 and 2.125, respectively. Thus, for this implementation of the conditional error principle, the final z-score boundary is somewhat more palatable. Of course there is a tradeoff: the larger we make the boundary at $t = 0.75$, the smaller the boundary at $t = 1$ will be.

The breadth of possible changes that can be used in conjunction with the conditional error principle is staggering! Friede, Parsons, and Stallard (2012) used it in the context of subgroup selection. Müller and Schäfer point out that the principle can even be used to change the primary endpoint, test statistic, or hypothesis. This is both amazing and frightening. Remember that clinical trialists tend not to react well to major changes in the protocol. Still, sometimes unexpected things happen; in those cases, the conditional error principle can be useful.

11.3.6 Criticisms of Adaptive Methods Based on Treatment Effect

The conditional error principle of Müller and Schäfer (2004) shows how drastically one could stray from the pre-specified trial design while still preserving the type I error rate. Theoretically, one could change the sample size, population, and primary outcome all at once. Before making any major change, think carefully about how the clinical trial community will react. Unless such changes are absolutely necessary, resist the temptation to make them.

Several arguments have been lodged against adaptive methods based on the treatment effect. One issue is that such methods can be inefficient. See, for example, Jennison and Turnbull (2003) or Jennison and Turnbull (2006). Some insight can be gained by consideration of the z-score combination function $(Z_1 + Z_2)/\sqrt{2}$, where the sample size recalculation occurs at the planned halfway point. Equally weighting the two z-scores is a very sensible thing to do if the sample size is not changed, but not if n_2 is increased so much that n_1 is a tiny fraction of the total sample size, $n_1 + n_2$. If this were a non-adaptive trial with sample size $n_1 + n_2$, where $n_1/(n_1 + n_2)$ is tiny, the usual z-score at the end would give almost no weight to Z_1. This big discrepancy between the weight attached to Z_1 and Z_2 in an adaptive versus non-adaptive trial means that a large Z_1 based on a small amount of data could drive results in the adaptive trial. However, there are obvious practical limitations to dramatically increasing the planned sample size. In realistic settings, the sample size will be increased by a relatively modest amount.

A closely related concern is that adaptive methods can exhibit strange behavior. Burman and Sonesson (2006) point out that the critical value c for the usual z-statistic at the end of the trial can, in extreme cases, be negative even for a one-tailed test that would reject for a positive z-score in the fixed sample size case. It would be hard to argue that a negative z-score provides strong evidence of treatment benefit! Consider again the above example with the z-score combination function $(Z_1 + Z_2)/\sqrt{2}$ and a sample size recalculation at the planned halfway point. Suppose that $Z_1 = 3.5$ and n_2 is increased to $99n_1$. Of course, this is an insane thing to do. Why increase n_2 99-fold when the first stage z-score is large? Nonetheless, it is a theoretical possibility. Then $(Z_1 + Z_2)/\sqrt{2} \geq 1.96$ as long as $Z_2 \geq 1.96\sqrt{2} - 3.5 = -0.728$. If $Z_2 = -0.70$, the result will be declared statistically significant even though the usual overall z-score is

$$\frac{\sqrt{n_1}Z_1 + \sqrt{99n_1}Z_2}{\sqrt{100n_1}} = \sqrt{1/100}(3.5) + \sqrt{99/100}(-0.70) = -0.35.$$

In fact, Proschan and Hunsberger (1995) already showed that c could be negative in incredibly unrealistic settings like the one above. Because of the possibility of strange critical values, Proschan and Hunsberger stressed the need to take numerous factors into account, including the critical value for the overall z-score, when deciding the final sample size.

Another complaint against adaptive methods based on the treatment effect is that the sample size might be increased to detect a clinically meaningless treatment effect. Bear in mind that if the smallest clinically meaningful treatment effect were known, the trial would have been sized to detect it. These methods are intended to be used when there is a complete dearth of information when the trial begins. Also, while it is theoretically possible to try to detect very small effects, that would require unrealistically large sample sizes.

A more compelling concern is raised by Tsiatis and Mehta (2003). They show that for each adaptive design that allows up to K different sample sizes $n_1, \ldots, n_k$, there is a more powerful group-sequential design with analyses after $n_1, n_2, \ldots, n_k$. The idea is that a group-sequential method with given cumulative crossing probabilities by time t_i, $i-1, \ldots, K$, may be viewed as a likelihood ratio test. Of course, the group-sequential test that beats the adaptive test requires the same number of analyses as the number of sample sizes allowed in the adaptive design. Most clinical trials have no more than 10 analyses. Nonetheless, the power properties of a group-sequential trial with a large number of equally-spaced analyses may be well approximated by a group-sequential trial with fewer equally-spaced analyses. Therefore, it is often the case that for a given adaptive sample size trial, there is a more powerful group-sequential design.

The general consensus is that starting with a very large sample and using group-sequential monitoring boundaries is preferable to starting with a smaller sample size and allowing it to be increased. A counterargument is that specifying a very large maximum sample size may not be palatable. Consider an emerging infectious disease such as COVID-19. So little information was known and there was an imperative to find an effective treatment quickly. Pre-specifying a very large maximum sample size implies an upfront willingness to continue to that sample size. There is a psychological attraction to planning a more modest sample size and increasing it only after seeing concrete evidence that treatment works. Additionally, some statisticians who previously advocated for starting big have since shown that efficient adaptive designs that start small can be constructed (Jennison and Turnbull, 2015). The debate on the usefulness of adaptive designs examining the treatment effect will no doubt continue.

11.4 Unplanned Changes before Breaking the Blind

A key component of adaptive methods is that the potential and plan for design modification are specified before the trial begins. By contrast, decisions on how to analyze data from an observational study are often driven by the data themselves. Our statistical training teaches us to check assumptions and modify the analysis accordingly. If normality is violated, for example, we may change from a t-test to a Wilcoxon rank sum test. If we discover a potential confounder, we might emphasize results that adjust for this confounder, even if that was not originally planned. But there is a difference between hypothesis generating studies, like observational studies, and definitive studies like clinical trials. If we allow arbitrary data-driven changes in clinical trials, there is a danger of bias from changing to an analysis that accentuates the benefit of treatment. This can happen with or without bad intent. For example, investigators might genuinely believe that their changes to the original analysis plan are necessary to understand hidden meanings in the data. Because of the recognized potential for drawing misleading conclusions from 'massaging' data, unplanned changes in clinical trials are frowned upon.

Even though unplanned changes are discouraged, it is not always possible to anticipate all contingencies. For example, during the coronavirus pandemic beginning at the end of 2019, many clinical trials were disrupted. Non emergency appointments were postponed, including follow-up and other visits for clinical trials. Investigators had difficult decisions to make. One trial that originally planned to stop early only if benefit was established decided to allow early stopping for noninferiority. Other contingency plans included censoring data during the pandemic and 'restarting the clock' after the pandemic ended. The need for improvisation is not confined to medical emergencies like a pandemic. In one tuberculosis trial, a blinded review of lung x-rays revealed that the original primary endpoint could not be measured. There was no choice; the primary endpoint had to be changed. A more common problem is that the overall event rate is so low that power is severely compromised. A statistically significant result might be literally impossible with the given number of events. That is, even if all events were in one arm, a test of proportions would not be statistically significant. If there is a compelling secondary endpoint that has many more events, why not make it the new primary endpoint? In this section, we review a very important technique for making changes to the design of a trial before the treatment blind has been broken. We will see that in such cases, re-randomization tests can save what would otherwise be an unsalvageable trial.

Remember that a key idea of re-randomization tests is that they condition on the data, so only the treatment assignments remain random. This remains true even if design changes are made before breaking the blind. For instance, consider the above example concerning changing the primary endpoint after all data are in. A re-randomization test on a given endpoint conditions on all of the outcomes for that endpoint and generates the null reference distribution by re-randomizing according to the original scheme. If treatment truly has no effect, the outcomes should offer no evidence about the treatment assignments. Likewise, under the stronger null hypothesis that treatment has no effect on any of the endpoints being considered, knowledge of outcomes of all endpoints should tell us nothing about the treatment assignments. But before getting too excited about changing endpoints, consider the following variant of a provocative example of Posch and Proschan (2012).

Example 11.6. Posch and Proschan (2012) Suppose we are considering which of three possible endpoints to deem as primary in a trial comparing active drug to placebo for treatment of hospitalized patients with coronavirus disease (COVID-19). The possible endpoints are (1) mortality, (2) progression to ventilation or death, or (3) whether the patient has a therapeutic level of study drug in the blood. Of course, no one would actually use the third endpoint, but ignore that for the moment. Examining data on all three endpoints unblinds us to the treatment assignments. Having full knowledge of treatment assignments allows us to compute the z-statistics for endpoints 1 and 2 and pick the larger of the two. A re-randomization test on the larger of the two z-statistics will inflate the type I error rate if that endpoint is treated as if it had been pre-selected. The problem is exacerbated by considering a huge number of possible endpoints, one of which is whether the patient has a therapeutic level of drug in the blood. □

What goes wrong in Example 11.6? Actually, nothing! Remember that by examining many possible endpoints, we are testing a very strong null hypothesis that treatment has no effect on **any** of the endpoints, singularly or in combination. Thus, even if we settle on endpoint 2, for example, the proper conclusion when we reject the null hypothesis is that treatment has an effect on **at least one** endpoint under consideration. Rejection of the strong null hypothesis of no effect on any endpoint is not a type I error because treatment does indeed have an effect on at least one endpoint, namely endpoint 3. The punishment meted out for inclusion of endpoint 3 is that rejection of the null hypothesis tells us only what we already knew: treatment increases the level of study drug in the blood!

Example 11.6 is extreme, but it alerts us to the potential dangers of overly broad adaptations. There are more subtle examples in which information about treatment assignments can be conveyed unwittingly. For instance, suppose that the three endpoints being considered are all reasonable clinical endpoints (unlike endpoint 3 in Example 11.6), but we decide to use the amount of missing data to help guide the decision of which endpoint to choose. If all three endpoints are reasonable choices and one has less missing data than the others, it should be selected as primary, right? The problem with this strategy is that the amount of missing data could be giving information about the treatment assignments. There may be more missing data in the treatment arm, for instance. Any amount of unblinding can potentially inflate the type I error rate, albeit not nearly to the same degree as in Example 11.6.

For simplicity, we have discussed the case of an unplanned change made at the end of the trial, but the same principles apply if the change is made earlier; the only caveat is that the re-randomization test should be stratified by before, versus after, the change was made. We hope that the reader will never need to make a major unplanned trial alteration, but it is reassuring to know that a re-randomization test can be used in such an emergency.

Exercises

1. Consider a clinical trial of a continuous endpoint, but the variance is unknown. You are considering whether to use a blinded or unblinded sample size re-calculation.

   (a) Name an advantage of blinded over unblinded recalculation.

   (b) Name an advantage of unblinded over blinded sample size calculation.

2. In a small vaccine trial with a single investigator, that investigator sees immune responses. Explain how that might complicate sample size recalculation, even if it is done using the lumped variance of all observations.

3. Why are adaptive methods based on the treatment effect potentially problematic?

4. Use Equation (11.9) to compute the inflation of the blinded standard deviation method for treatment effects of size one-quarter and three-quarters of a standard deviation.

5. Suppose that a blinded group of investigators decides to increase their sample size on the basis of the overall (lumped) event rate. The Data and Safety Monitoring Board (DSMB) can see that the treatment effect is much larger than expected, so

no sample size increase is needed. Should they convey that information to the study team? Explain your answer.

6. Prove the adaptation principle for z-scores (Z_1, Z_2). Remember that we have already shown that the null joint distribution of p-values from stages 1 and 2 are iid uniform in the adaptive setting.

7. The $100(1 - \alpha)\%$ t-confidence interval for the difference $\mu_1 - \mu_2$ of means with n observations per arm is

$$\bar{Y}_{Tn} - \bar{Y}_{Cn} \pm t_{2(n-1),\alpha/2}\sqrt{2s_n^2/n}, \tag{11.37}$$

where s_n^2 is the pooled sample variance at the end of the trial and $t_{2(n-1),\alpha/2}$ is the $(1 - \alpha/2)$th quantile of the t-distribution with $2(n - 1)$ degrees of freedom.

(a) Before the trial starts, can you choose n to guarantee that the width of confidence interval (11.37) is no greater than 1 regardless of the true standard deviation?

(b) **Confidence intervals of fixed width** Stein's method computes the following confidence interval for $\mu_1 - \mu_2$:

$$\bar{Y}_{Tn} - \bar{Y}_{Cn} \pm t_{2(n_1-1),\alpha}\sqrt{2s_{n_1}^2/n}, \tag{11.38}$$

where $s_{n_1}^2$ is the pooled sample variance at the end of the first stage with n_1 observations per arm and $t_{2(n_1-1),\alpha/2}$ is the $(1-\alpha/2)$th quantile of the t-distribution with $2(n_1-1)$ degrees of freedom. You are now at the end of the first stage, so $s_{n_1}^2$ is a constant. Give a formula for n that guarantees that the width of confidence interval (11.38) is no greater than 1.

11.5   Summary

1. Adaptive methods are pre-specified methods of using accumulating data from the trial to make changes in design.

2. The most accepted adaptive methods are based on looking at nuisance parameters rather than the treatment effect, and before breaking the treatment blind.

3. Adaptive sample size changes based on the treatment effect generate controversy and should be avoided in most trials.

(a) In many cases, a preferable approach is to begin with a large sample size and use group-sequential monitoring to stop early.

4. In rare cases when a major unplanned change must be made, a re-randomization test remains a valid tool if the change was made before breaking the treatment blind. In that case, the re-randomization test should be stratified by pre- versus post-change.

References

1. Armitage, P., McPherson, C.K., and Rowe, B.C. (1969). Repeated significance tests on accumulating data. *JRSS A.* **132**, 235–244.

2. Appel, L.J., Moore, T.J, Obarzanek, E., et al. for the DASH Collaborative Research Group (1997). A clinical trial of the effects of dietary patterns on blood pressure. *New England Journal of Medicine* **336**, 1117–1124.

3. Baker, S.B. and Kramer, B.S. (2003). A perfect correlate does not a surrogate make. *BMC Medical Research Methodology* **3**, 16.

4. Barnard G.A. (1945). A new test for 2×2 tables. *Nature* **156**, 177.

5. Barthel, F.M, Parmar M.K., and Royston, P. (2009). How do multi-stage, multi-arm trials compare to the traditional two-arm parallel group design–a reanalysis of 4 trials. *Trials* 10:21.

6. Basu, D. (1980). Randomization analysis of experimental data: The Fisher randomization test. *Journal of the American Statistical Association* **75**, 575–582.

7. Bauer, P, Köhne, K. (1994). Evaluations of experiments with adaptive interim analyses. *Biometrics* **50**, 1029–1041.

8. Begg, C. (1990). On inferences from Wei's biased coin design for clinical trials. *Biometrika* **77**, 467–473. See also commentary immediately following article.

9. Benkeser, D., Díaz, I., Luedtke, A., Segal, J., Scharfstein, D., and Rosenblum, M. (2020). Improving precision and power in randomized trials for COVID-19 treatments using covariate adjustment, for binary, ordinal, and time-to-event outcomes. *Biometrics* September 26: https://doi.org/10.1111/biom.13377.

10. Berger, J.O. and Berry, D.A. (1988). Statistical analysis and the illusion of objectivity. *American Scientist* **76**, 159–165.

11. Berry, S.M., Carlin, B.P., Lee, J.J., and Müller, P. (2010). *Bayesian Adaptive Methods for Clinical Trials*. CRC Press, New York.

12. Birkett, M.A. Day, S.J. (1994). Internal pilot studies for estimating sample size. *Statistics in Medicine* **13**, 2455–2463.

13. Blichert-Toft, M., Rose, C., Andersen, J.A., Overgaard, M., Axelsson, C.K., Andersen, K.W., Mouridsen, H.T. (1992). Danish randomized trial comparing breast conservation therapy with mastectomy: six years of life-table analysis. *Journal of the National Cancer Institute* **11**, 19–25.

14. Boschloo, R.D. (1970). Raised conditional level of significance for the 2×2-table when testing the equality of two probabilities. *Statistica Neerlandica* **24**, 1–35.

15. Branson, Z. and Bind, M.A. (2019). Randomization-based inference for Bernoulli trial experiments and implications for observational studies. *Statistical Methods in Medical Research* **28**, 1378–1398.

16. Bretz, F., Posch, M., Glimm, E., Klinglmueller, F., Maurer, W., and Rohmeyer, K. (2011). Graphical approaches for multiple comparison procedures using weighted Bonferroni, Simes, or parametric tests. *Biometrical Journal* **53**, 894–913.

17. Burman, C.F. and Sonesson, C. (2006). Are flexible designs sound? *Biometrics* **62**, 664–669.

18. Buyse, M., Molenberghs, G., Burzykowski, T., Renard, D., and Geys, H. (2000). The validation of surrogate endpoints in meta-analyses of randomized experiments. **1**, 49–67.

19. Cardiac Arrhythmia Suppression Trial (CAST) Investigators (1989). Preliminary report: effect of encainide and flecainide on mortality in a randomized trial of of arrhythmia suppression after myocardial infarction. *New England Journal of Medicine* **321**, 406–412.

20. Casella, G. and Berger, R.L. (2002). *Statistical Inference*, 2nd ed., The Wadswoth Group, Pacific Grove, CA.

21. Chen, Y.H., DeMets, D.L., and Lan, K.K. (2004). Increasing the sample size when the unblinded interim result is promising. *Statistics in Medicine* **23**, 1023–1038.

22. Chi, G.H. and Liu, Q. (1999). The attractiveness of the concept of a prospectively designed two-stage clinical trial. *Journal of Biopharmaceutical Statistics* **9**, 537–547.

23. Clopper, C. and Pearson, E.S. (1934). The use of confidence or fiducial limits illustrated in the case of the binomial. *Biometrika* **26**, 404–413.

24. Coffey, C.S. and Muller, K.E. (1999). Exact test size and power of a Gaussian error linear model for an internal pilot study. *Statistics in Medicine* **18**, 1199–1214.

25. COMMIT Investigarors (1995). Community intervention trial for smoking cessation (COMMIT): II. Changes in adult cigarette smoking prevalence. *American Journal of Public Health* **85**, 193–200.

26. Conover, W. J. (1999). *Practical Nonparameteric Statistics, 3rd ed.* John Wiley & Sons, New York.

27. Cox, D.R. and Reid, N. (2000). *Theory of the Design of Experiments*. Chapman & Hall/CRC.

28. Denne, J.S. and Jennison, C. (2000). A group sequential t-test with updating of sample size. *Biometrika* **87**, 125–134.

29. Dixon, D.O. and Pennello, G. (2001). Coping with multiplicity. *Controlled Clinical Trials* **22**, 548-550.

30. Efron, B. (1971). Forcing a sequential experiment to be balanced. *Biometrika* **58**, 403–417.

31. Einstein, A. (1956). *Investigations on The Theory of The Brownian Movement*. Dover Publications (reproduction of a translation of a manuscript originally published in 1926).

32. Evans, S.R., Li, L., and Wei, L.J. (2007). Data monitoring in clinical trials using prediction. *Drug Information Journal* **41**, 733–742.

33. Fay, Michael P. and Hunsberger, Sally A. (2021). Practical valid inferences for the two-sample binomial problem. *Statistics Surveys* **15**, 72–110.

34. Fay, M.P. and Proschan, M.A. (2010). Wilcoxon-Mann-Whitney or t-test? On assumptions for hypothesis tests and multiple interpretations of decision rules. *Statistical Surveys* **4**, 1–39.

35. Fayers, P.M., Ashby, D., and Parmar, M.K. (1997). Tutorial in biostatistics: Bayesian data monitoring in clinical trials. *Statistics in Medicine* **16**, 1413–1430.

36. Fine, J.P. and Gray, R.J. (1999). A proportional hazards model for the subdistribution of a competing risk. *Journal of the American Statistical Association* **94**, 496–509.

37. Fisher, R.A. (1925). *Statistical Methods for Research Workers*. Oliver and Boyd (Edinburgh). ISBN 0-05-002170-2.

38. Fisher, R.A. (1935). *The Design of Experiments*. Oliver and Boyd, Edinburgh. (Sixth edition in 1951).

39. Fleming, T. R., Prentice, R. L., Pepe, M. S. and Glidden, D. (1994). Surrogate and auxiliary endpoints in clinical trials, with potential applications in cancer and AIDS research. *Statistics in Medicine* **13**, 955–968.

40. Flynn, M.N., Forthal, D.N., Harro, C.D., et al. (2005). Placebo-controlled phase 3 trial of a recombinant glycoprotein 120 vaccine to prevent HIV-1 infection. *Journal of Infectious Diseases* **191**, 654–665.

41. Ford, B.N. (1983). An overview of hot deck procedures. In *Incomplete Data in Sample Surveys, vol II: Theory and Annotated Bibliography* (W.G. Madow, I. Olkin, and D.B. Rubin, Editors). Academic Press, New York.

42. Fowler, M.G., Qin, M., Fiscus, S.A., et al. for the IMPAACT 1077BF/1077FF PROMISE Study Team (2016). Benefits and risks of antiretroviral therapy for perinatal HIV prevention. *New England Journal of Medicine* **375**, 1726–1737.

43. Frangakis, C.E. and Rubin, D.B. (2002). Principal stratification in causal inference. *Biometrics* **58**, 21–29.

44. Freedman, L.S., Graubard, B.I., and Schatzkin, A. (1992). Statistical validation of intermediate endpoints for chronic diseases. *Statistics in Medicine* **11**, 167–178.

45. Freedman, L.S. and Spiegelhalter, D.J. (1989). Comparison of Bayesian with group sequential methods for monitoring clinical trials. *Controlled Clinical Trials* **10**, 357–367.

46. Freeman, T.B., Vawter, D.E., Leaverton, P.E., et al. (1999). Use of placebo surgery in controlled trials of a cellular-based therapy for Parkinson's disease. *The New England Journal of Medicine* **341**, 988–992.

47. Friede, T., Parsons, N., and Stallard, N. (2012). A conditional error function approach for subgroup selection in adaptive clinical trials. *Statistics in Medicine* **31**, 4309–4320.

48. Goodman, S. N. (1992). A Comment on replication, p-values and evidence. *Statistics in Medicine*, **11**, 875–879.

49. Gould, A. (1992). Interim analyses for monitoring clinical trials that do not materially affect the type I error rate. *Statistics in Medicine* **11**, 55–66.

50. Gould, A.L. Shih, W.J. (1992). Sample size re-estimation without unblinding for normally distributed outcomes with unknown variance. *Communications in Statistics (A)* **21**, 2833–2853.

51. Greenland, S. (2019). Valid p-values behave exactly as they should: some misleading criticisms of p-values and their resolution with s-values. *The American Statistician* **73**, 106–114.

52. Gutjahr, G., Brannath, W., and Bauer, P. (2011). An approach to the conditional error rate principle with nuisance parameters. *Biometrics* **67**, 1039–1046.

53. Hallstrom, A.P., McAnulty, J.H., Wilkoff, B.L., Follmann, D., et al. and the Antiarrhythmics Versus Implantable Defibrillator (AVID) Trial Investigators (2001). Patients at lower risk of arrhythmia recurrence: A subgroup in whom implantable defibrillators may not offer benefit. *Journal of the American College of Cardiology* **37**, 1093–1099.

54. Haybittle, J.L. (1971). Repeated assessment of results in clinical trials of cancer treatment, *British Journal of Radiology* **44**, 793—797.

55. Henao-Restrepo, A.M., Camacho, A., Longini, I.M. et al. (2017). Efficacy and effectiveness of an rVSV-vectored vaccine in preventing Ebola virus disease: final results from the Guinea ring vaccination, open-label, cluster-randomised trial (Ebola Ca Suffit!). *Lancet* **389**, 505–518.

56. Hochberg, Y. (1988). A sharper Bonferroni procedure for multiple tests of significance. *Biometrika* **75**, 800-802.

57. Hoeffding, W. (1951). A combinatorial central limit theorem. *Annals of Mathematical Statistics* **22**, 558–556.

58. Hollander, M. and Wolfe, D.A. (1973). *Nonparametric Statistical Methods*. John Wiley & Sons, New York.

59. Holm, S. (1979). A simple sequentially rejective multiple test procedure. *Scandinavian Journal of Statistics* **6**, 65–70.

60. Hommel, G. (1988). A stagewise rejective multiple test procedure based on a modified Bonferroni test. *Biometrika* **75**, 383–386.

61. Hu, F. and Rosenberger, W.F. (2006). *The Theory of Response-Adaptive Randomization in Clinical Trials*. Wiley, New York.

62. Hulley, S., Grady, D., Bush, T., et al. (1998). Randomized trial of estrogen plus progestin for secondary prevention of coronary heart disease in postmenopausal women. *Journal of the American Medical Association* **280**, 605–613.

63. Hung, H,M, Wang, S.J., and O'Neill, R. (2007). Statistical considerations for testing multiple endpoints in group sequential or adaptive clinical trials. *Journal of Biopharmaceutical Statistics* **17**, 1201–1210.

64. Hwang, I.K., Shi, W.J., and DeCani, J.S. (1990). Group sequential designs using a family of type I error probability spending functions. *Statistics in Medicine* **9**, 1439–1445.

65. Jatoi, I. and Proschan, M.A. (2005). Randomized trials of breast-conserving therapy versus mastectomy for primary breast cancer: A pooled meta-analysis. *American Journal of Clinical Oncology* **28**, 289–294.

66. Jennison, C. and Turnbull, B.W. (2000). *Group Sequential Methods with Applications to Clinical Trials.* Chapman & Hall/CRC, Boca Raton, Florida.

67. Jennison, C. and Turnbull, B.W. (2003). Mid-course sample size modification in clinical trials based on the observed treatment effect. *Statistics in Medicine* **22**, 971–993.

68. Jennison, C. and Turnbull, B.W. (2006). Adaptive and nonadaptive group sequential tests. *Biometrika* **93**, 1–21.

69. Jennison, C. and Turnbull, B.W. (2015). Adaptive sample size modification in clinical trials: start small then ask for more? *Statistics in Medicine* **34**, 3793–3810.

70. Kallmes, D.F., Comstock, B.A., Heagerty, P.J., et al. (2009). A randomized trial of vertebroplasty for osteoporotic spinal fractures. *New England Journal of Medicine* **361**, 569–579.

71. Karlin, S. and Taylor, H.M. (1975). A First Course in Stochastic Processes, 2nd ed.. Academic Press, New York.

72. Kenward, M.G., Molenberghs, G. (2009). Last observation carried forward: A crystal ball? *Journal of Biopharmaceutical Statistics* **9**, 872–888.

73. Kim, K. (1989). Point estimation following group sequential tests. *Biometrics* **45**, 613–617.

74. Kim, K. and DeMets, D.L. (1987). Design and analysis of group sequential tests based on the type I error rate spending function. *Biometrika* **74**, 149–154.

75. Knatterud, G.L., Bourassa, M.G., Pepine, C.J., et al. (1994). Effects of treatment strategies to suppress ischemia in coronary artery disease patients: 12 week results of the Asymptomatic Cardiac Ischemia Pilot (ACIP). *Journal of the American College of Cardiology* **24**, 11–20.

76. Korn, E.L. and Friedlin, E.L. (2011). Outcome-adaptive randomization: Is it useful? *Journal of Clinical Oncology* **29**, 771–776.

77. Kuznetsova, O.M. and Tymofyeyev, Y. (2012). Preserving the allocation ratio at every allocation with biased coin randomization and minimization in studies with unequal allocation. *Statistics in Medicine* **31**, 701–723.

78. Lakatos, E. (1986). Sample size determination in clinical trials with time-dependent rates of losses and noncompliance. *Controlled Clinical Trials* **7**, 189–199.

79. Lakatos, E. (1988). Sample size based on the logrank statistic in complex clinical trials. *Biometrics* **44**, 229–241.

80. Lan, K.K. and DeMets, D.L. (1983). Discrete sequential boundaries for clinical trials. *Biometrika* **70**, 659–663.

81. Lan, K.K., Simon, R., and Halperin, M. (1982). Stochastically curtailed tests in long-term clinical trials. *Communications in Statistics-Sequential Analysis* **1**, 207–219.

82. Lan, KK and Wittes, J. (1988). The B-value: A tool for monitoring data. *Biometrics* **44**, 579–585.

83. Lan, K.K. and Zucker, D.M. (1993). Sequential monitoring of clinical trials: The role of information and Brownian motion, *Statistics in Medicine* **12**, 753–765.

84. Lee, J.J. and Chu, C.T. (2012). Bayesian clinical trials in action. *Statistics in Medicine* **31**, 2955–2972.

85. Li, L., Evans, S,R., Uno, H., et al. (2009). Predicted interval plots (PIPS): A graphical tool for data monitoring of clinical trials. *Statistics in Biopharmaceutical Research* **1**, 348–355.

86. Lindley, D.V. and Phillips, L.D. (1976). Inference for a Bernoulli process (a Bayesian view). *The American Statistician* **30**, 112–119.

87. Little, R.J. and Rubin, DB (2019). *Statistical Analysis with Missing Data*, 3rd edition. John Wiley & Sons, New York.

88. Luepker, R.V., Raczynski, J.M., Osganian, S., et al. for the REACT Study Group (2000). Effect of a community intervention on patient delay and emergency medical service use in acute coronary heart disease: the Rapid Early Action for Coronary Treatment (REACT) trial. *Journal of the American Medical Association.* **284**, 60–67.

89. Magirr, D., Jaki, T., and Whitehead, J. (2012). A generalized Dunnett test for multi-arm multi-stage clinical studies with treatment selection. *Biometrika* 99, 494–501

90. Mantel, N. (1966). Evaluation of survival data and two new rank order statistics arising in its consideration. *Cancer Chemotherapy Reports* **50**, 163–170.

91. Marcus, R., Peritz, E., and Gabriel, K.R. (1976). On closed testing procedures with special reference to ordered analysis of variance. *Biometrika* **63**, 655–660.

92. McNemar, Q. (1947). Note on the sampling error of the difference between correlated proportions or percentages. *Psychometrika* **12**, 153–157.

93. Melfi, V.F. and Page, C. (2000). Estimation after adaptive allocation. *Journal of Statistical Planning and Inference* **87**, 353–363.

94. Moore, T.J. (1995). *Deadly Medicine: Why Tens of Thousands of Heart Patients Died in America's Worst Drug Disaster*. Simon & Schuster, New York.

95. Moseley, J.B., O'Malley, K., Petersen, N.J., et al. (2002). A controlled trial of arthroscopic surgery for osteoarthritis of the knee. *The New England Journal of Medicine* **347**, 81–88.

96. Müeller, H.H. and Schäfer, H. (2004). A general statistical principle for changing a design any time during the course of a trial. *Statistics in Medicine* **23**, 2497–2508.

97. Murray, E.J. and Hernán, M.A. (2016). Adherence adjustment in the Coronary Drug Project: A call for better per-protocol effect estimates in randomized trials. *Clinical Trials* **13**, 372–378.

98. Nason, M. and Follmann, D. (2010). Design and analysis of crossover trials for absorbing binary endpoints. *Biometrics* **66**, 958–965.

99. Noether, G.E. (1949). On a theorem by Wald and Wolfowitz. *Annals of Mathematical Statistics* **20**, 455–458.

100. O'Brien, P.C. and Fleming, T.R. (1979). A multiple testing procedure for clinical trials. *Biometrics* **35** 549–556.

101. O'Brien, P.C., Zhang, D., and Bailey, K.R. (2005). Semi-parametric and non-parametric methods for clinical trials with incomplete data. *Statistics in Medicine* **24**, 341–358.

102. Pagano, M. and Gauvreau, K. (20000). *Principles of Biostatistics, 2nd ed.* Duxbury, Pacific Grove, California.

103. Pampallona, S., Tsiaitis, A.A., and Kim, K. (2001). Interim monitoring of group sequential trials using spending functions for the type I and type II error probabilities. *Drug Information Journal* **35**, 1113–1121.

104. Parzen, E. (1960). *Modern Probability Theory And Its Applications.* John Wiley & Sons, New York.

105. Pawitan, Y. and Hallstrom, A. (1990). Statistical interim monitoring of the Cardiac Arrhythmia Suppression Trial. *Statistics in Medicine* **9**, 1081–1090.

106. Peto, R. and Peto, J. (1972). Asymptotically efficient rank invariant test procedures. *Journal of the Royal Statistical Society, Series A* **135**, 185–207.

107. Pocock, S.J. (1977). Group sequential methods in the design and analysis of clinical trials. *Biometrika* **64**, 191–199.

108. Pocock, S.J. and Simon, R. (1975). Sequential treatment assignment with balancing for prognostic factors in the controlled clinical trial. *Biometrics* **31**, 103–115.

109. Posch, M. and Proschan, M.A. (2012). Unplanned adaptations before breaking the treatment blind. *Statistics in Medicine* **31**, 4146–4153.

110. Potter, G.E. (2020). Dismantling the fragility index: A demonstration of statistical reasoning. *Statistics in Medicine* **39**, 3720–3731.

111. Prentice, R.L. (1989). Surrogate endpoints in clinical trials: definition and operational criteria. *Statistics in Medicine* **8**, 431–440.

112. Proschan, M., Brittain, E., and Kammerman, L. (2011). Minimize the use of minimization with unequal allocation. *Biometrics* **67**, 1135–1141.

113. Proschan, M. and Follmann, D. (2008). Cluster without fluster: The effect of correlated outcomes on inference in randomized clinical trials. *Statistics in Medicine* **27**, 795–809.

114. Proschan, M.A., Dodd, L.E., and Price (2016). Statistical considerations for a trial of Ebola virus disease therapeutics. *Clinical Trials* **13**, 29–48.

115. Proschan, M.A., Follmann, D.A., and Waclawiw, M.A. (1992). Effect of assumption violations on type I error rate in group sequential monitoring. *Biometrics* **48**, 1131–1143.

116. Proschan, M., Ford, C., Cutler, J., et al. for the ALLHAT Collaborative Research Group (2013). How much effect of different antihypertensive medications on cardiovascular outcomes is attributable to their effects on blood pressure? *Statistics in Medicine* **32**, 884–897.

117. Proschan, M., Glimm, E. and Posch, M. (2014). Connnection between permutation and t-tests: relevance to adaptive methods. *Statistics in Medicine* **33**, 4734–4742.

118. Proschan, M.A., Hunsberger, S.A. (1995). Designed extension of studies of studies based on conditional power. *Biometrics* **51**, 1315–1324.

119. Proschan, M.A., Lan, K.K., and Wittes, J.T. (2006). *Statistical Monitoring of Clinical Trials: A Unified Approach.* Springer, New York.

120. Proschan, M.A., McMahon, R.P., Shih, J.H., Hunsberger, S.A., Geller, N.L., Kantterud, G., and Wittes, J. (2001). Sensitivity analysis using an imputation method for missing binary data in clinical trials. *Journal of Statistical Planning and Inference* **96**, 155–165.

121. Proschan, M.A. and Shaw, P.A. (2016). *Essentials of Probability Theory for Statisticians.* CRC Press, Boca Raton, Florida.

122. Proschan, M.A. and Waclawiw, M.A. (2000). Practical guidelines for multiplicity adjustment in clinical trials. *Controlled Clinical Trials* **21**, 527–539.

123. Proschan, M. and Waclawiw, M. (2001). Reply. *Controlled Clinical Trials* **22**, 550–552.

124. Randles, R.H. and Wolfe, D.A. (1979). *Introduction to the Theory of Nonparametric Statistics.* John Wiley & Sons, New York.

125. Raynaud Treatment Study Investigators (2000). Comparison of sustained-release nifedipine and temperature biofeedback for treatment of primary Raynaud phenomenon. Results from a randomized clinical trial with 1-year follow-up. *Archives of Internal Medicine* **160**, 1101–1108.

126. Robertson, D.S., Lee, K.M., López-Kolkovska, B.C., and Villar, S.S. (2020). Response-adaptive randomization in clinical trials: from myths to practical considerations. *arXiv:Methodology* 2005.00564v1 1 May 2020.

127. Rosenbaum, P.R. (2007). Interference between units in randomized experiments. *Journal of the American Statistical Association* **102**, 191–200.

128. Rosenberger, W.F. and Lachin, J.M. (2016). *Randomization in Clinical Trials: Theory and Practice, 2nd ed.* John Wiley & Sons, New York.

129. Rosner, G.L. (2005). Bayesian monitoring of clinical trials with failure-time endpoints. *Biometrics* **61**, 239–245.

130. Rothman, K.J. (1990). No adjustments are necessary for multiple comparisons. *Epidemiology* **1**, 43–46.

131. Royston P., Parmar, M.K., and Qian, W. (2003). Novel designs for multi-arm clinical trials with survival outcomes with an application in ovarian cancer. *Statistics in Medicine* **22**, 2239–2256

132. Rubin, D.B. (1976). Inference and missing data. *Biometrika* **63**, 581–592.

133. Rubin, D.B. (1978). Multiple imputations in sample surveys. *American Statistical Association Proceedings of the Survey Research Methods Section*, 20–34.

134. Sarkar, S. (1998). Some probability inequalities for ordered MTP2 random variables: A proof of the Simes conjecture. *Annals of Statistics* **26**, 494–504.

135. Satterthwaite, F.E. (1946). An approximate distribution of estimates of variance components. *Biometrics Bulletin* **2**, 110–114.

136. Senn, S.J. (2001). Two cheers for p-values. *Journal of Epidemiology and Biostatistics* **6**, 193–204.

137. Senn, S.J. (2002). Letter to the editor re: Goodman 1992. *Statistics in Medicine* **21**, 2437–2444.

138. Serfling, R.J. (1980). *Approximation Theorems of Mathematical Statistics*. Wiley, New York.

139. Simes, R.J. (1986). An improved Bonferroni procedure for multiple tests of significance. *Biometrika* **73**, 751–754.

140. Simon, R. and Simon, N.R. (2011). Using randomization tests to preserve type I error with response-adaptive and covariate-adaptive randomization. *Statistics and Probability Letters* **81**, 767–772.

141. Slud, E. and Wei, L.J. (1982). Two sample repeated significance tests based on the modified Wilcoxon statistic. *J. Am. Statist. Assoc.* **77**, 862–868.

142. Stampfer, M.J., Willett, W.C, Colditz, G.A., et al. (1985). A prospective study of postmenopausal estrogen therapy and coronary heart disease. *New England Journal of Medicine* **313**, 1044–1049.

143. Stein, C. (1945). A two-sample test for a linear hypothesis whose power is independent of the variance. *Annals of Mathematical Statistics* **16**, 243–258.

144. Tamhane, A.C., Mehta, C.R., and Liu, L. (2010). Testing a primary and a secondary endpoint in a group sequential design. *Biometrics* **66**, 1174–1184.

145. Taves, D.R. (1974). Minimization: A new method of assigning patients to treatment and control groups. *Clinical Pharmacology and Therapeutics* **15**, 443–53.

146. The ALLHAT Officers and Coordinators for the ALLHAT Collaborative Research Group (2002). Major outcomes in high-risk hypertensive patients randomized to angiotensin-converting enzyme inhibitor or calcium channel blocker vs diuretic: The Antihypertensive and Lipid-Lowering Treatment to prevent Heart Attack Trial (ALLHAT). *Journal of the American Medical Association* **288**, 2981–2997.

147. The Coronary Drug Project Research Group (1980). Influence of adherence to treatment and response of cholesterol on mortality in the Coronary Drug Project. *New England Journal of Medicine* **303**, 1038–1041.

148. The INSIGHT START Study Group (2015). Initiation of Antiretroviral Therapy in Early Asymptomatic HIV Infection. *New England Journal of Medicine* **373**, 795–807.

149. The PREVAIL II Writing Group, for the Multi-National PREVAIL II Study Team (Davey, R.T., Dodd, L., Proschan, M.A., et al.) (2016). A randomized, controlled trial of ZMapp for ebola virus infection. *New England Journal of Medicine* **375**, 1448–1456.

150. Thernau, T.M. (1993). How many stratification factors are "too many" to use in a randomization plan? *Controlled Clinical Trials* **14**, 98–108.

151. Thompson, W.R. (1933). On the likelihood that one unknown probability exceeds another in view of the evidence of two samples. *Biometrika* **25**, 285–294.

152. Tsiatis, A.A., Davidian, M., Zhang, M., and Lu, X. (2008). Covariate adjustment for two-sample treatment comparisons in randomized clinical trials: A principled yet flexible approach. *Statistics in Medicine* **27**, 4658–4677.

153. Tsiatis, A.A. and Mehta, C. (2003). On the inefficiency of the adaptive design for monitoring clinical trials. *Biometrika* **90**, 367–378.

154. UK Collaborative ECMO Clinical Trial Group (1996). UK collaborative randomised trial of neonatal extracorporeal membrane oxygenation. The Lancet **348**, 75–82.

155. van der Vaart, A.W. (1998). *Asymptotic Statistics*. Cambridge University Press. Cambridge, U.K.

156. Vermuelen, K., Thas, O., and Vansteelandt, S. (2015). Increasing the power of the Mann-Whitney test in randomized experiments through flexible covariate adjustment. *Statistics in Medicine* **34**, 1012–1030.

157. Villar, S.S., Bowden, J., and Wason, J. (2018). Response-adaptive designs for binary responses: How to offer patient benefit while being robust to time trends? *Pharmaceutical Statistics* **17**, 182–197.

158. Wald, A. and Wolfowitz, J. (1944). Statistical tests based on permutations of the observations. *Annals of Mathematical Statistics* **15**, 358–372.

159. Wang, S.K. and Tsiatis, A.A. (1987). Approximately optimal one-parameter boundaries for group sequential trials. *Biometrics* **43**, 193–199.

160. Wason, J. and Jaki, T. (2012). Optimal design of multi-arm multi-stage trials. *Statistics in Medicine* **31**, 4269–4279.

161. Waters, D., Alderman, E., Hsia, J., et al. (2002). Effects of hormone replacement therapy and antioxidant vitamin supplements on coronary atherosclerosis in postmenopausal women: A randomized controlled trial. *Journal of the American Medical Association* **288**, 2432–2440.

162. Wei, L.J. (1988). Exact two-sample permutation tests based on the randomized play-the-winner rule. *Biometrika* **75**, 603–606.

163. Wei L.J., and Durham, S. (1978). The randomized play-the-winner rule in medical trials. *Journal of the American Statistical Association* **73**, 840–843.

164. Welch, B.L. (1937). On the z-test in randomized blocks and Latin squares. *Biometrika* **29**, 21–52.

165. Welch, B.L. (1947). The generalization of "Student's" problem when several different population variances are involved. *Biometrika* **34**, 28–35.

166. Wilk, M.B. (1955). The randomization analysis of a generalized randomized block design. *Biometrika* **42**, 70–79.

167. Wittes, J., Brittain, E. (1990). The role of internal pilot studies in increasing the efficiency of clinical trials. Statistics in Medicine 9, 65–72.

168. Wittes, J., Lakatos, E., and Probstfield, J. (1989). Surrogate Endpoints in clinical trials: cardiovascular diseases. *Statistics in Medicine* **8**, 415–425.

169. Wittes, J., Schabenberger, O., Zucker, D., Brittain, E., and Proschan, M. (1999). Internal pilot studies I: Type I error rate of the naive t-test. *Statistics in Medicine* **18**, 3481–3491.

170. Writing Group for the Women's Health Initiative Investigators (2002). Risks and benefits of estrogen plus progestin in healthy postmenopausal women: principal results from the Women's Health Initiative randomized controlled trial. *Journal of the American Medical Association* **288**, 321–333.

171. Yusuf, S., Peto, R., Lewis, J., Collins, R., and Sleight, P. (1985). Beta blockade during and after myocardial infarction: An overview of the randomized trials. *Progress in Cardiovascular Disease* **27**, 335–371.

172. Zhang, L., Hu, F., Cheung, S.H. and Chan, W.S. (2011). Immigrated urn models– theoretical properties and applications. *Annals of Statistics* **39**, 643–671.

173. Zucker, D.M, Wittes, J.T., Schabenberger, O., and Brittain, E. (1999). Internal pilot studies II: Comparison of various procedures. *Statistics in Medicine* **18**, 3493–3509.

Index

Printed in the United States
by Baker & Taylor Publisher Services